Notes for the DCH

Notes for the DCH

N J Gilbertson

MBChB, MRCP
Consultant Paediatrician, Royal Cornwall Hospital, Truro
(Previously Senior Registrar in Paediatrics, Charing Cross Hospital,
London)

S J Walker

MBBS, MRCGP, DCH
General Practitioner, Wiltshire

EDITORIAL ADVISORS

David Harvey MB, FRCP, DCH

Consultant Paediatrician, Queen Charlotte's and Chelsea Hospital,
London

Ilya Kovar MB, FRCP, FRCPC, FAAP

Consultant Paediatrician, Chelsea and Westminster Hospital and
Charing Cross Hospital, London

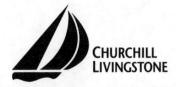

CHURCHILL
LIVINGSTONE

EDINBURGH LONDON MADRID MELBOURNE AND
NEW YORK 1993

CHURCHILL LIVINGSTONE
Medical Division of Pearson Professional Limited

Distributed in the United States of America by Churchill
Livingstone Inc., 650 Avenue of the Americas,
New York, N.Y. 10011, and by associated companies, branches
and representatives throughout the world.

First published 1993
  Reprinted 1996

ISBN 0-443-04375-2

British Library Cataloguing in Publication Data
A catalogue record for this book is available from the British Library

The
publisher's
policy is to use
**paper manufactured
from sustainable forests**

Produced by Longman Singapore Publishers Pte Ltd
Printed in Singapore

Preface

Recent Government proposals redefining national health objectives and strategies highlight the scope for reduction of preventable ill health in pregnant women, infants and children. Emphasis is placed on the importance of general paediatric practice collaborating with other community-based services in the provision of an integrated Child Health Service.

Children form 22% of the total population and their care constitutes one of the most demanding aspects of the family doctor's practice.

This book was written primarily to help General Practitioners preparing for the Diploma in Child Health; we hope that other members of the primary health care team and junior hospital doctors may also find it of use. Whilst the book is not intended to be comprehensive, we have tried to include paediatric problems commonly encountered in general practice together with an outline of the hospital-based management of less common and more severe childhood illnesses, emphasizing the GP's role in the care of children with such problems and their families.

NJG
SW

Contents

1. Demography

Definitions

1. *Epidemiology*. Study of patterns and determinants of disease in a population.

2. *Demography*. Study of population statistics.

Uses: to study the pattern of disease distribution within a community and thus compare the incidence or prevalence of disease between geographical areas or different groups within a population.

3. *Mean*. Total of the observed values divided by the number of observations.

4. *Mode*. The value which occurs most frequently in all observations.

5. *Median*. The value which is exactly half way in a range of observations.

6. *Normal distribution*. A bell-shaped curve which represents the range of continuously variable values, usually biological, about a population mean (Fig. 1). For such distributions, the scatter of observations around the mean is described by the standard deviation (SD) which is useful for interpreting data in terms of probability. 1 SD above and below the mean includes 68% of the population being studied, 2 SD include 95%, and 3 SD above and below 99.73% of the observations.

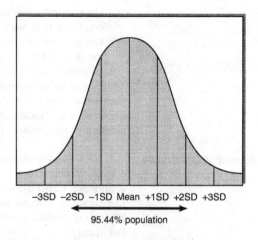

−3SD −2SD −1SD Mean +1SD +2SD +3SD

95.44% population

Fig. 1 Chart of normal distribution (Gaussian curve)

Incidence/prevalence
The number of new cases of a disease in an area is determined by the frequency of occurence of new cases and the duration of the disease (from which there will be either recovery or death).

1. *Incidence.* The number of new cases of a condition occurring during a specified period in a defined population.

2. *Prevalence.* The number of cases of a condition at any particular time (point prevalence) or during a specified period in a defined population.

Both incidence and prevalence are usually expressed as a rate per 1000 of the population. Therefore an acute illness with a quick recovery, e.g. rubella, will have a high incidence but low prevalence, whereas for a chronic illness, e.g. diabetes, the annual incidence is very much lower than the prevalence.

Mortality rates
1. *Perinatal mortality.* Number of stillbirths and deaths within the first week of life per 1000 total births. Good indicator of quality of health services available. Gradual decline in the UK over recent years (see p000).

2. *Stillbirth rate.* Number of stillbirths per 1000 total births.

3. *Neonatal mortality rate.* Deaths of live born babies up to 1 month of age per 1000 live births.

4. *Infant mortality rate.* Deaths of all children under 1 year of age per 1000 live births.

Types of epidemiological studies
1. *Descriptive* (cross-sectional). Determine the frequency of a disease or a symptom in different populations or samples of a population.

2. *Analytical.* Test hypotheses as the cause of a disease, e.g.

(a) Case–control studies comparing people with a chosen condition to those without it.
(b) Cohort studies comparing groups of people exposed to the factor of interest to groups not exposed to it.

3. *Experimental.* Test whether or not the frequency of a disease can be decreased by preventing the suspected cause. Prevention may be primary, i.e. to prevent the illness occurring at all, e.g. vaccination, or secondary, i.e. to prevent progression or recurrence of disease.

Sources of information
1. *Office of Population Census Surveys (OPCS).* There is a full census every 10 years in England and Wales. Information is obtained about the size of the population, sex distribution, marital status, occupation, housing conditions, and occasionally about specific questions asked of a sample of the population only.

2. *Death and birth certificates.*

3. *Hospital Activity Analysis (HAA)*. Includes information about hospital admissions, treatment and consultant, as well as discharge date or cause and date of death. Processed regionally, theoretically available 3–6 monthly. Event-, not person-based.

4. *Hospital Inpatient Enquiry (HIPE)*. Based on a 10% sample of hospital discharges across the country. Analyses personal, administrative and clinical data (as coded by the International Classification of Disease — ICD). Event- not person-based. Accuracy of coding variable; processed centrally at the OPCS and data released at 3–4 year intervals.

5. *Infectious diseases notifications*. Data collected by OPCS (often incomplete, especially for less serious diseases).

6. *Notification of congenital malformations*. Some Regional Health Authorities keep congenital malformation registers, with the aims of:

— audit of perinatal screening programmes
— identification of regional clusters
— provision of database for epidemiological studies

7. *Malignancy*. Registers of cases of malignant disease are kept by OPCS and also by the UK Childhood Cancer Research Group.

8. *Rare conditions*. The British Paediatric Surveillance Unit, sponsored by the British Paediatric Association (BPA), uses monthly notifications by paediatricians to monitor the incidence of rare conditions in childhood.

9. Consultant responsible for community child health will have details of *paediatric referrals* where data are needed about children with possible special educational needs.

10. Local authorities have a *register of the physically and mentally handicapped*.

Screening

Before mass screening for any condition is introduced a number of criteria must be observed:

(a) Disease must be important for the community in terms of prevalence and severity.

(b) Early diagnosis must result in improved prognosis through treatment, for which facilities must be available.

(c) Definition of a 'case' must be precise.

(d) The natural history of the condition must be known and adequate follow-up available, in order to assess the benefits of screening.

(e) The screening test must:

— be safe and acceptable, repeatable, specific (few false positives) and sensitive (few false negatives)
— be cheap and easy to perform. Calculation of the true cost should include money saved by detection of disease at an early stage. Costs can be reduced by

selective screening of known high-risk populations — give a high yield. A prevalence of 1 in 10 000 is considered an acceptable yield

Epidemics

Definition A temporary pronounced rise in the incidence or prevalence of a disease above the normal endemic level.

Types 1. *Common source*, i.e. all cases due to exposure of susceptible persons to same infection or toxin, e.g. recent cases of Legionnaire's disease around a London shopping centre.
2. *Propagated*, i.e. one case infects another, leading to a gradual rise in the incidence.

Control (a) Identify and treat all known cases and look for undiagnosed cases by informing local doctors.
(b) Obtain as much information as possible about the infectious agent from the laboratory.
(c) Identify and investigate the population at risk, i.e. those exposed to the source of infection.
(d) Take necessary measures to prevent further spread, e.g. inform public of known risks, isolate cases, stop sale of suspected contaminated food.

2. The newborn infant

Preparation for parenthood

Perceptions of parenting skills are formed initially from children's experiences with their own parents. Such experiences, whether favourable or adverse, then form the basis for a person's expectations of the likely rewards, and demands, of parenting.

Preparation for parenting should be part of the educational system, along with sex education, basic child development and 'design for living' courses.

Pre-pregnancy counselling and parentcraft teaching are important aspects of preventative care, which can be provided in the community by the primary care team. There is a role for pre-conception clinics where parents with concerns because of family history, recurrent abortion or previous abnormal babies can be referred for expert genetic, obstetric and paediatric advice.

Objectives of antenatal care

(a) To provide information and support to counter fear and anxiety about child-bearing.
(b) To achieve the optimal level of maternal and infant health by early identification of risk factors and anticipation of potential problems.
(c) To encourage parents' informed involvement in decisions about the pregnancy and delivery.
(d) Parentcraft teaching.
(e) To build a relationship in the antenatal period which will provide a basis of trust for future communication.

Since antenatal care was established as a therapeutic and preventative branch of medicine at the beginning of this century, there has been a marked reduction in perinatal and infant mortality.

Perinatal mortality

Stillbirths and babies dying in the first 7 days of life per 1000 total births (8.7 per 1000 total births in the UK in 1988). Major causes include:

— congenital abnormality
— prematurity
— birth asphyxia

Policies aiming to reduce perinatal mortality rate (PNMR):

— improvement of general health of population
— education about avoidable risk factors e.g. teratogens

— better maternity services
— selection of high-risk patients for delivery in units with specialized monitoring facilities and neonatal care
— reduction of preterm labour
— intrapartum fetal monitoring and active management of labour
— screening for fetal anomalies
— advances in neonatal care

Maternal risk factors associated with increased perinatal mortality and morbidity (can be identified in 50% of perinatal deaths):

— age >35 years
— ethnic origin — highest PNMR in Pakistani mothers (may be explained by higher rates of low birth weight (LBW) infants or congenital abnormalities)
— short stature
— medical
  • malnutrition
  • cyanotic heart disease
  • chronic renal disease
  • hypertension
  • diabetes mellitus
  • anaemia, including sickle cell disease
  • smoking
  • alcoholism
  • drug dependence

— socioeconomic
  • malnutrition
  • low socioeconomic class

— obstetric
  • parity (first or fourth)
  • birth interval (PNMR highest if interval <12/12 and lowest if 18–36/12)
  • hypertension in pregnancy
  • diabetes
  • anaemia
  • rhesus antibodies
  • intrauterine growth retardation (IUGR) ⎫ proportion of LBW
  • preterm labour ⎬ infants has major effect on PNMR ⎭
  • malpresentation
  • postmaturity
  • multiple pregnancy
  • hydramnios
  • adverse obstetric history, e.g. ectopic pregnancy, abortion, antepartum haemorrhage, preterm labour, previous Caesarian section, perinatal death or congenital anomaly

Prenatal diagnosis

Prenatal diagnosis with selective termination of pregnancy became an option for parents in the UK with the Abortion Act of 1967. This, in conjunction with important advances in human genetics, has markedly increased the need for genetic counselling services.

In the UK, under the Congenital Disabilities (Civil Liability) Act of 1976, legal action can be brought against a person whose breach of duty to parents results in a child being born disabled, abnormal or unhealthy.

It is essential that all doctors are able to give potentially affected parents valid and up-to-date information, or to refer them to someone who can, about the risk of fetal abnormality in a future pregnancy and the possibility of prenatal diagnosis. The *Report on Prenatal Diagnosis and Genetic Screening* by the Royal College of Physicians (1989), indicates that genetic counselling should be offered to many more people than at present receive it. Prenatal diagnosis for genetic conditions is presently indicated in 8% of all pregnancies. In practice, 93% of prenatal screening tests are negative, providing reassurance for the parents.

Prenatal diagnostic techniques

— maternal serum screening, e.g. alphafetoprotein (AFP)
— imaging: ultrasonography, radiography
— amniocentesis
— fetoscopy
— fetal blood sampling — either under fetoscopic or US guidance by cordocentesis
— chorionic villus biopsy

Maternal serum AFP (MSAFP)

Increased in:

— fetal abnormality, including
  • anencephaly
  • open neural tube defect (NTD)
  • anterior abdominal wall defect
  • Turner's syndrome
— multiple pregnancy
— fetal distress or death
— placental haemangioma
— underestimated fetal age

Decreased in Down's syndrome (<25th centile suggests increased risk).

The antenatal detection rate is improved if MSAFP is interpreted in conjunction with maternal age and changes in maternal serum unconjugated oestriols and human chorionic gonadotrophin (HCG). Using all these predictor factors, it is possible to predict six of 10 babies likely to have Down's syndrome, whereas offering amniocentesis based on maternal age alone detects <30% of Down's babies antenatally. Work is in progress to identify other biochemical markers, e.g.

neutrophil alkaline phosphatase, which may further improve detection rates.

Ultrasound   Diagnostic ultrasound, using a narrow beam of high frequency (2–5 MHz) pulsed sound waves, is an essential tool in modern obstetrics. Among its uses are assessment of gestational age, delineation and monitoring of fetal growth and detection of fetal abnormalities.

Fetal anomaly may be suspected from initial ultrasound scan (usually done around 16 weeks gestation to confirm dates, identify multiple pregnancies and localize the placenta). If so, or if there is another reason to consider the pregnancy at high risk for anomaly (e.g. family history, raised MSAFP, abnormal growth pattern, hydramnios, exposure to teratogen), then the patient is referred to a tertiary centre for high resolution scan by a skilled sonologist.

Major fetal anomalies detectable by US:
1. *Central nervous system*

— anencephaly, encephalocele, microcephaly
— spina bifida, hydrocephalus

2. *Cardiac*

— severe congenital heart disease (abnormality detected in 2 per 1000 pregnancies on four-chamber view at 16 weeks)

3. *Renal*

— Potter's syndrome
— polycystic kidney, hydronephrosis
— bladder outflow obstruction

4. *Gastrointestinal*

— omphalocele
— gastroschisis
— diaphragmatic hernia
— duodenal atresia
— ascites

5. *Musculoskeletal*

— severe dwarfing conditions
— osteogenesis imperfecta
— limb reduction deformities

Radiography   Occasionally indicated for prenatal diagnosis of skeletal dysplasias. Optimal time 20 weeks.

Amniocentesis   Usually performed at 16–18 weeks (when ratio of viable: non-viable cells is maximal).
(a) Anti-D is given if Rhesus negative.
(b) Abortion rate following amniocentesis is 0.5–1%.

(c) Indications:

— maternal age >40 years
— previous baby with: Down's, NTD, inborn errors of metabolism (IEM)
— family history (first degree relative with above abnormalities)
— mother carrying X-linked disorder
— Rhesus immunization (from 26 weeks)
— to assess fetal pulmonary maturity by lecithin: sphingomyelin (L:S) ratio if induction planned

Tests on amniotic fluid cells and supernatant:

— fetal sexing (results available in 3 h)
— fetal karyotyping (2–3 weeks; 1.5% cells fail to grow)
— fetal enzyme assay (3–6 weeks)
— amniotic fluid biochemistry
  • AFP
  • 17α-hydroxyprogesterone
  • glycosaminoglycans
  • alkaline phosphatase isoenzymes
— fetal DNA analysis (extracted from cells either directly or after culture. As DNA can be extracted from chorionic villi without prior culture, chorionic villus biopsy is usually preferred)

Chorionic villus biopsy First reported in 1968 and now available in most major obstetric centres.
(a) Performed at 8–11 weeks gestation.
(b) Aspiration of villi from placental edge by cannula passed under US guidance either trans-cervically or -abdominally (the latter probably carries less risk of infection).
(c) Procedure-related abortion risk is 2–3%
(d) Tests on chorionic villi:

— fetal sexing
— fetal karyotyping (24 h)
— biochemical tests (1–2 weeks)
— fetal DNA analysis

As it allows earlier diagnosis in first trimester, the *advantages* of this technique are:

— abortion technique simpler
— less parental bonding to fetus
— only parents need know about the pregnancy

Fetoscopy Endoscopic visualization of the fetus.
(a) Performed from 17 weeks gestation.
(b) Allows fetal blood sampling, skin or liver biopsy.
(c) Procedure-related abortion rate is 3–5%.

Indications are declining since the availability of chorionic villus sampling and newer techniques for fetal blood sampling by cordocentesis under US control.

Biochemical apects There are about 200 inherited IEM; prenatal diagnosis is possible for over 70 of them. Some of the more common enzyme deficiencies which can be diagnosed prenatally include:

1. *Lipid metabolism*

— Tay–Sachs
— Gaucher
— Niemann–Pick
— metachromatic leucodystrophy

2. *Mucopolysaccharidoses*

— Hunter's syndrome
— Hurler's syndrome

3. *Amino acid metabolism*

— methylmalonic aciduria
— homocystinuria
— cystinosis
— maple syrup urine·disease

4. *Carbohydrate metabolism*

— galactosaemia
— glycogen storage disease (types 2, 3, 4)

5. *Other*

— Lesch–Nyhan
— Refsum's disease

Gene probe linkage analysis Variation in DNA nucleotide sequences is common and occurs randomly throughout the human genome. These changes in base sequence mean that the fragments produced by a particular restriction enzyme will vary in length in a population — restriction fragment length polymorphism (RFLP) — and can be recognized by altered mobility of the restriction fragments on gel electrophoresis.

The use of DNA probes to identify these DNA polymorphisms, and thence to detect genes located near the polymorphisms, has been a major advance in the antenatal diagnosis of single gene disorders.

A probe is a radiolabelled DNA or RNA fragment used to identify a complementary sequence. It is made using an endonuclease enzyme which cleaves DNA at sequence-specific sites (the recognition site) into fragments which can then be replicated by incorporating them into bacterial plasmids (recombination technique). The fragment is then cloned (reproduced by mitotic division from a single cell) and radiolabelled. The radioactive fragment probe can then be used to identify complementary fragments of DNA (the RFLP) if these are present in the leucocytes of the individual being investigated.

Duchenne muscular dystrophy in 1982 was the first genetic disorder to which a DNA probe was linked. There has since been dramatic progress in cloning and mapping disease genes, permitting identification of gene carriers and antenatal diagnosis of an increasing number of single gene disorders, including:

— thalassaemia (α and β)
— haemophilia A and B
— sickle cell anaemia
— cystic fibrosis
— Huntingdon's disease
— muscular dystrophy (Becker and Duchenne)
— tuberous sclerosis
— phenylketonuria
— neurofibromatosis
— myotonic dystrophy
— lethal osteogenesis imperfecta
— α1-antitrypsin deficiency

Prenatal diagnosis should be considered if the following criteria apply:

— maternal age >35 years
— severe disorder anticipated, e.g. raised MSAFP
— previous child with chromosomal abnormality
— parental chromosome abnormality
— family history of genetic disorder
— X-linked disorders to detect fetal sex
— either prenatal treatment possible or termination acceptable to parents

Future prospects   Pre-implantation embryo biopsy can be done with a pre-embryo produced by IVF and subsequently implanted if genetic testing shows it to be normal. Such techniques rely on selective abandonment of affected embryos and raise many ethical and legal questions.

Fetal therapy   In utero treatment has been successful in some antenatally diagnosed conditions e.g. direct intravascular infusion for treatment of Rhesus iso-immunization, ultrasound-guided insertion of shunts for drainage of fetal hydrocephalus, obstructive uropathy or ascites.

Assessment of fetal well-being

Antenatally   — clinical examination: maternal weight gain, fundal height, amniotic fluid volume and fetal activity
— fetal movement chart
— serial US scans (fortnightly)

— serial placental function tests: human placental lactogen
— oestriols
— cardiotocography (CTG) (2–3 times/week)

Intrapartum monitoring for
fetal distress
— continuous CTG
— fetal blood sampling

Causes of fetal hypoxia
— obliterative vascular lesions in the placenta
— long-standing placental insufficiency
— placental separation and haemorrhage
— acute compression of the cord
— fetal anaemia or haemorrhage
— maternal shock or hypoxia
— uterine spasm

Signs (a) CTG

— flat trace (loss of beat-to-beat variability, normally 5–10 beats/min)
— non-reactive trace (no acceleration in heart rate on palpation or fetal movement)
— tachycardia (>160)
— bradycardia (<120)
— decelerations:
  • *type 1* (with contractions) rapid recovery of heart rate. Common in 2nd stage, particularly if cord around neck)
  • *type 2* (persisting after contractions) unprovoked (unassociated with contractions)

(b) Fetal scalp blood pH <7.25 (obtained endoscopically when cervix >3 cm dilated)

(c) Passage of meconium.

Resuscitation of the newborn

About 5% of babies do not establish respiration until >3 min after delivery, and 53% of neonatal deaths occur within this group. It is essential that wherever babies are delivered, including at home, there is a person of adequate skill in resuscitation immediately available.

It is possible to predict 70% of infants who will require resuscitation.

Deliveries where the need for resuscitation should be anticipated
— fetal distress
— prematurity/IUGR
— suspected major congenital anomaly
— multiple birth
— breech presentation
— Caesarian section/mid-forceps/ventouse
— Rhesus isoimmunization
— antepartum haemorrhage (APH)
— severe toxaemia
— prolonged rupture of membranes/maternal fever
— maternal medical problems, e.g. diabetes mellitus

Resuscitation procedure   (a)   Before delivery

— prepare and check equipment
— familiarize yourself with history
— introduce yourself to parents

(b)   At delivery, under a radiant heater:

— assess baby whilst drying rapidly with a warm towel, thus providing gentle stimulation
— if *meconium* or other particulate matter present in the airway, clear by suction and inspect to make sure no meconium around vocal cords
— if *centrally cyanosed* give O_2 by facemask.

Babies with *primary apnoea* (i.e. centrally cyanosed but with a heart rate >100 and good tone) will usually respond to bag and mask O_2, but if no spontaneous respirations by 1 min or heart rate falling, intubate and ventilate.

Babies with *terminal apnoea* (i.e heart rate <60, limp, pale, no reflex response to stimulation) must be intubated and intermittent positive pressure ventilation applied with an infant bag with a spring-loaded pressure limiting blow-off valve set at 30 cmH_2O (e.g. Laerdal bag).

Preterm babies <28–30 weeks may be electively intubated.

The *Apgar score* is used in many units to record the condition of the infant at birth:

Clinical state	0	1	2
Heart rate	0	<100	>100
Respiration	Absent	Irregular	Regular
Muscle tone	Limp	Some flexion	Good
Reflex irritability	Nil	Grimace	Cough
Colour	White	Blue	Pink

The score is recorded at 1 and 5 min.

(c)   If the baby fails to respond, consider the following possibilities:

Problem	*Management*
• Gas cylinder empty/tubing disconnected	Restore gas flow
• Endotracheal tube incorrectly placed	Re-intubate
• Maternal drug effect	Naloxone
• Tension pneumothorax	Drain
• Meconium aspiration syndrome	Ventilate ± paralyse
• Sepsis	Antibiotics

• Diaphragmatic hernia	Ventilate Volume expanders Inotropes Nasogastric tube (8F) — Replogle Head up Don't bag Treat persistent pulmonary hypertension Surgery
• Hypoplastic lungs	?Potter's facies Ventilate Assess renal function, etc.

(d) If no apex beat or heart rate <50 and falling at any time, commence external cardiac massage by encircling infant's chest with both hands, apposing thumbs at midsternum. Compress ~80 times/min.

If severe bradycardia persists, adrenaline (intratracheal or i.v.) should be given. Sodium bicarbonate 4.2% and calcium gluconate if no response to adrenaline.

Once cardiac output has restarted, further inotropic support may be required.

(e) Give the baby to the parents as soon as possible after any resuscitation and reassure them about the baby's progress.

About 6 per 1000 liveborn infants sustain significant asphyxia but only one-third of these suffer permanent neurological damage.

Examination of the newborn

All babies should be checked soon after birth; usually by the midwife following uncomplicated term delivery. If called to the delivery the doctor should make a rapid assessment of the baby after any necessary resuscitation. The purposes of the initial examination are:

(a) To detect any major abnormalities which require immediate attention or explanation to the parents.

(b) To detect any effects of an adverse intrauterine environment (e.g. infection) or of a difficult delivery (birth asphyxia or trauma).

(c) To answer questions parents may have about the baby's appearance, e.g. minor skin blemishes.

Full examination of the baby must be performed during the first week, ideally in a warm, well-lit room with the mother present so that any questions she has may be answered. Avoid examining the baby just before or after feeding.

(a) Familiarize yourself with the mother's medical, obstetric and social history first from notes and nursing staff.

(b) Introduce yourself and explain what are you doing.
(c) Discuss any relevant features noted in the maternal history.
(d) Ask the mother if she has any concerns about the baby. At the same time observe her attitude to the baby and try to establish rapport.

Suggested order   If the baby is quiet initially take the opportunity to observe the infant at rest, feel the fontanelles, listen to the heart and palpate the abdomen with as little disturbance to the baby as possible. This accomplished, the baby is examined from head to toe, although it is probably a good idea to leave the hips until last as it is invariably unpopular.

1. *General observations*

   — behaviour: posture, reactions, cry, movements
   — skin: colour, rashes
   — respiratory pattern
   — nutritional state

2. *Head*

   — scalp
   — skull: shape, sutures, fontanelles, trauma
   — ears
   — facies: eyes, nose, mouth including palate
   — neck

3. *Auscultate* heart, check peripheral pulses.
4. *Undress* baby.
5. *Chest*

   — shape, clavicles, breast tissue
   — movement, asymmetry
   — palpate for heaves, thrills, apex beat

6. *Abdomen*

   — observe, palpate: asymmetry, masses, herniae
   — external genitalia, anus
   — check baby has passed urine and meconium

7. *Femoral pulses.*
8. *Limbs.*
9. *Turn* baby prone, examine back.
10. *Neurological* check: tone, movement, response to handling, cry.
11. examine *hips* (see p. 27).
12. check *OFC.*
13. assess *gestational age* if indicated

If examination is normal reassure the mother at the end that all is well; if any problems are discovered explain their nature and management and be prepared to return later to answer further questions.

Birth trauma

Cephalhaematoma   Fluctuant swelling due to localized subperiosteal collection of blood. Most commonly parietal, limited by sutures. May exacerbate jaundice. Usually disappears in 6 weeks–3 months.

Facial palsy   Unilateral LMN VII nerve palsy usually due to forceps. Eye drops should be instilled to protect the cornea. Usually resolves by 3 weeks.

Intracranial injury   May be due to asphyxia or mechanical trauma:

1. *Hypoxic–ischaemic encephalopathy* (HIE). In the distressed neonate circulatory depression, hypotension and impaired cerebral autoregulation result in cerebral ischaemia. Oedema and/or intracranial haemorrhage may increase intracranial pressure and further reduce perfusion pressure, causing further ischaemia.

In the first 12 h after such insult the baby appears lethargic and hypotonic. Seizures may occur within the first 24 h and by the end of day 1 the baby seems more alert with staring eyes. Apnoea and jitteriness may be apparent.

Over the next 2–3 days in severe cases the infant becomes comatose with evidence of brain-stem dysfunction. If the baby survives this stage, gradual improvement may begin during the next few weeks and months, although abnormal neurological signs usually persist, with residual motor and/or cognitive deficit.

2. *Intracranial bleeding.*

(a) *Subarachnoid haemorrhage (SAH)*. Unlike the dramatic arterial bleeds seen in adults, SAH in the newborn usually originates from small bridging veins in the subarachnoid space and may cause few clinical signs. Sometimes seizures follow, usually from the second day. In the absence of severe preceding trauma or co-existent HIE, outcome is usually good.

(b) *Subdural haemorrhage (SDH)*. Results from laceration of major veins or sinuses. Four types:

— tentorial lacerations
— occipital diastasis
— falx laceration
— rupture superficial cerebral veins

Following major SDH, prognosis is poor. Frequently there is co-existent HIE; injuries may be fatal and hydrocephalus is common in survivors.

3. *Periventricular haemorrhage.* Predominantly occurs in preterm LBW infants (see p. 33).

Subconjunctival haemorrhage   Common. Resolves in 1–2 weeks. No significance.

Sternomastoid tumour   Non-tender swelling palpable within the sternocleidomastoid muscle, usually detected from first 2 weeks. Some, but not all, follow breech or difficult forceps deliveries. Due to haemorrhage and/or oedema and muscle necrosis after pressure on the neck during birth, leading to muscle fibrosis. Contracture of sternocleidomastoid and torticollis may follow, with resultant asymmetric facial development and often associated plagiocephaly.

Passive stretching exercises from 6 weeks may reduce chance of torticollis developing; tenotomy is occasionally necessary in the first 1–2 years.

Fractures   Bones most often broken during difficult deliveries are the clavicle, humerus and femur. Usually heal rapidly. Important to record that they are due to birth trauma as the detection of a healed fracture at a later stage may lead to erroneous suspicions as to the cause.

Brachial plexus lesions   1. *Erb's palsy.* Due to contusion of the upper trunk of the plexus (roots C5, C6) causing paralysis of shoulder abductors, elbow flexors and supinator, resulting in 'waiter's tip' position.

2. *Klumpke's palsy.* Upward traction on the arm may damage the lower trunk of the plexus (C8, T1), causing paralysis of intrinsic muscles of the hand and flexors of wrist and fingers ('claw hand').

Most of these lesions heal spontaneously with full movement returning within a few months.

Newborn screening

Guthrie test for phenylketonuria (1 in 7–10 000)   Detects elevated levels of phenylalanine by a bacterial inhibition assay. An anti-metabolite analogue of phe–ala is used to render the growth of *Bacillus subtilis* dependent on the concentration of phe–ala in the blood spot (see p. 283). Performed worldwide.

Heel prick capillary blood is taken by the midwife, usually on day 6 (>48 h after start of milk feeds)
Note: antibiotics interfere with assay.

Hypothyroidism (1 in 3500)   Most countries use thyroid stimulating hormone (TSH) assay (see p. 276). Performed on same filter paper heel prick blood as Guthrie test.

Tests suitable for mass newborn screening have been developed for a number of other IEM, including galactosaemia (1 in 60 000) and MSUD (1 in 250 000). These can be done on the Guthrie filter paper test but are only thought to be justifiable in selected communities.

Haemoglobinopathies   This screening is controversial. Experience from the USA, where this has been in progress since the early 1970s, shows a significant reduction in case fatality from pneumococcal septicaemia and in the overall mortality rate in children with sickle cell disease diagnosed in the neonatal period. The effectiveness of such programmes however demands:

— high quality controlled methodology
— efficient recall mechanisms
— available and accessible treatment and follow-up care
— culturally specific education and counselling programmes, including genetic counselling
— confidentiality of results

In Britain screening for haemoglobinopathy is routinely performed in some health regions where incidence is high. The test is performed on a filter paper blood spot taken at the same time as the Guthrie, using isoelectric focusing techniques. Regional counselling centres have been set up with doctors and health visitors trained in haemoglobinopathy counselling, and paediatric haematology follow-up is coordinated locally.

Minor problems   These may present in the first few days.

Peripheral cyanosis   Providing the baby is centrally pink and warm, this is of no significance.

Stork marks
— seen in 30–50% of normal babies
— macular capillary haemangioma
— common sites: bridge of nose, nape of neck, eyelids
— fade by 1 year (usually sooner)

Mongolian blue pigmentation
— bluish-black colouration of skin usually over lumbosacral spine and buttocks
— more common in dark-skinned races (90%) though also seen in 1–5% of Caucasian babies
— fades within 2 years

Milia
— tiny white spots mainly around nose in 40% of babies
— sebaceous retention cysts
— similar spots along the hard palate of many babies ('Epstein's pearls')
— disappear in 2–3 weeks

Urticaria neonatorum (Erythema toxicum)
— blotchy red rash with sterile white pustular centres containing eosinophils
— occurs in one-third of babies between 2 and 7 days and disappears within 48 h

Portwine stain (Naevus flammeus)
— purple non-blanching discolouration of skin due to permanent capillary dilatation
— may be anywhere on the skin though facial lesions are most common (rarely occur in distribution of trigeminal nerve as part of the Sturge–Weber syndrome)

Strawberry naevus
— occurs anywhere on the body
— due to cavernous haemangioma

— generally not evident at birth but develops over first few weeks. Enlarges for first 6 months then regresses completely by 7 years

— no treatment necessary (unless rarely very large and associated with thrombocytopaenia)

Sticky eye   (a) A *slight* exudate from the eyes in the first 24 hours is common (5–10% of neonates), usually non-infective and clears spontaneously.

(b) *Sticky* discharge with redness or swelling of the eyes may be due to bacterial conjunctivitis, most often staphylococcal. Mild cases settle with bathing of the eyes with sterile swabs. If discharge persists or there is associated oedema, antibiotic eye drops are needed, e.g. chloramphenicol.

(c) A *profuse* purulent discharge, usually presenting within 24 h of delivery may be due to gonococcal infection (*Ophthalmia neonatorum*). Uncommon in the UK but in many parts of the world 1% silver nitrate is used as prophylaxis against this serious infection, which is a major cause of blindness. Treat with topical and systemic penicillin for 7 days.

(d) *Chlamydial* conjunctivitis presents later, towards the end of the first week. Occurs in infants whose mothers have cervical or pelvic inflammatory disease due to *Chlamydia trachomatis*. Also risk of subsequent chlamydia pneumonia at 2–4 months, so treatment with chlortetracycline eye ointment and systemic erythromycin (10 days) is advised.

(e) *Gonococcal* and *chlamydial* eye infections in the newborn are notifiable.

Breast engorgement   — common and harmless

— due to hormonal stimulus. May lactate (witches' milk)

— spreading erythema, purulent discharge or pyrexia indicate mastitis and require treatment with systemic antibiotics

Vaginal discharge ± bleeding   Common in female infants due to maternal hormones. Maximum at 3–5th day, settles by the second week.

Red urine   Brick-red staining on nappy is due to urate excretion. May be mistaken for haematuria but is harmless.

Umbilical hernia   — common especially in LBW and black infants

— Due to failure of closure of extra-abdominal coelom, often associated with diastasis recti

— usually asymptomatic although incarceration can rarely occur (i.e. retention of contents of hernia outside abdomen)

— most disappear spontaneously by 1 year

— surgery is hardly ever required (unless the hernia strangulates or becomes progressively larger, persisting beyond the age of 3–5 years).

Hydrocele — common
— due to persistence of communication between tunica vaginalis and peritoneum
— most disappear spontaneously in first few months so surgery should be delayed until over 1 year (unless associated hernia found)

Inguinal hernia — common, especially in preterm infants
— congenital indirect inguinal hernia results from persistence of the processus vaginalis
— elective herniotomy performed as there is a significant risk of incarceration which may cause intestinal obstruction or strangulation, i.e venous obstruction, leading to gangrene. Risk highest in first 3 months

Undescended testes Normally descend around 36 weeks gestation Descended in 98% of boys by term. In remaining 2%, majority descend within first month. Surgery will be needed by 5 years if descent has not occurred by 1 year (0.5%); boys should be referred before the age of 18 months as early surgery may improve fertility

Hypospadias Opening of the external meatus on the under surface of the penis; may be associated with a curvature of the penis (chordee) and may interfere with normal micturition and sexual intercourse when older.

In mild cases where the opening is on the glans, operation is not usually necessary but in more severe cases corrective surgery, usually in two stages, is generally undertaken after the child is continent but before school age. Parents must be warned that circumcision is contraindicated as preputial skin will be required for the repair. Any associated cryptorchidism should be investigated, e.g. 17-ketosteroid assay, IVP and sex chromosome studies.

Circumcision The only grounds for circumcision in the newborn are religious (required by Jews on day 8 and customary in Moslems between 3–15 years).

Medical indications which may develop later are:

— recurrent balanitis
— true phimosis causing ballooning of foreskin during micturition and poor stream

Congenital abnormalities One child in every 30 has a congenital malformation. Some are isolated, others are part of complex dysmorphic syndromes. Single minor abnormalities are common. They are of no serious medical or cosmetic consequence to the child but may serve as indicators of altered morphogenesis, occurring with increased frequency in children with major malformations.

— 14% of newborn babies have a single minor malformation

— 0.5% of newborn babies have three or more malformations; 90% of these have one or more major defect as well

Incidence of minor anomalies	Single palmar crease	4% unilateral
		1% bilateral
	Upslanting palpebral fissures	4%
	Epicanthic folds	4%
	5th finger clinodactyly	9%
	Syndactyly 2nd/3rd toes	1.6%

Aetiology of major anomalies Genetic or pre-conceptual causes account for 80% of major congenital anomalies, chromosomes or conceptual (cell division) causes for 8% and environmental causes for ~10%.

— drugs, e.g. thalidomide, phenytoin, methotrexate, warfarin, alcohol
— infection, e.g. rubella, syphilis, toxoplasma, cytomegalo-virus
— maternal metabolic disturbance, e.g. diabetes, thyroid disorders, phenylketouria
— intrauterine moulding, e.g. oligohydramnios, amniotic bands
— maternal diet, e.g. vitamin D deficiency, ? other vitamin deficiencies (see p. 24)

Fetal alcohol syndrome Alcohol is the most common environmental teratogen to which the fetus is likely to be exposed. Studies in N. America and France have revealed an incidence of >1 in 1000.

Fetal effects from alcohol exposure vary according to intake. With an intake of 2 units of alcohol per day, slight reduction in birth weight may result; most children with the fetal alcohol syndrome are born to chronically alcoholic mothers taking >8–10 drinks per day.

Variables features of fetal alcohol syndrome include:

— prenatal onset growth deficiency
— mental deficiency (IQ 50–80 range)
— microcephaly
— short palpebral fissure
— short nose
— smooth philtrum with thin upper lip
— ± joint, cardiac and renal anomalies

Incidence of major malformations		per 1000 births
	Anencephaly	3.9
	Spina bifida	3.4
	Hydrocephalus	1.2
	Congenital Heart Disease	8.0
	Cleft lip and/or palate	1.3
	Down syndrome	1.3

Congenital dislocation of the hip   10.0
Diaphragmatic hernia   0.5

Cleft lip and palate   This may be unilateral or less commonly bilateral and of variable severity. In some cases there is a positive family history; exposure to maternal anticonvulsant drugs is also a risk factor but in most cases the aetiology is unknown.

Most parents will need much reassurance and support in accepting and dealing with the baby's problems: feeding, speech, cosmetic.

Parents should be shown photographs of successful repairs. The Cleft Lip And Palate Association (CLAPA) is a useful source of advice and support. Feeding can usually be managed with specially modified big teats or spoon feeds. Palatal obturator plates are sometimes fitted and some babies manage to breast fed. Timing of surgery varies. Some surgeons prefer to repair the cleft in the first few days of life, in other centres repair of the lip is undertaken at 3 months and palate at 12–18 months.

With careful otological supervision, orthodontic care and speech training, results are generally very good.

Spina bifida   CNS malformations, including anencephaly, spina bifida and hydrocephalus, constituted up to one-fifth of all congenital malformations in the early 1970s, but their incidence has been steadily decreasing since. This fall is due in part to the widespread introduction of screening procedures such as MSAFP and US.

Spina bifida occulta   This is seen in 5–10% of spines, usually as an incidental finding on X-ray. There may be an overlying patch of hair or dermal sinus, which is usually asymptomatic. Rarely may be associated with underlying tethering or splitting of the cord (diastematomyelia).

Spina bifida cystica   1. *Meningocele*. Constitutes 5–10% of spina bifida cystica cases. Dorsal vertebral laminae are absent with a skin-covered lesion containing only CSF without underlying neurological involvement. Hydrocephalus develops in ~10%. Operative closure is performed when convenient and most survive without handicap.

2. *Myelomeningocele*. In these cases with absent dorsal laminae of vertebral arches there is a defect over the spine, usually covered by just a transparent membrane, which may have neural tissue adherent to its inner surface and through which CSF may leak. In the most severe cases (rachischisis), the neural plaque may lie open on the surface for several segments.

The neurological deficit depends on the level and nature of the lesion:

(a) *hydrocephalus*. Develops in 90% of affected children, most often due to associated Arnold–Chiari malformation (downward displacement through the foramen magnum into the vertebral canal of the cerebellar tonsils, 4th ventricle and medulla oblongata).

(b) *paralysis*. Mixed UMN and LMN lesions are seen. Usually flaccid but spastic paraplegia is not uncommon. The resulting muscle imbalance may cause deformities such as dislocated hips and talipes.

(c) *sensory loss*. Predisposes to trophic lesions especially at pressure sites.

(d) *defective bladder innervation*. Most commonly causes retention with overflow incontinence. There may be dribbling with a palpable distended bladder. Urinary tract infection and hydronephrosis may be additional problems.

(e) *anal sphincter incompetence*. Demonstrated by patulous anus with absent anal reflex.

Early management Every baby with spina bifida must have a full and expert assessment as soon as possible after birth, to determine the extent of the neurological deficit, the degree of spinal deformity and the coexistence of hydrocephalus or another major congenital anomaly (which occurs in 5% of babies with myelomeningocele, usually those most severely affected).

After a full discussion with the parents about their baby's condition, likely problems and potential, a decision must be made about treatment.

Babies with a poor prognosis may be identified by the following adverse features (the Lorber criteria) which are generally accepted as relative contraindications to active management;

— a thoraco-lumbar or thoraco-lumbosacral lesion
— severe paralysis of the legs
— grossly enlarged head (OFC at least 2 cm above 90th centile)
— other severe abnormalities, e.g. cardiac, chromosomal
— cerebral injury

These criteria will generally exclude 50% of cases from early surgery. (Non-treatment rates vary between centres from 25% to 75%.) Active treatment , if indicated in the neonatal period, usually consists of closure of the spinal lesion and insertion of a shunt (e.g. Spitz–Holter, Pudenz, Hakim), if there is progressive hydrocephalus (~70%). Either ventriculo-atrial or ventriculo-peritoneal drainage may be preferred: complications are common, particularly blockage and infection.

The mortality rate of untreated patients is about 90%, whilst the survival rate of treated cases has increased to over 80%.

Long-term   See p. 104.
problems/management   Quality of life in children over 5 years after surgery (Lorber):

— 18% mild/moderate physical handicap and normal IQ
— 49% severe physical handicap and normal IQ
— 33% severe physical handicap and borderline or subnormal IQ

The recurrence risk after one baby with a NTD is 5% and after two 10%.

Prevention   There is some evidence to suggest that peri-conceptional vitamin supplements may reduce the incidence of NTDs. A trial undertaken by Smithells et al in 1980 compared the incidence of NTDs in women who had a history of NTD in a previous pregnancy given a combination of folate and vitamins with the incidence in an unsupplemented group with similar history. A reduction in incidence was seen in the treatment group, but the trials were not randomly controlled and did not establish which vitamin(s) in the mixture was important. Further studies are in progress under the aegis of the MRC.

Diaphragmatic hernia
(1 in 2000)   Herniation of the stomach and intestine into the chest through a defect in the hemi-diaphragm (patent pleuro-peritoneal canal). More common on the left (~80%), through the foramen of Bochdalek.

In two-thirds of cases the lung on the affected side fails to develop and displacement of the mediastinum may cause the other lung to be hypoplastic as well. There may be other associated major congenital abnormalities.

Presentation   As swallowed air inflates the small bowel in the chest the lungs are further compressed and the infant presents with marked cyanosis and tachypnoea; signs of mediastinal shift, unequal air entry and a scaphoid abdomen suggest the diagnosis. If suspected:

(a) Pass nasogastric tube (8F) and place on continuous suction.
(b) Intubate and ventilate (paralysis usually necessary) (do *not* use facemask — this will increase gastric distension and worsen respiratory distress)
(c) Chest X-ray to confirm diagnosis.
(d) May be pulmonary hypertension: treat with tolazoline.
(e) Monitor arterial blood gases and treat metabolic acidosis.
(f) Transfer to neonatal surgical unit.

Repair is undertaken via the abdominal or thoraco-abdominal route, either by direct suture of defect or by patching.

Survival rate is 60%. Long-term lung function in survivors is usually normal though some develop bronchopulmonary dysplasia (BPD) ± cor pulmonale, and there is an increased incidence of respiratory infection in the first few years.

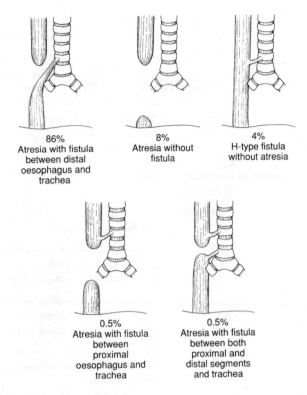

Fig. 2 Atresia and fistula

Oesophageal atresia ± tracheo-oesophageal fistula (1 in 3000)	Due to anomalous differentiation of the oesophagus and trachea from the laryngo-tracheal sulcus between the 3rd and 6th week of gestation (Fig. 2). Other major anomalies (in 50% of affected infants) also occur around this stage.
Diagnosis	(a) US in utero.
	(b) Suspected because of polyhydramnios:

— occurs in >50% cases
— 1 in 14 infants of mothers with hydramnios have oesophageal atresia

(c) Suspect if neonate presents with frothy secretions and drooling, choking or cyanotic attacks or abdominal distension.

Confirm diagnosis by passing a 10 FG radio-opaque catheter. In oesophageal atresia, this will be held up at 9–10 cm and X-ray will confirm the tube is stuck in the oesophageal pouch at level T2–T4. If gas is present in bowel, coexistence of fistula is confirmed.

Management (a) Continuous aspiration of oesophageal pouch by Replogle tube.

(b) Supportive, e.g. antibiotics if possible, aspiration.

(c) Transfer to neonatal surgical unit.

Primary oesophageal anastomosis is usually possible, with division of fistula and feeding gastrostomy until anastomosis is healed. If the gap between the oesophageal segments is too great, cervical oesophagostomy, closure of fistula and feeding gastrostomy is performed, with oesophageal reconstruction using colon delayed until the infant reaches ~6 kg. Survival rate is ~80%.

Duodenal obstruction (1 in 6000)

May be due to atresia, stenosis, diaphragm or annular pancreas.

Diagnosis

(a) US in utero.

(b) Suspected because:

— maternal polyhydramnios occurs in 30%
— Down's syndrome

(c) Suspected if neonate presents with:

— recurrent vomiting, often bile-stained
— abdominal distension ⎫ in some
— delayed passage of meconium ⎭ cases

Confirm diagnosis by erect abdominal X-ray, which will show a 'double bubble' sign of gas in the stomach and dilated proximal bowel.

Management

(a) Correct fluid and electrolyte disturbance

(b) Duodeno-jejunostomy

(c) Parenteral feeding until enteral feeding can be re-established when anastomosis healed.

Exomphalos (1 in 6–10 000)

Herniation of gut through umbilical hiatus covered by an avascular membrane. Ranges from minor defect (abdominal wall opening <5 cm) to exomphalos major (large defects with stomach, intestine and sometimes other viscera outside the abdomen).

Up to 50% of cases are associated with other abnormalities, mainly genitourinary or gastrointestinal. Occasionally (5%) seen as part of Weidemann–Beckwith syndrome:

— macroglossia
— exomphalos
— macrosomia
— hypoglycaemia (up to 50% of cases)
— linear grooves on ear lobes

Gastroschisis

Herniation of intestine through a para-umbilical defect in the abdominal wall. Associated malformations are uncommon.

Management

Similar for exomphalus and gastroschisis.

(a) Immediately after delivery cover the exposed bowel with a sterile moist towel and place the infant's lower body in a drawstring bag pulled round the axillae to minimize evaporative heat loss.

(b) Pass nasogastric tube and place on continuous suction.
(c) Correct fluid and electrolyte disturbance if necessary.
(d) Transfer for surgery.

Primary repair is possible for a minor defect. If large amounts of bowel are extruded or the abdomen is contracted the bowel is enclosed in a silastic bag stitched to the edge of the defect or skin flaps mobilized to cover the defect. Over some weeks the contents can gradually be returned to the growing abdominal cavity and the defect closed.

Imperforate anus/rectal atresia (1 in 5000)

Usually noted at birth. The rectum may terminate high, above the pelvic floor (supralevator) or low (infralevator). Confirm diagnosis by antero-posterior and lateral abdominal X-ray with position of anus marked — it may help to invert the baby.

Management

(a) With *low* lesions an anal canal can be created by incision and dilation or a cutback procedure.
(b) *High* anomalies are usually treated with a defunctioning colostomy followed by pull-through operation at 6–9 months, utilizing the pubo-rectalis sling to assist with sphincter control.

Congenital dislocation of the hip (CDH)

Incidence of unstable hips at birth is 1.7%, of which about 10% are dislocated and 90% are dislocatable:

— more common in females (6:1)
— more common on left side (55%)
— other associated factors:
  • family history CDH
  • first child
  • breech presentation (30–50% of infants with CDH)
  • history of maternal oligohydramnios
  • other deformities, e.g. talipes

Examination

1. *Ortolani manoeuvre*: detects a *dislocated* hip. With baby quiet and relaxed, hips and knees in 90° flexion, examine hips one at a time. Grasp baby's thigh with middle finger tip over greater trochanter and thumbs along the medial aspect of the femur. Pull the thigh gently forward with simultaneous abduction. If the hip is dislocated the femoral head will be felt to 'clunk' forward into the acetabulum.

2. *Barlow's test*: detects a *dislocatable* hip. With baby relaxed, hips are flexed to 90° and adducted. The femoral head is then gently pressed posteriorly whilst internally rotating it ~25°. If the hip is dislocatable the head will be felt to 'clunk' back over the rim of the acetabulum. (Some authorities consider this part of the test to be potentially harmful.)

If these tests are positive some form of abduction splintage is employed to allow the hip to stabilize in the correct position (e.g. Aberdeen, Pavlik or Van Rosen splint), usually for about 6 weeks. X-rays are unhelpful before 6 weeks.

Clinical and radiological follow-up at 3, 6 and 12 months will show most hips to have stabilized. Very rarely persistent instability will require open reduction. This is more likely if treatment is delayed.

Despite the introduction of routine testing of the hips of neonates, the incidence of established dislocation in the UK has not decreased; some series show an increasing incidence. Screening may fail because:

(a) Neonatal instability is overlooked by the inexperienced clinician.
(b) May be a clinically silent predislocation stage (e.g. due to a shallow acetabulum), which progresses to dislocation only when weight-bearing begins.
(c) Dislocation may be acquired later in infancy consequent on certain nursing practices such as swaddling babies with legs adducted and extended.

Recent studies suggest US screening would aid in the detection of some of these abnormal hips and help to avoid the unnecessary splinting of normal babies.

Hips should be re-examined at 6 weeks, 6–9 months, 18–24 months and school entry. (Ortolani–Barlow manoeuvre not appropriate after 3 months.)

Late presentation of CDH
— asymmetry of skin folds
— limited abduction of hips
— shortening of the thigh: knees at different levels with patient supine, legs flexed (Galeazzi sign)
— limping

Foot deformities
(1 in 250)

Talipes calcaneo-valgus

Common neonatal finding. May be related to intrauterine moulding. Most correct with gentle foot manipulation. (Differentiate from congenital vertical talus by lateral X-ray of foot if in doubt.)

Talipes equino-varus
(club foot)

Foot inverted and supinated with adducted forefoot and internally rotated heel (twice as common in boys).

Mild cases are easily corrected by stretching and strapping in the correct plantigrade position. *Severe* cases are treated with serial strapping or casts. In over one-third surgery will be needed. Start treatment early as foot ligaments start to tighten up within a few days of birth.

Ambiguous genitalia

Disorders of sexual development may be classified into three groups:

1. *Male pseudohermaphroditism*

— XY karyotype
— testes present
— inadequate virilization

2. *Female pseudohermaphroditism*

— XX karyotype
— ovaries present
— Virilization

3. *True pseudohermaphroditism*

— dysgenetic gonads
— both testicular and ovarian tissue present
— variable karyotype: 60% XX, 10% XY, 30% mosaic.

1. Male pseudohermaphroditism

(a) *Impaired testosterone synthesis.* At least five enzyme defects may impair the synthesis of testosterone in both the testis and fetal adrenals. Defective steroid synthesis may also cause cortisol deficiency with risk of hypoglycaemia (these are types of congenital adrenal hyperplasia, see p. 279).

(b) *Impaired peripheral testosterone responsiveness.* Partial or complete (testicular feminization syndrome).

Testosterone levels are normal but there is a defect in androgen binding receptors. Neonates look like normal females but may diagnosed if positive family history (X-linked or autosomal recessive) or if gonads palpable in groin.

(c) *Dysmorphic syndromes.*

2. Female pseudohermaphroditism

(a) *Congenital adrenal hyperplasia.* Most common cause of virilized female.

This is an autosomal recessive IEM affecting cortisol synthesis in the adrenal gland. Near normal levels of cortisol may be achieved due to raised ACTH levels leading to adrenal hyperplasia. However, this also results in increased androgenic cortisol precursors, causing masculinization of females (see p. 279).

(b) *Maternal androgen excess.* Seen after oral synthetic progestogens given to mothers in the 1950s to prevent recurrent abortion. Androgen-secreting maternal tumour is seen very rarely.

(c) *Dysmorphic syndrome.*

3. True pseudohermaphroditism

Dysgenetic gonads are removed (risk of malignancy) and gender assignment is usually female.

Management of baby with ambiguous genitalia

(a) Do *not* guess the baby's gender.

(b) Explain to parents that their baby's sex is uncertain but that it will be established after investigation. (It may help in dealing with family and friends to suggest they are told simply that some tests are needed and that the parents prefer not to discuss the baby's progress for a while. Also explain to parents that there is no connection between their baby's problem and any form of deviant behaviour.)

(c) Review the history and examination for clues (e.g. BP, pigmentation, palpable gonads).

(d) Establish genetic sex as quickly possible by karyotype (buccal smear is occasionally unrealiable in first few days; may be negative in XX females).

(e) Other investigations as indicated by clinical findings, e.g. plasma 17α-hydroxyprogesterone, plasma and urinary electrolytes, US, 'genitogram', plasma aldosterone, gonadal biopsy.

Low birth weight baby

Low birthweight (LBW) infants are those weighing 2.5 kg or less and very low birthweight (VLBW) infants those weighing 1.5 kg or less. LBW infants constitute 7.1% of all babies born in England and Wales (OPCS 1988).

A LBW infant may be:

— small for gestational age (SGA), i.e. birthweight below the tenth centile
— preterm, i.e. born before 37 weeks gestation
— both

SGA baby

Factors associated with growth retardation include:

— placental insufficiency
— smoking
— maternal illness, e.g. chronic renal failure, cyanotic heart disease
— multiple pregnancy
— maternal heroin use
— intrauterine infections
— congenital malformations

Problems

1. *Intrapartum asphyxia.* Increased risk because of limited stores of cardiac and hepatic glycogen. Also increased risk of meconium aspiration following hypoxia.

2. *Hypoglycaemia.* Monitor with BM stix 2, 6, 12, 24, 36 and 48 h of life. Prevent by early feeding (see p. 41).

3. *Impaired thermoregulation.* Increased risk of hypothermia because of high surface area: weight ratio and low fat stores.

4. *Polycythaemia.* Packed cell volume (PCV) >70. May cause respiratory distress, cardiac failure, convulsions, jaundice.

5. *Pulmonary haemorrhage.* Usually at 2–4 days following other insults, e.g. birth asphyxia. Probably due to left heart failure.

Preterm baby

The cause of preterm labour is unknown in many cases; a small number are associated with, for example, cervical incompetence, infection or another maternal complications of pregnancy. 6–7% of infants are born prematurely.

Problems   1. *Idiopathic respiratory distress syndrome (RDS)*. Major cause of mortality among preterm babies: occurs in 50% of neonates of <32 weeks' gestation. More common and more severe in boys.

Caused by deficiency of surfactant, a complex phospholipid which reduces surface tension and thus prevents collapse of small airways. Synthesized in granular (type II) pneumocytes, which appear at about 20 weeks with gradual increase in production until a surge between 30 and 34 weeks. Synthesis is inhibited by cold, hypoxia and acidosis. Glucocorticoids accelerate production though this effect is mainly seen between 30 and 34 weeks.

Chest X-ray shows diffuse granularity ('ground glass appearance') and air bronchogram.

Management
(a) Humidified O_2 in headbox may suffice.
(b) Continuous positive airways pressure (CPAP) to keep small airways open may help babies failing to maintain PaO_2 >8 kPa in 60% O_2. Delivery by nasopharyngeal prong, nasal cannula, face mask or endotracheal tube.
(c) Ventilation, usually intermittent positive pressure ventilation (IPPV) is required if:

— infant failing to maintain adequate oxygenation despite CPAP and 70% O_2
— $PaCO_2$ rising (>7.8 kPa)
— failure to establish satisfactory respiration after resuscitation on labour ward

The need for ventilation should be anticipated before the baby deteriorates acutely. Sedation and paralysis may be necessary to achieve satisfactory compliance.

Exogenously administered surfactant reduces neonatal mortality rates in preterm infants with proven RDS. The optimal preparation and administration schedules, the effect on the incidence of chronic lung disease and the role of surfactant in treatment of infants with other respiratory problems are not yet clear; many multicentre trials are in progress to try and answer such questions.

Pulmonary complications include:

— pneumonia
— air leaks: pneumothorax, pneumomediastinum, pulmonary interstitial emphysema
— bronchopulmonary dysplasia (BPD)

2. *Jaundice*. There is a higher incidence of jaundice among preterm infants because of transient deficiency of glucuronyl

transferase, the liver enzyme responsible for bilirubin conjugation. Preterm infants, particularly if hypoxic or acidotic, may have a lower bilirubin binding capacity so that kernicterus may develop at lower levels of unconjugated hyperbilirubinaemia than in more mature infants (see p. 39).

3. *Apnoea.* Many normal term infants have periodic breathing, i.e. regular respirations separated by periods of cessation of breathing for up to 10 seconds. Apnoeic attacks are defined as absence of breathing for >10 seconds and are very common in preterm babies. During such attacks the infant may become cyanosed and bradycardiac.

Apnoea may be a manifestation of immature central control of respiration with in some cases a poor ventilatory response to changes in $PaCO_2$. In such cases a good response to methylxanthines is usually found.

However, other possible causes for apnoea should always be considered. A preterm infant's tendency to apnoea may be increased by:

— anaemia
— handling
— changes in incubator temperature
— feeding
— airway obstruction, e.g. nasal tubes
— more frequent during rapid eye movement (REM) sleep

Apnoea may be a presenting sign of:

— septicaemia
— HMD or other lung disease
— heart failure
— intracranial haemorrhage
— upper airway obstruction
— anaemia
— convulsions
— metabolic disturbance, e.g. hypoglycaemia, hypocalcaemia

4. *Impaired thermoregulation.* Cold stress in a baby is countered by non-shivering thermogenesis from metabolism of brown fat distributed at the base of the neck, between the scapulae and around the kidneys and adrenals. It accounts for 2–6% of the birth weight of a term baby but, like the SGA baby, the preterm neonate has small reserves of brown fat in relation to body weight.

Even mild cold stress reduces survival of LBW infants. Adverse effects of cold stress include:

— increased O_2 consumption
— increased energy expenditure
— increased risk of: infection, haemorrhage, RDS

Both core and peripheral temperature should be monitored and baby nursed in the thermoneutral range, which is the environmental temperature range in which O_2 consumption is minimal. It is influenced by birth weight, gestation and nursing conditions. Heat loss may be reduced by clothing, including bonnets, humidification, heat shields and incubators.

Causes of:

— *hypothermia*: sepsis, brain damage, hypoxia, hypoglycaemia
— *hyperthermia*: ambient temperature too high, brain damage, phototherapy, over-swaddling, sepsis, dehydration

5. *Infection*. Preterm infants are more vulnerable to infection because of immaturity of defence mechanisms:

(a) Reduced numbers of T-lymphocytes with mixed functional abilities.

(b) Very low levels of IgG (most of which is transplacentally acquired in last trimester).

(c) Low levels of IgM and A (do not cross placenta, but increased production after birth even in preterm babies.)

(d) Low levels of complement components, particularly C1q, C2, C3 and C4.

(e) Reduced polymorphonuclear phagocytosis, primarily due to defective opsonization.

Many of the sickest and most preterm infants must be nursed in intensive care units which contain a wide selection of pathogenic organisms which colonize the baby. It is essential that scrupulous attention is paid to prevention of cross-infection by such measures as hand-washing and avoidance of equipment sharing or overcrowding.

6. *Periventricular haemorrhage (PVH)*. Occurs in about 40% of infants with birth weight <1500 g or gestational age <35 weeks. Usually develops within first 72 h. In preterm infants haemorrhage usually originates in the capillaries of the subependymal germinal matrix, which is richly perfused but fragile. This germinal matrix resolves in a caudorostral direction with increasing gestational age and has disappeared by term in most infants. Residual matrix may uncommonly be the site of PVH in term infants; in other term infants the choroid plexus is the site of origin.

Bleeding may extend into the lateral ventricles and in severe cases haemorrhage is seen in the cerebral parenchyma which may resolve to leave a porencephalic cyst.

Many infants survive a small germinal matrix or intra-ventricular haemorrhage with no neurological sequelae. Hydrocephalus may follow, more often after moderate or severe PVH; if serial US scans demonstrate progressive ventricular dilatation, shunt insertion is considered. There is also a high incidence of cerebral palsy, particularly with occipital porencephalic cysts.

The presence of flare-shaped echo-dense areas adjacent to the angles of the lateral ventricles may indicate cerebral ischaemia (periventricular leukomalacia) and predict the development of spastic diplegia due to damage mainly to the descending motor fibres to the lower limbs.

7. *Necrotising enterocolitis* (NEC). Affects up to 15% of LBW infants, usually in first 2 weeks of life. About 10% of cases occur in term infants, sometimes in clusters.

The aetiology is probably multi-factorial, with bowel hypoxia/ischaemia and secondary infection important contributory factors in most cases. Risk factors include:

— low end-diastolic flow on antenatal Doppler studies
— birth asphyxia
— HMD
— polycythaemia
— PDA
— exchange transfusion
— umbilical catheters

Usually sporadic, but organisms associated with outbreaks have included: *Escherichia coli, Klebsiella, Salmonella, Clostridia, Rotavirus, coronavirus.*

Diagnosis: suspect if neonate develops signs of sepsis and/or abdominal distension with blood in the stools.

Abdominal X-ray: dilated loops ± bowel wall oedema. In severe cases, intramural gas (Pneumatosis intestinalis), free fluid, portal venous gas.

Management

— conservative
  • NBM, NG suction
  • intravenous fluids, total parenteral nutrition (TPN)
  • antibiotics
  • analgesics
— surgical: for perforation or obstruction

Prognosis: mortality rate 20–30%. Long-term complications include late stricture (10% cases).

8. *Retinopathy of prematurity (ROP).* Commonest cause of blindness acquired in neonatal period in the UK. Susceptibility related to gestation, birth weight, duration of exposure to high oxygen tensions and blood transfusion requirement. Very rare in infants over 32 weeks' gestation. Trials of vitamin E (which protects cell membranes against oxidative damage) suggest possible benefit in the early proliferative stages of the disease but are still being evaluated. Cryotherapy may prevent progression to the later cicatricial (scarring) stages where permanent damage is likely.

Outcome in LBW infants

Centres throughout the world have reported an increased neonatal survival rate, particularly of VLBW infants (birthweight <1500 g), attributable in part to improved standards of perinatal care. Survival rates vary between centres but average figures are:

Birth weight (g)	Survival %
500–600	15
600–800	35
800–1000	55
1000–1500	80
1500–2000	90
2000–2500	95

Surviving LBW infants with handicap:

Birth weight (g)	Major handicap (%)
<1000	25
1000–1500	15
>1500	8

Longterm problems of LBW infants may include:

— cerebral palsy (4–10%)
— visual handicap (1–2%)
— sensorineural deafness (1–2%)
— minor motor dysfunction
— specific learning difficulties

Common neonatal problems

Feeding problems

Individual babies vary greatly in their requirements but as a general guide a term baby needs about 150 ml/kg by the 5th day of life. Babies fed on demand usually take 6–8 feeds/day. Most babies take about 15–20 minutes per feed. Breast-fed babies usually feed for about 10 minutes at each breast by the end of the first week.

Parents worried about feeding can often be reassured by explaining the normal variations in feeding patterns and demonstrating that the baby is growing normally. A home visit may be helpful and the health visitor is usually the best person to offer advice and reassurance. (Test weighing is inaccurate and is likely to increase maternal anxiety.)

1. *Reluctance to feed*
(a) may be a sign of serious illness, e.g. sepsis
(b) may be tired, e.g. small preterm baby
(c) poor suck
   • exclude submucous cleft palate
   • micrognathia

- underlying neurological problem, e.g. cerebral palsy

2. *'Always hungry'*

(a) Underfed: check quantity and constitution of feeds being offered if formula-fed. In breast-fed infants, consider adequacy of lactation, maternal depression, sore nipples?

(b) Thirsty: may need increased fluid particularly in hot weather.

(c) Crying for other reasons (see below).

3. *Possetting/small vomits*

(a) Air swallowing.

(b) Inadequate winding.

(c) Overfeeding (rare in breast-fed babies. Occasionally due to incorrect preparation of powdered milks. Some mothers add cereal to milk in the hope that baby will sleep longer).

(d) Gastro-oesophageal reflux (see p. 188).

(e) Consider pathological causes of vomiting (see below).

4. *Poor weight gain.* Most babies lose weight initially but regain their birthweight by 10 days. Initial losses of up to 10% of the birthweight may be due to physiological fluid adjustment; infants losing in excess of 10% should be carefully assessed, particularly if they are symptomatic, e.g. reluctant to feed, vomiting, diarrhoea.

The crying baby   Most mothers are adept at interpreting the cause of their baby's cry. Appropriate response to relieve the child's distress strengthens the relationship of confidence between mother and baby. Inability to recognize the cause of a baby's persistent crying leads to maternal anxiety and self-doubt.

Usual causes include hunger, boredom, tiredness, wind, wet nappy, teething or other discomfort. However, persistent excessive crying must be investigated to exclude a pathological cause and to relieve the parents. Consider:

— infections
— strangulated hernia
— intussusception
— torsion of the testis
— intestinal obstruction
— CMP allergy
— child abuse

Vomiting   Regurgitation of small amounts of milk is normal ('possetting'), but vomiting must never be assumed to be normal if:

(a) Baby is *unwell*, e.g. lethargic, off feeds, irritable. Consider:

— sepsis
— raised intracranial pressure
— IEM

(b) Associated *bowel disturbance*:

— watery stools may indicate
  • infective diarrhoea
  • NEC
  • septicaemia
  • IEM
— signs of obstruction, e.g. abdominal distension, visible peristalsis, bile-stained vomitus, may be due to
  • functional ileus
  • bowel atresia
  • meconium ileus
  • Hirschsprung disease
  • NEC

(c) *Blood-stained vomiting*. Consider:

— HDN
— gastric erosions
— swallowed maternal blood
— hiatus hernia

(d) *Persistent vomiting*. May be due to:

— sepsis
— neurological damage
— hiatus hernia
— pyloric stenosis
— cow's milk allergy
— intracranial SOL

Nappy rash   (See also Chapter 21)
Common causes

— ammoniacal dermatitis
— candidiasis
— seborrhoeic dermatitis

Other

— eczema
— psoriasis

Perianal excoriation   May be due to diarrhoea or acid stools. May accompany change from breast to formula feeds. If severe, investigate cause, e.g. disaccharide intolerance or infection. Expose and protect with barrier cream.

Jaundice   Becomes clinically apparent when SBr >85 mmol/1. Occurs in up to 50% of neonates. In majority it is 'physiological', i.e. occurs after 24 h, rises to a peak on 3rd–4th day (SBR <220 mmol/1) and then resolves by 7th–10th day. Well babies with jaundice following the above pattern do not need investigation.

Jaundice should be considered *abnormal* if:

— it occurs within first 24 h
— the baby is ill
— the rate of rise is >85 mmol/day
— it recurs after initial improvement
— it reaches a level of >220 mmol/1 in term babies or
                              >250 mmol/1 in preterm babies
— it is prolonged beyond 10 days in term babies or 14 days
  in preterm babies

Causes of neonatal jaundice before 24 h:

— haemolysis • Rhesus incompatibility
              • ABO incompatibility
              • red cell defects
— polycythaemia
— congenital infections

Causes of jaundice can be divided into those causing unconjugated and those causing conjugated hyperbilirubinaemia.
Many of the latter, particularly cases due to obstructive
causes (e.g. biliary atresia), are more likely to present with
prolonged jaundice after the baby has been discharged from
hospital, so it is important for health visitors and family
doctors to appreciate the possible significance of prolonged
jaundice and refer babies back for investigation.

Unconjugated
hyperbilirubinaemia

1. Haemolytic disorders
   — iso-immune: Rhesus/ABO/rare, e.g. Duffy, Kell
   — other: glucose-6-phosphate dehydrogenase deficiency,
     congenital spherocytosis
2. Infection.
3. Hypoxia.
4. Hypothyroidism.
5. Hypoglycaemia.
6. Galactosaemia, fructosaemia.
7. Dehydration.
8. Meconium retention.
9. High intestinal obstruction, e.g. pyloric stenosis.

Conjugated
hyperbulirubinaemia

1. Hepatocellular disease, including neonatal hepatitis.
2. Biliary hypoplasia.
3. Extrahepatic biliary atresia.
4. Choledochal cysts.
5. Infections: septicaemia, UTI, syphilis, toxoplasmosis,
viral (e.g. CMV, hepatitis, rubella, herpes simplex).
6. Metabolic: α1-antitrypsin deficiency, cystic fibrosis,
tyrosinaemia, some storage disorders, prolonged TPN.
7. Endocrine: hypothyroidism, hypopituitarism, hypo-
adrenalism.

Bilirubin toxicity Free unconjugated bilirubin is lipid soluble and readily diffuses across brain-cell membranes. When bilirubin in the brain reaches toxic levels, symptoms of *kernicterus* develop:

— poor feeding
— irritability, hypertonicity, opisthotonus
— high pitched cry
— apnoea, convulsions

Necropsy shows yellow bilirubin staining of the brainstem nuclei, basal ganglia, hippocampus + VIII N. If baby survives, residual effects may include:

— choreoathetoid cerebral palsy
— high frequency nerve deafness
— paralysis of upward gaze
— mental retardation

Rare in term infants if SBr does not exceed 380 mmol/1 but in preterm infants or in presence of acidosis, sepsis or hypoxia kernicterus may occur at much lower levels.

Management Graphic guidelines varying with gestation are available for management of jaundice in neonates but levels for intervention must be reviewed in the light of the clinical state of each infant.
(a) Ensure adequate hydration.
(b) Phototherapy. Narrow spectrum blue light of wavelength 450–475 nm causes photo-isomerization and photo-oxidation of bilirubin to less lipophilic pigments. Adverse effects include:

— diarrhoea
— increased fluid loss
— rashes
— thermal stress
— physical separation from mother
— possible retinal damage

(c) Exchange transfusion. For hyperbilirubinaemia use '2 volume' exchange, i.e. twice the infant's blood volume = 160 ml/kg. Will reduce SBr by up to 50%.

Respiratory distress Physical signs of respiratory distress include tachypnoea, grunting, cyanosis, sternal retraction and recession.
Conditions presenting with respiratory distress can usually be differentiated on the basis of the history, examination and chest X-ray. They include:

— pneumonia (especially Group B strep.)
— RDS (surfactant deficiency, see p. 31)
— aspiration syndromes: meconium, amniotic fluid, milk
— pneumothorax
— transient tachypnoea of the newborn

— congenital heart disease
— cardiac failure
— pulmonary haemorrhage
— congenital malformations
- diaphragmatic hernia
- tracheo-oesophageal fistula
- pulmonary hypoplasia, e.g. Potter syndrome
- choanal atresia
— persistent fetal circulation (PFC)
— hydrops ± pleural effusions
— Metabolic acidosis, e.g. asphyxia, haemorrhage, metabolic disorders
— neuromuscular disorders, e.g. myasthenia gravis, myotonic dystrophy

Convulsions   Occur in neonatal period in at least 1% of all live births. May be subtle (with tonic deviation of eyes, rhythmic sucking or cycling of limbs) or present as focal or generalized tonic–clonic seizures, sometimes with accompanying apnoea or cyanosis.

Causes

1. *Haemorrhagic ischaemic encephalopathy:*
   — perinatal asphyxia
   — subarachnoid haemorrhage
   — subdural haemorrhage
   — cerebral oedema
   — PVH

2. *Metabolic:*
   — hypoglycaemia
   — hypocalcaemia, hypomagnesaemia
   — hypernatraemia
   — rare IEM (e.g. pyridoxine deficiency)
   — kernicterus

3. *Infections:*
   — meningitis
   — septicaemia
   — congenital infection

4. Congenital malformation.
5. Drug withdrawal.
6. Idiopathic.

Investigations   In all cases:

— blood glucose
— infection screen
— serum electrolytes, calcium, magnesium
— blood gases

± further investigations as indicated by the clinical picture, e.g. cerebral US, toxicology screen, EEG, metabolic screen, skull X–ray, CT scan.

Management

(a) Check airway clear, O_2 if cyanosed.
(b) Check BM stix. If <2.2, draw blood for lab. glucose, then give i.v. dextrose 0.5 g/kg stat.
(c) Anticonvulsants if fitting continuing and not hypoglycaemic, e.g. phenobarbitone, paraldehyde, phenytoin.
(d) Investigate and treat for underlying cause as above.

Hypoglycaemia

Blood glucose falls rapidly in the first few hours of life and the infant draws on hepatic glycogen stores laid down in the last trimester. Alternative fuels such as lactate can be utilized to compensate for a low blood glucose temporarily but if the blood glucose remains low (<2.6 mmol/L), symptoms of neuroglycopenia may occur.

Up to 50% of symptomatic infants have severe neurological sequele, including mental retardation and spastic quadriplegia.

At risk babies should have regular capillary glucose checks at 3–4 hourly intervals. Early feeding should be started; if feeds have to be delayed for other reasons (e.g. RDS), then i.v. dextrose infusion should be commenced.

Causes of increased risk of hypoglycaemia

— prematurity
— SGA infants
— infant of diabetic mother
— asphyxia
— infection
— haemolytic disease
— hypothermia

Infection

The newborn infant is particularly susceptible to infection because of reduced defence mechanisms. Limited ability to localize infection means that local sepsis is likely to become generalized.

Presenting features may be subtle and non-specific:

— change in behaviour noted by parents or nurses
— poor feeding
— unstable temperature
— vomiting
— diarrhoea
— respiratory distress
— apnoea, bradycardia
— jaundice
— jitteriness, convulsions
— rash
— purpura
— pseudoparalysis

Increased risk of infection is associated with:

— prematurity or LBW
— traumatic delivery

— male sex
— PROM (>24 h)
— fetal distress
— maternal pyrexia/infection
— admission to NICU
— multiple invasive procedures, eg. indwelling catheters, drain insertion, etc.

Congenital infections	Intrapartum pathogens	Postnatal pathogens
Toxoplasma	*E. Coli*	*E. Coli*
Rubella	*N. gonorrhoea*	*Klebsiella*
CMV	*Group B strep.*	*Pseudomonas*
Herpes	*Chlamydia*	*Group B strep.*
Enterovirus	*Listeria monocytogenes*	*Staph. aureus*
Varicella	*H. simplex*	*Staph. epidermidis*
Syphilis	Hepatitis B	Candida
TB	CMV	
HIV		

If infection is suspected after delivery, a sepsis screen is performed, including:

— FBC, differential WBC, film, platelet count
— blood cultures
— surface swabs: ear, umbilicus
— gastric aspirate
— urine analysis and clean catch or SPA urine microscopy and culture
— stool culture
— blood glucose
— CXR

Other investigations which may be indicated include:

— CSF microscopy, culture, glucose and protein
— total IgM, TORCH titres, specific IgM
— Urine: CMV, rubella
— throat swabs ⎫
— stools   ⎬ for isolation of viruses
— skin vesicle fluid: EM for herpes virus
— clotting screen: PT, PTT, TT, FDPs
— skull X-ray (looking for calcification)
— ECG
— AXR if NEC suspected
— eye swab for Gram stain and culture for gonococcus
— Acute phase reactants: C-reactive protein is the most reliable of those evaluated so far and results can be rapidly available. Used in conjunction with other investigations, it may be useful indicator of neonatal bacterial infection
— counter current immuno-electrophoresis or latex agglutination for bacterial antigens in plasma or CSF

Management   1. *Broad spectrum antibiotics*. Initial choice will depend on presentation and age of onset but first-line antibiotics for onset of infection within 48 h of birth usually include e.g. penicillin and an aminoglycoside. Regimen is modified according to subsequent isolation of organism and sensitivities.

2. *General supportive treatment*:

(a) Ventilatory support for respiratory distress, apnoea, etc.

(b) Correct hypotension with FFP 10 ml/kg (will also aid opsonization).

(c) Transfuse if anaemic.

(d) Check for DIC, treat with vitamin K, FFP, platelet transfusions.

(e) Correct fluid, electrolyte and glucose imbalance.

(f) Correct metabolic acidosis by treating underlying cause as above + sodium bicarbonate 4.2% may be required.

(g) Intravenous immune globulin (IVIG) may be a useful adjunctive treatment in infected newborns but results of large studies regarding its safety and efficacy are needed.

(h) Nutritional support: iv alimentation often required.

(i) Exchange transfusion of fresh whole blood may be of value for severe septicaemia.

Congenital infections   Up to 5% of babies have congenital infections but the majority are asymptomatic. The commonest non-bacterial organisms infecting the fetus are toxoplasma, rubella, CMV and herpes (the TORCH infections).

Clinical symptoms	Toxoplasma	Rubella	CMV	Herpes	Enterovirus
Growth retardation	+	+	+	+	+
Jaundice	+	+	+	+	+
Hepatosplenomegaly	+	+	+	+	+
Pneumonitis	+	+	+	+	+
Petechiae	+	+	+	+	+
Exanthems	+	–	–	+	+
CNS					
Meningoencephalitis	+	+	+	+	+
Microcephaly	+	–	++	+	–
Intracranial calcification	++	–	++	–	–
Paralysis	–	–	–	–	++
Myocarditis	+	+	–	+	++
Eye					
Glaucoma	–	++	–	–	–
Chorioretinitis	++	++	+	+	–
Cataract	+	++	–	+	–

CMV   Commonest congenital viral infection: rate of primary CMV infection in pregnancy 2–3%; carries 30% risk of transmission to the fetus.

Incidence in UK 3–4 cases in 1000 births. Up to 95% of these infants are asymptomatic, although a small number develop neurological deficit later in life. The remainder may present with severe multisystem disease: these cases are usually due to primary maternal infection rather than re-activation.

Confirm diagnosis by culture of throat swab and urine for CMV and demonstrating CMV-specific IgM in infant's serum.

In those with severe neonatal disease, mortality rate is 20–30% and many survivors will have neurological sequelae, including microcephaly, cerebral palsy, deafness and visual impairment.

In the 1970s, infants were found to have acquired CMV from blood transfusions and some developed a fatal pneumonitis. To reduce this risk transfusion services now provide screened CMV-negative blood for neonates.

Toxoplasmosis   Toxoplasma gondii is a protozoon which has its sexual cycle in the cat and can be transmitted to humans by the ingestion of material (usually meat from other animals) contaminated with oocysts from cat faeces.

About 75% of the UK population are susceptible to toxoplasmosis but the rate of primary infection in pregnancy is low (about 2 cases in 1000 pregnancies). Patients may be asymptomatic or have a 'flu' or glandular fever type illness. In only 10% of cases is the fetus damaged; 12–15 cases of congenital toxoplasmosis per annum are reported to the Clinical Diseases Surveillance Unit (CDSU). The classic presentation is a small-for-dates baby with hydrocephalus, diffuse intracranial calcification and chorioretinitis.

For women found to have seroconverted in pregnancy, spiramycin may reduce the risk to the fetus. For the affected neonate alternate courses of spiramycin with pyrimethamine plus sulphadiazine may reduce morbidity.

Rubella   Despite routine vaccination of girls between 11 and 13 years, up to 15% of females are still susceptible to rubella at the time of pregnancy.

In the first 4 weeks chance of congenital damage is 50%, at 8 weeks 25%, and at 12 weeks 15%. In later pregnancy, leads to hearing defects alone in approx. two-thirds.

Clinical features   May cause stillbirth or SGA infant with active infection (purpura, hepatosplenomegaly, jaundice, encephalitis) ± congenital anomalies (congenital rubella syndrome) including:

— cataract, retinopathy, micropthalmia, glaucoma
— cardiac defect (PDA, ASD, PS)
— deafness
— microcephaly, cerebral palsy, mental retardation
— osteitis

Now rare (<20 cases per annum). Must be notified to the Congenital Rubella Surveillance Programme.

No specific treatment available. Rubella-susceptible women should be immunized in the puerperium with live attenuated rubella vaccine.

(Infants with congenital CMV or rubella may shed the virus for several years and should be segregated from pregnant members of staff.)

Herpes simplex (Types 1 and 2)   Causes a serious neonatal infection. 61 confirmed cases notified to the BPSU in UK between July 1986 and December 1990.

Usually acquired by intrapartum contact with maternal genital herpes, though transplacental transmission rarely occurs. Overt primary genital herpes at term is an indication for delivery by Caesarian section.

There are three forms of neonatal illness:

— localized oral, cutaneous or ophthalmic lesions
— localized CNS disease
— disseminated disease. May cause overwhelming infection with hypotension, renal failure, DIC, pneumonitis, meningoencephalitis

Mortality rate in disseminated herpes is up to 90%.

Treatment   I.V. acyclovir for 14 days.

Varicella zoster   Congenital infections are very rare; reported in mothers developing chickenpox before 20 weeks gestation; infants have cutaneous scars, limb hypoplasia, fits and cortical atrophy. Most women with first trimester varicella either abort spontaneously or have a normal baby at term.

If a mother develops chickenpox within 2–3 weeks of delivery, 20% of infants develop neonatal chickenpox. Those born within 5 days of the appearance of the rash often develop chickenpox at 5–10 days, have a high mortality and should receive a dose of zoster immune globulin (ZIG) as soon after delivery as possible. If any signs of illness develop in these babies they should be treated with acyclovir for at least 10 days.

Hepatitis   Infections hepatitis in the newborn period may be associated with congenital infections including those discussed above.

1. *Hepatitis A*: transplacental infection not reported. Does not cause congenital abnormalities.

2. *Hepatitis B*: Hepatitis B surface antigen HB_sAg, the marker for the hepatitis B carrier state, is present in up to 15% of the population in some tropical countries.

Transplacental passage is uncommon but perinatal infection due to leak of maternal blood into infant's circulation, or its ingestion at birth, is an important route of infection.

A small number of infected infants are unwell with neonatal jaundice; some develop fulminating hepatitis and die with massive hepatic necrosis. The majority remain well but HB$_5$Ag appears in their blood between 6 weeks and 4 months after birth and usually persists. They become chronic carriers and are at long-term risk of chronic liver disease and primary hepatic carcinoma in adulthood.

Management

In Britain a national surveillance programme of hepatitis B immunoglobulin administration is in progress.

The serology of carriers whose infants are at high risk is either HB$_e$Ag positive, or HB$_e$Ag negative and anti-HB$_e$ negative. Passive-active immunization of infants of carrier mothers is recommended.

Schedule: Hep B Ig 200 mg i.m. within 48 hours of delivery + Hep B virus vaccine 0.5 ml i.m. at:
- birth
- 1 month
- 7 months

The course may be hastened by giving the third dose at 3 months with a booster at 1 year. Serology should be checked at 1 year.

HIV infection

(see p. 149)

Syphilis

Congenital syphilis is now rare in the UK; screening in the first trimester has significantly contributed to its decline. As the fetus is not infected before the 4th month of pregnancy the results of treatment in early pregnancy are excellent for both mother and fetus. Cases may occasionally be missed, however, due to late booking, failure of treatment or re-infection.

The clinical features may appear at birth or later, between 2nd and 6th week:

— skin eruptions (coppery maculopapular rash)
— hepatosplenomegaly
— purulent or sanguinous nasal discharge
— lymphadenopathy
— rhagades (radiating fissured scars around the mouth)
— saddle nose
— genital condylomata
— osteochondritis
— CNS: meningitis, hydrocephalus

Diagnosis

Positive IgM FTA (may be false positive if mother positive, therefore if no clinical signs repeat test in 3 months.

Treatment

Penicillin for 14 days.

Listeriosis

Listeria monocytogenes is a Gram positive coccus commonly found in the environment and in food. The upward trend in food poisoning in general has been the focus of much recent concern. Foods implicated in outbreaks of Listeriosis have included coleslaw, milk, soft cheeses and meat paté. The epidemiology of the disease is currently under study by the CDSU.

Fetal infection in 1st trimester can cause abortion (may be recurrent) and in the 3rd trimester can cause preterm delivery of a very ill neonate with disseminated infection. Clinical features include pneumonia, hepatomegaly and meningitis. Widespread granulomatous lesions in skin, lung, liver and nervous system may be found at autopsy (Granulomatosis infantisepticum).

Perinatal and late onset listeriosis usually present with meningitis ± septicaemia.

Treatment   Ampicillin and gentamicin.

Tuberculosis   Maternal TB is now rare in pregnancy in Britain but if it does occur the infant has no transmitted immunity and must be protected by prophylactic treatment with isoniazid for 3 months. Isoniazid-resistant BCG must be given.

Advances have been made in prevention of some congenital infections, notably rubella, and also in recognition of other microbial pathogens which are emerging as potential causes of fetal morbidity such as parvovirus, cryptosporidium and borrelia burgdorferi, the tick-borne spirochete which causes Lyme disease. New forms of adjunctive immunotherapy may help to improve survival in the sick, infected neonate.

3. Infant feeding and nutrition

Breast feeding   All mothers should be encouraged to breast feed for the first 4–6 months of life.

Advantages

(a) Breast feeding is enjoyable and facilitates bonding.

(b) Breast milk is more convenient. It is supplied pre-prepared, pre-heated, and sterile. The baby can take as much as he wants and leave the rest for later.

(c) It has an ideal protein:fat ratio. Fore milk has relatively more protein, hind milk has more fat.

(d) It is more interesting for the baby as the maternal diet changes the taste.

(e) In the first 2 days of life colostrum is a good source of carbohydrate and antibody. Secretory IgA protects the gut directly from bacterial and viral infection.

(f) Macrophages in breast milk produce complement, lacto-peroxidase and lysozymes to destroy microorganisms.

(g) Breast milk contains lactoferrin, an iron binding protein which inhibits pathogenic *Escherichia coli* and promotes growth of lactobacilli in the gut.

(h) Structural changes take place in the baby's gut in response to feeding due to the stimulation of secretion of gut hormones such as insulin, enteroglucagon and motilin.

(i) Breast milk contains cyclic AMP and GMP which are important for the regulation processes of maturation.

(j) Breast milk contains higher concentrations of some substances which may be important for development, e.g. taurine, long-chain fatty acids. Recent studies suggest breast-fed infants have a higher IQ than those fed on formulae.

(k) Studies suggest reduction in the incidence of eczema in breast-fed infants of atopic parents compared with formula fed infants.

(l) Full breast feeding provides good contraception via prolactin suppression of ovulation.

Bottle feeding   Compared to breast milk, cow's milk has:

— more protein, sodium, phosphate and other minerals (i.e. more solute)

— less lactose and polyunsaturated fatty acids (PUFA)

— higher casein:whey ratio

— higher energy density

The processes involved in making cow's milk suitable for babies involve, therefore, reducing the curd protein to make it more easily digested, or adding carbohydrate and fat to reduce solute load by dilution.

There is a wide range of modified milks on the market. If bottle feeding is started at birth, the choice is usually determined by the hospital stocks of pre-packed bottled milks, which the mother will continue to buy. Otherwise the health visitor or GP may be approached and tend to advise their own particular favourite, but there is no evidence to suggest that any one formula will suit a baby better than another. Mothers tend to blame the formula used if the baby is especially unsettled but should be advised not to keep changing brands as this is rarely the cause.

Formula milks

Commonly used formula milks are of four basic types.

1. *Whey-based formulae* in which casein is demineralized by electrodialysis. Minerals, vegetable oils and lactose are then added. The casein:whey ratio of 40:60 is equal to that of human milk, e.g. Wyeth SMA Gold Cap, Cow & Gate Premium, Farley's Osterfeed.

2. *Casein-based formulae* with vegetable fat replacing animal fat and addition of carbohydrate (maltodextrins) to reduce solute load. The casein:whey ratio is 80:20 (equivalent to cow's milk) and the renal solute load is higher, e.g. Wyeth SMA White Cap, Cow & Gate Plus, Farley's Ostermilk complete.

3. *Hydrolysed casein formulae*. The breakdown of casein renders it less antigenic and more easily digested. These milks are suitable for babies with allergic problems or malabsorption, e.g. Pregestimil, Prejomin, Nutramigen.

4. *Soya-based formulae*. Soya protein replaces animal protein, with vegetable fats and non-lactose sugars added, e.g. Wyeth Wysoy, Cow & Gate Formula S.

Other specialized infant formulae are available for specific indications. These are usually nutritionally complete, e.g.

(a) Lactose-free milks for lactose intolerance (contain sucrose or glucose), e.g. Pregestimil, Wysoy.
(b) Glucose-free milks for glucose–galactose intolerance (contain fructose), e.g. Galactomin 19.
(c) Low calcium feeds for use in hypercalcaemia (e.g. Cow & Gate Locasol).
(d) Specific formula milks for use in disorders of amino acid metabolism, e.g. Lofenalac for phenylketonuria.
(e) High energy density milks are often used for LBW and premature babies.

Milk feeds should be made up according to the manufacturer's instructions (generally one level scoop to 1 fl. ounce/30 ml of water). The daily requirement is about 150 ml/kg/day in divided feeds. Bottle-fed babies can be fed 3–4 hourly or on demand. All utensils must be sterilized by immersion for at least half an hour in a sodium hypochlorite solution or by steam sterilization for 10 min. Sterilizers are now available for use in microwave ovens.

Advantages

(a) Enables another person to feed the baby. Important if mother is ill or has more than one baby.
(b) Volume of milk taken can be measured accurately.
(c) Type of feed can be changed if necessary, e.g. milk allergy, low birth weight, disorders of amino acid metabolism.
(d) Formula milks have added vitamins, iron and minerals.

General advice about feeding

- A common complaint of new mothers is about the surfeit of advice received on the subject of feeding! The GP and health visitor are in an ideal position to make early contact and advise on correct feeding practices.
- All mothers should be visited at home around the 11th day postnatally (the midwife attends until day 10). Observation of feeding is the easiest way to establish that there is good maternal–infant bonding and no problems breast feeding, or in making up formula feeds.
- Inverted nipples are not a reason to discourage breast feeding as most babies will draw out the nipple well once latched on.
- Breast feeding should begin at birth or shortly after, as soon as the mother is able.
- Breast feeding should be on demand, or at least 4 hourly. Some babies will feed every hour. The best stimulus to milk production is frequent suckling and breast emptying.
- Advise the mother to eat a sensible diet with plenty of fresh fruit and vegetables. Dairy produce is a good source of calcium and calories. Calorie-restricted, weight-reducing diets are inadvisable at this time. In general, appetite will increase and the extra calories necessary for milk production will be taken without planning. The extra daily requirement is about 500 kcal.
- Breast milk production is very dependent on a happy relaxed frame of mind. An anxious mother will produce less milk, or find that the let-down reflex, which is stimulated by oxytocin release, is inhibited. With persistence, most mothers can breast feed successfully.
- Check position of baby at the breast to minimize air swallowing and therefore regurgitation and colic.
- Babies taking large amounts of milk often pass soft, even liquid, stools several times a day. They may, alternatively, only pass a single stool every few days. Mothers should be reassured that both these extremes are normal.
- Regular weighings at a weekly well-baby clinic provide mothers with an opportunity to discuss worries and make

important social contacts. It also allows the health visitor to monitor the baby's progress and refer to the GP at the earliest opportunity should problems arise.

Increased surveillance may be necessary of babies with poor intrauterine growth or those at high risk of sudden infant death. There is some evidence that daily weighing combined with advice from the health visitor and early medical checks in the case of suspected illness may reduce the number of babies dying from sudden infant death syndrome (see p. 316).

11. The Department of Health recommends that vitamin supplements are given to all breast-fed babies. Abidec (Parke Davies) drops (0.6 ml) contain:

Vitamin A 4000 iu
Vitamin C 50 mg
Vitamin D 400 iu
Vitamin B6 0.5 mg
Riboflavine 0.4 mg
Nicotinamide 5 mg

Feeding problems in the neonate   See Chapter 2.

Weaning   Current recommendations are that solids should not be introduced before the age of 3–4 months. (Few mothers actually wait this long. The 1985 OPCS study found 89% of babies aged 4 months had already started on solids.) Early introduction of solids may cause allergic reactions due to increased permeability of the intestinal mucosa to a variety of food antigens (e.g. gluten) in the first 3 months.

(a) New foods should be introduced singly so any adverse reaction can be observed.

(b) Start with rice cereal mixed with breast or formula milk, given on a teaspoon. Subsequently add in fruit purees and vegetables. As the amount of solids taken increases, reduce the milk feeds and offer water or fruit juices. These can be given in a 'teacher beaker' with a spout and handles.

(c) Add iron-containing foods (meat, dark green vegetables and iron fortified cereals) at around 6 months.

(d) Avoid eggs and wheat until at least 6 months.

(e) Increase the amount of solids gradually up to 3 meals a day.

(f) Foods should be pureed up to 6–7 months. After this most babies start chewing. This is an important developmental stage and should be encouraged by offering mashed foods and 'finger foods'.

(g) By 1 year should be feeding themselves using a spoon and eating ordinary family meals cut into small pieces.

(h) Breast milk or infant formulae should be continued (up to 600 ml/day) with the weaning diet until 1 year of age.

(i) 'Doorstep' milk can be safely given to children after the age of 1 year. Full cream milk is recommended for all children until age 5 years as it is an important source of calories and fat-soluble vitamins.

Feeding the older child

Many children aged 1–3 years are 'fussy eaters' and mothers frequently complain about poor appetite. Studies have shown however that, if offered a variety of foods, children will take a balanced diet over a period of time but not at every meal.

• Continue intake of 300 ml of milk daily.
• Children at risk of nutritional deficiency include vegetarians, those in large families with low incomes, and some immigrant families.
• Average calorie requirements in childhood:
  0–3 months 530 kcal/day
  4–6 months 675 kcal/day
  7–9 months 795 kcal/day
  1 year 1000 kcal/day
  3 years 1300 kcal/day
  4–6 years 1500–1800 kcal/day
  Teenagers may need as many calories as a manual labourer (up to 3500 kcal/day).
• When giving dietary advice remember the differences in diet of ethinic populations:

  — Kosher Jews exclude pork, rabbit and shellfish. They eat Kosher meat only, not to be consumed at the same time as dairy produce
  — Hindus and Sikhs exclude beef and pork
  — Halal moslems exclude pork. Halal meat only
  — vegetarians exclude meat, chicken and fish
  — vegans exclude all animal produce and products including eggs, honey and milk. These children are at high risk of failure to thrive, with protein, vitamin and calcium deficiency. Pulses and nuts are however a good source of nutrients and if taken in reasonable quantities provide a satisfactory protein intake. B12 supplements are usually required

Obesity

Definition   >30% over ideal weight. This is the commonest form of malnutrition in developed countries.

Aetiology   Genetic and environmental factors play a part. There is a high concordance rate in studies of monozygotic twins, including those raised apart.

Less than half of all overweight infants remain overweight as adults but the older the child, the more likely it is that the problem will continue into adult life. Most overweight adults were overweight as children.

Gross obesity in childhood is very difficult to treat. Prevention is the best management and involves identifying those children who are mildly obese and monitoring progress closely.

Diagnosis   (a) Take a full dietary history, including mealtime and snacking behaviour.

(b) Plot height and weight on a centile chart.

(c) Examine the child for signs of pathological causes for obesity. All obese healthy children are tall for their age (with an advanced bone age). In short obese children look for signs of:

— Cushing's syndrome
— hypothyroidism
— Prader–Willi syndrome
— Lawrence–Moon–Biedl syndrome.

(d) Measure skinfold thickness.

Management   (a) Successful weight reduction is most likely if the child recognizes the problem and wants to solve it.

(b) The whole family should be involved in supporting the child, and should follow a healthy eating programme.

(c) See children weekly for weighing and encouragement.

(d) Suggest strategies for coping with unhealthy snacking habits; increasing physical activity is ideal as it decreases the amount of time available for eating and increases energy expenditure.

(e) Children under 10 years should aim to maintain weight with increasing age.

(f) Over the age of 10 years reduce calorie intake to aim at a loss of 0.5–1.0 lb weekly.

(g) Calorie intake should not be less than 6 kcal/cm for girls and 8 kcal/cm for boys. For school age children, allow a total of 800–1400 kcal/day, depending on height and degree of obesity.

(h) 'Calorie counting' is a good way of involving parent and child and allows the child to exercise a degree of choice. Children do not like to be different at school and choose appropriate foods from what is on offer with occasional 'treats' to boost morale.

There is a strong social stigma attached to obesity and children are usually teased about it. This may result in feelings of shame, rejection and low self-esteem. Direct discussion with the child about these issues and positive reinforcement of how they can change the situation helps even in young children.

Malnutrition
There are over 150 million malnourished children in the world. 'Malnourished' is defined as more than 2 SD below the desirable weight for age. Malnutrition may be due to poverty, disease or lack of knowledge about the special feeding needs of young children.
- major forms are *marasmus* and *kwashiorkor*.
- classification is related to weight for age, weight for height and height for age.
- onset is commonest after weaning between the ages of 9 months and 2 years.
- Presentation varies with age and duration.
- Interference with normal development will result if it becomes severe.

Marasmus
This is the commonest form of malnutrition. Caused by inadequate calorie intake or chronic diarrhoea and malabsorption. The former may be due to:
— inadequate breast milk (often because of maternal malnutrition during famine)
— feeding problems (e.g. LBW infants tire easily with feeding, etc.)
— maternal deprivation

Features
— weight loss, failure to thrive with muscle and tissue wasting and marked growth retardation
— alert but irritable
— hungry
— sparse hair, abdominal distension
— impaired immune function

Treatment
(a) High calorie, high protein diet (calories — 100 kcal/kg/day; protein 3 g/kg/day based on expected weight). Feed 2 hourly if very ill.
(b) Exclude infection/parasites.
(c) Weekly weighing until full recovery.

Kwashiorkor
This is more common among older children. Aetiology is poorly understood but possible association with mycotoxin from Aspergillus sp. in contaminated food.

Results from a diet low in protein but low or normal in calorie intake. This causes disturbance of protein, water and electrolyte metabolism. Occasionally seen in British children fed on 'macrobiotic' diets.

Presentation
— oedema (due to low serum protein and/or increased sodium retention), with ascites
— reduction in growth rate (not as marked as in marasmus)
— nutritional anaemia
— diarrhoea
— vitamin deficiencies, e.g. rickets, xerophthalmia

— dermatoses on arms and legs, look like burns with irregular pigmentation and desquamation
— hair loss (may see 'flag sign' bands of different colours in hair due to past periods of malnutrition)
— anorexia
— drowsy, apathetic
— can be rapidly fatal in some children. Death is usually due to complications, e.g. dehydration, septicaemia, hypoglycaemia, hypothermia, hypokalaemia

Investigations
— serum proteins, cholesterol, potassium and magnesium all low
— serum cortisol and growth hormone levels increased
— somatomedins low, increase as nutrition improves

Treatment
(a) Treat infections.
(b) Correct fluid and electrolyte disturbances.
(c) Start with low calorie/low protein diet, ~80 kcal/kg/day, supplement with magnesium, potassium, folic acid. No iron, as low tranferrin gives risk of toxicity. Hourly nasogastric or i.v. feeding if necessary. Increase after 5 days to 100 kcal/kg/day.
(d) May need lactose-free milk.
(e) Parenteral vitamin K, plus vitamin A and D supplements.
(f) Blood transfusion if very anaemic.
(g) Gradually introduce mixed diet appropriate to locality.

Vitamin A deficiency
Daily requirement of vitamin A is 500 µg in children under 4 years. Food sources: liver, dark green vegetables, carrots, wheat. (Deficiency common in parts of the world where the staple food is rice, with little animal fat.)

Presentation
— night blindness
— xerophthalmia: dryness of the eyes with corneal cloudiness and scarring (keratomalacia) leading to blindness. This is the major preventable cause of childhood blindness in the world

Treatment
Severe deficiency: i.m. vitamin A 3000 µg/kg to start, followed by the same dose orally for 5 days, then 1500 µg daily until the eyes are normal.

Scurvy
Due to deficiency of vitamin C which is essential for the formation of healthy collagen. Minimum daily requirement 20–35 mg. Food sources: citrus fruits, green vegetables, potato skins, breast milk and supplemented formula milks.

Presentation
Any age but commonly between 6–24 months. Deficiency causes increased capillary fragility resulting in:

— petechiae, bruising and bleeding especially from gums

and subperiosteally (resulting in the typical 'pseudo-paralysis'). A hypochromic anaemia may develop
— anorexia
— fever
— slow wound healing

Diagnois   (a) Clinical.
        (b) Characteristic X-ray changes:
           — decalcification
           — atrophy of bony trabeculae
           — dense cortical bone unaffected
           — epiphyseal separation
           — superiosteal haemorrhages calcify
        (c) Vitamin C levels in buffy layer of centrifuged blood.

Treatment   200 mg vitamin C orally.

Iron deficiency   See p. 288.

4. Preventive paediatrics

Child health surveillance　The Government child health surveillance (CHS) programme in general practice is carried out by family doctors who have satisfied the Family Health Services Committee that they are competent to provide such services. Parents must decide whether to attend their GP or the local community clinic, staffed by Community Medical Officers (CMOs), in order to establish accountability for the checks over the child's first 5 years.

Aims　(a) Early detection of significant problems in infancy.
(b) Health education. Advice about:

— infant feeding/weaning
— normal development
— routine immunisation
— recognition of illness in babies

(c) Formation of a relationship with the mother and child. Provides opportunity to see the child when in good health and to observe the interaction between mother and child.

Examinations are generally carried out at the following ages (correction should be made for prematurity):

— neonatal
— 6 weeks
— 8 months
— 18 months
— 3 years

At each examination a detailed history is taken. The physical examination should include all areas of development:

— gross motor
— fine motor
— vision
— hearing and speech
— social

Neonatal examination　See p. 14.

6-week check　About 5% of babies will be found to have a developmental or physical problem at 6 weeks.

History　(a) Antenatal and birth history, including birth weight, gestation and any neonatal problems.

(b) Family and social history, including mother's current mental and physical health.
(c) Baby's progress. Ask about:

— feeding problems
— weight gain
— bowels
— sleep
— parental worries, particularly concerns regarding vision and hearing

Physical examination   Weight, length and head circumference (plot on centile chart). Note:

— dysmorphic features
— skull: size, shape, fontanelles, sutures
— mouth: palate, sucking reflex, monilia
— spine: dimples, dermal sinus
— CVS: murmurs, femoral pulses, palpable liver
— RS: look for tachypnoea, recession, cyanosis
— abdomen: herniae, visceromegaly
— external genitalia: note position of testes in boys
— skin, e.g. jaundice, naevi, milia, cradle cap
— limbs: check for congenital dislocation of hips
— eyes: check for squint, red reflex, fixation, proptosis, nystagmus
— hearing: difficult to assess reliably at 6 weeks. If in high-risk category for hearing loss, refer for testing.

Development   1. *Motor.* Observe nature and symmetry of spontaneous movements. Asymmetry may suggest hemiplegeia, brachial plexus injury, fracture or joint infection.

Supine posture: Full term 6-week-old infant lying supine has limbs semiflexed; when head turns to one side, arm and leg on that side are extended (asymmetric tonic reflex (ATNR)). Normally present from 2 weeks and lost by 5 months; persistence beyond this age suggests neurological abnormality, e.g. cerebral palsy.

Prone: Intermittent semi-extension of the hips when awake.

Ventral suspension: Head held briefly in same plane as rest of body with hips partially extended and knees and elbows semiflexed. In contrast the hypotonic infant hangs limply with head down and limbs extended.

Head control: Lifts head briefly when prone, turning face to side.

2. *Inherent reflexes. Moro*: Rapid release of the head in a supine infant produces abduction and extension of the arms with opening of the hands, followed by adduction of the arms. It is a vestibular response initiated by the sudden cervical movement. Present from birth to about 4 months; persistence after 6 months abnormal. Diminished in hypertonia, absent in severe hypotonia. Asymmetry suggests

brachial plexus injury, fractured clavicle or humerus, hemiplegia.

Grasp: The hands should be intermittently open. Reflex gripping occurs when palm or sole is stimulated (with head in mid-line). Disappears by 3 months; persistence suggests spasticity.

Primary walking: Supporting baby upright with soles of feet pressing against table produces stepping movements. Present from birth to about 6 weeks (longer if performed with neck extended). Abnormal if still present by 6 months. May be difficult to elicit after breech presentation.

Oral reflexes: When the baby's cheek touches the breast he searches or 'roots' for milk. Sucking and swallowing reflexes are present at birth in term babies, and in preterm babies from about 34 weeks' gestation.

3. *Vision*

— fixes, follows
— defensive blink
— shuts eyes to bright torch

4. *Hearing*

— startles or stills to sound
— reflex eye movements or attempt to turn head to voice

5. *Social*

— smiles in response to mother's face. Delay after 8 weeks is significant in a full-term infant
— vocalization: coos and gurgles start about 2 weeks after first smiles. (Note: deaf children may do this as well but babble diminishes with time)

8-month check

History

From mother if possible:

(a) Baby's *general condition*: any recent illnesses, hospital admissions, etc.
(b) Enquire about any other relevant *family* or *environmental problems*.
(c) *Feeding*. Chewing should be well established, providing that the infant has been given solid foods to try. He should be able to hold a biscuit alone and eat it. Mentally retarded children are late in learning to chew.

   Discuss details of weaning diet. Advise on nutritional requirements.
(d) *Sleeping*. Most babies of this age will have settled into a routine and be sleeping through the night. Teething can cause problems at this age.
(e) *Immunisations* (see p. 67).
(f) *Development*. Ask whether the child can sit, crawl, pull to stand, roll over, grab toys voluntarily and transfer from

hand to hand. This is important because, although the examination will test for these, an uncooperative child may not perform as well as he is able. The history and examination taken together can be used to decide whether the child should be recalled at a later date.

(g) *Parental concerns.* Ask specifically about vision and hearing.

Physical examination

— Observe responsiveness, smiling, interest in surroundings
— measure weight, length, head circumference. Plot on centile chart and compare with previous recordings
— listen to vocalization; should be babbling, e.g. da-da, ga-ga
— examine skin, e.g. haemangiomas may not have been present at 6 week check
— skull shape, fontanelles
— mouth and palate: check erupting teeth
— respiratory system
— cardiovascular system
— check abdomen for masses, herniae, testicular descent in boys
— examine hips, looking for symmetry of skin creases in thighs and buttocks and range of abduction
— check spine for scoliosis
— eyes: squint, cataracts
— note any congenital abnormality

Development

1. *Gross motor. Head control*: No lag on pulling to sit (full head control at 4–5 months).

Sitting: Most babies will be able to sit unsupported for a few seconds.

Rolling: Learn to roll prone to supine first and should have progressed to rolling supine to prone by 8 months.

Weight bearing: If trunk supported. May stand holding on.

Crawling: Average age of crawling is 10 months. 'Bottom shufflers' tend not to want to lie prone but sit and wriggle and in so doing move forward. Babies can become so proficient at this that walking can be delayed until 18 months or more. Thus there are a variety of normal methods of progression but no mobility by 10 months is cause for concern.

2. *Reflexes. Parachute*: This appears at 6–9 months and persists for life. Sudden lowering of the baby head first towards the ground causes the arms to extend as if to protect him from falling. In cerebral palsy this reflex is weak or absent. In hemiplegia it is asymmetrical.

Propping reactions: Present from about 6 months. With the baby sitting, tilting him to one side will cause the arm on that side to extend as if to protect him from falling sideways. May be absent in cerebral palsy.

Neonatal reflexes (moro, grasp, stepping) should have disappeared.

3. *Fine motor. Reaching*: By 8 months, can reach out and grasp toys accurately with either hand. Handedness should not be present at this age. Hand preference suggests weakness of the other hand and should be investigated.

No voluntary release yet. If offered a second toy, the first will be either dropped or transferred to the other hand.

All objects taken to mouth for exploration at 6–12 months. Persists beyond 13 months in retarded children.

Intermediate grasp: Index finger approach and finger-thumb apposition develop at 9–10 months.

4. *Vision*

— observe visual interest in objects; look for squint, head tilt or wandering eye movements
— test for fixing on small objects such as 'hundreds and thousands'
— preferential looking tests and the Catford drum are also used to test visual acuity by orthoptists, to whom children should be referred for further testing if concern arises

5. *Hearing and speech.* Hearing tests are difficult to carry out in a clinic. Distraction tests are reliable *if performed correctly*, by two specially trained examiners. One distracts the child, while the other produces test sounds at the correct frequency and amplitude. This is best done using calibrated machines producing 35 dB warble tones at different frequencies. Other suitable stimuli include *gentle* swirling of a Manchester rattle or a quiet 's' consonant. (Rustling paper and tinkling spoons in cups are unreliable and unacceptable methods.) Baby only passes if he responds with head turn (not just eyes) to each side.

6. *Social and general understanding*

— concept of permanence of objects. Looks for fallen objects
— understands 'no!'
— imitates sounds

Warning signs suggest developmental delay or emotional deprivation.:

— disinterest in surroundings
— infrequent smiles
— failure to imitate

18-month check

History (a) *General* health, behaviour and any sleeping or feeding problems. Tantrums common at this age.
(b) *Family* or *environmental* problems.

(c) *Immunizations*. The primary course of OPV, DPT and Hib and MMR should be complete.

(d) *Development*:

— ask about speech. Most use intelligible words by 18 months (first words usually about 11 months)
— ask when walked unaided (from 13 months)
— should be able to drink from a cup (from 15 months) and use spoon
— helps with undressing
— domestic mimicry
— indicates need for potty from 15 months. From 18 months may be dry by day
— Ask about behaviour with other children. Usually play alongside but not with each other at this age (parallel rather than interactive play). A history of lack of contact with other children may reveal maternal isolation or depression

(e) *Parental concerns*

Physical examination At this age this is sometimes difficult due to child's dislike of strangers and stethoscopes! Observe the child carefully while taking the history and examine him on the mother's knee to begin with.

— measure standing height, weight and head circumference. Plot on existing centile chart. A growth velocity chart may be started at this time if an accurate height measurement can be obtained
— repeat physical examination as at the 8-month check
— check teeth. This is a good time to educate parents about the importance of dental health. Encourage them to take the child for a first dental check up if not already performed

Development 1. *Gross motor. Gait*. Most children are walking alone by 18 months. Children who are not should be examined carefully for signs of cerebral palsy, muscle disorder or intellectual delay. Some may be 'bottom shufflers' who usually walk by 24 months. Congenital dislocation of the hip does not cause delay in walking (but look for signs of uneven gait and asymmetric skin creases).

2. *Fine motor*

— should have a well developed pincer grip, and release
— spontaneous straight scribbling with pencil held in palm
— builds a tower of 3 or 4 bricks
— enjoys looking at books, tries to turn pages two or more at once

Warning signs: Mouthing of objects and casting of toys to floor or any parental concerns.

3. *Hearing, speech and general understanding*

— knows and responds to own name
— test comprehension. Should be able to carry out simple commands, e.g. 'give me the shoe'
— will point to pictures of familiar objects in book, e.g. cat, ball, cup
— will identify object by using appropriate gesture, e.g. brushing hair
— speech should include at least three words with meaning, other than mummy and daddy. Many children have a well developed tuneful jargon which is incomprehensible but sounds as if they know what they are saying! It is a reassuring sign that normal speech will soon follow. 50% of children will have started to join words at this age. This is not very useful however as a screening test. The development of normal comprehension is a better guide to intelligence and development
— hearing tests are difficult to carry out at this age. Refer if not talking, parental concern about hearing or frequent ear infections

3-year check

History (a) Note any medical problems.
(b) Family or environmental problems.
(c) Ask about general behaviour, speech, social skills. Many children have started attending nursery school at 3 years. Most will settle comfortably into a daily routine having resolved initial separation anxiety. Starting to play with other children.

Most children are out of nappies during the day by 3 years of age, with about 50% dry at night as well. Failure to develop continence may be associated with developmental delay.

Physical examination — measure standing height and weight, plot on centile chart
— general system examination, as in earlier checks

Development 1. *Gross motor.*

— observe *gait*. Should walk with narrow stable gait and run easily in a straight line. Uses dominant hand (preference established from about 2 years). Climbs on and off chair with ease. Climbs up on chair to reach high objects
— can *stand* on one leg for a few seconds. Good screening test for mild hemiplegia
— *jumps* with two feet together
— *climbs* stairs one foot per step

2. *Fine motor.* Builds a tower of eight cubes and a bridge. Observe pencil grip and spontaneous drawing. The grip varies between an immature tripod grip held halfway along

shaft of pencil to a more mature writing grip. Spontaneous drawing usually takes the form of vertical and circular scribbles.

Ask child to copy horizontal line, circle and cross (usually copies circle at 3 years, cross at 4 years).

3. *Vision*

— five letter STYCAR matching test
— check for squint with cover test.
— screening by orthoptists performed in some parts of the UK at 3 years

4. *Hearing and language.* Assess speech. By 3 years most children are talking in sentences with frequent questions. Comprehension is usually ahead of expressive speech. Vocabulary is 200 words +.

Stuttering, indistinct speech and substitution of some speech sounds are all common at this stage, although referral for speech therapy is indicated if the speech pattern is not improving with age. Speech delay — see p. 100.

Miniature toys can be used to test verbal comprehension. The child should understand that the toys represent real objects and play with them meaningfully, following simple instructions, e.g. "put the baby on the chair". In the Six animal picture card test, check child recognizes animals, then withdraw to 10 ft and ask him to point to the pig, chick, etc.

Conditioning hearing tests can be done in the surgery. The child is asked to put a brick in the box every time he hears the word 'go'. The examiner sits 1 m away and repeats the word 'go' at progressively lower speech intensity levels with the mouth covered by a card. This test should ideally be done with a third person present who checks the decibel level of the sound with a calibrated meter. Children with hearing levels <45 dB should be referred for formal audiometry.

Any parental worries about hearing are a reason for referral for audiometric assessment. This is done by pure-tone audiometry with which most 3-year olds will cooperate well.

5. *Social skills and behaviour*

— most children can feed, wash and dress themselves at this age, providing they have been given the opportunity to learn
— dry by day and often at night
— behaviour in surgery should be appropriate
— interactive play with other children

School health service   After the age of 5 years the School Health Service takes over child health surveillance. All children are offered a full examination (including audiometry and vision testing) on state school entry and again before leaving primary school.

Established in 1907. *Objectives* (as outlined in the Court Report, 1967):

(a) To provide the understanding and practice of child health and paediatrics in relation to the process of learning.

(b) To provide a continuing service of health surveillance and medical protection.

(c) To recognize and ensure proper management of medical, surgical and neurodevelopmental disorders which may influence the child's learning and social development in school and at home.

(d) To ensure that parents and teachers are aware of such disorders and of their significance for the child's education and care.

(e) To give advice and services to the local education authority.

These services are provided by clinical medical officers (CMOs) under the leadership of the Consultant Community Paediatrician for the health district.

(a) The CMOs do not treat medical disorders and any necessary prescriptions must be given by the child's GP. Referral about developmental problems can, however, be made directly from the CMO to the paediatrician.

(b) The School Health Service ensures completion of immunisation, including Heaf testing and BCG vaccination or follow up where indicated. At present girls are still offered rubella vaccination at 11 years (as the MMR vaccine was only introduced in 1988); this will continue until the year 2000.

(c) Health education is undertaken by the school health team (CMO and school nurse) directly with individual children and as part of the school curriculum.

(d) Children with special needs are attending ordinary schools in increasing numbers. The school health team provides school staff with information and support in meeting the educational needs of such children.

Immunization Immunity can be induced:

1. *Actively* by using inactivated or attenuated organisms (or their antigenic products).

Live attenuated	Inactivated	Toxoid
Oral polio	Polio (injection)	Tetanus
MMR	Pertussis	Diptheria
BCG	Typhoid	

2. *Passively* by human immunoglobulin, which confers immediate protection which lasts only for a few weeks (e.g.

human normal immunoglobulin or specific immunoglobulins). Most vaccines work by stimulating antibody production. The first injection produces a slow IgM response —
the primary response. Further injections then accelerate IgG
antibody production — the secondary response. These levels
remain high for months or years and can be boosted by
further vaccine doses later.

Adjuvants are substances added to vaccines to stimulate antibody production, e.g. aluminium phosphate or hydroxide.

General contraindications   (a) Acute illness with systemic upset.
(b) Live vaccines should not be given in the following
situations:

— children with immunosuppression from disease or
therapy until at least 6 months after chemotherapy.
They must have immunoglobulin if exposed to
measles or chickenpox, and their siblings should
receive routine immunisation
— tumours of the reticuloendothelial system
— hypogammaglobulinaemia
— within 3 months following immunoglobulin injection
— children on high dose steroids (wait 3 months after
stopping treatment)

(c) Parental refusal. With full discussion and encouragement, this should rarely be a problem.

Schedule

Vaccine*	Age	Dose
DTP ⎫ Hib* ⎬ Oral polio ⎭	1st dose 2 months 2nd dose 3 months 3rd dose 4 months	DTP/Hib (given in different limbs) — 0.5 ml by deep s/c or i.m. OPV — 3 drops per dose
MMR	12–15 months	0.5 ml by deep s/c or i.m.
D/T&OPV booster	4–5 years	0.5 ml by deep s/c or i.m. OPV — 3 drops
Rubella (if MMR not given earlier)	10–14 years	0.5 ml s/c, girls only
BCG	Neonatal or 10–14 years	0.05 ml (neonates) 0.1 ml intradermally
Tetanus booster	15–18 years	0.5 ml s/c
OPV booster	15–18 years	3 drops

*Immunization against *H. influenzae* type b (Hib) added from October
1992 (see p. 71).

Pertussis   Pertussis vaccination was introduced in 1957 when there
were more than 100 000 cases of whooping cough annually
in the UK. By 1973, the vaccination rate was 80% and there

were only 2400 cases per year. Media reports of possible complications in the 1970s led to a fall in the vaccination rate to 30% and in 1978 there were 65 000 cases. In 1991, uptake was 88% and there were 5207 cases notified.

The vaccine is a suspension of killed *Bordetella pertussis* organisms. It is usually given as a triple vaccine combined with diphtheria and tetanus plus an adjuvant, DTPer/VAC/Ads, Trivax Ads. (It is preferable to use the adsorbed vaccine as it is more immunogenic and gives fewer systemic reactions.)

Efficacy: about 80%. Vaccinated children may occasionally develop the disease but are only mildly affected.

Contraindications   (a) General as for all vaccines, see p. 68.

(b) Severe local or general reaction to a previous dose:

— *local*: extensive area of redness and swelling involving most of circumference of upper arm
— *general*
  • fever >39.5°C within 48 h
  • anaphylaxis
  • prolonged screaming
  • convulsions within 72 h

Note: Stable neurological conditions such as cerebral palsy or spina bifida are not contraindications.

Children with a history of fits or idiopathic epilepsy in their immediate family may have a slightly increased risk of severe reaction but should usually still be vaccinated. Advice should be sought from a consultant paediatrician before withholding the vaccine on these grounds.

Immunisation of children with a history of febrile convulsions should proceed, with advice on prevention of fever given at time of immunisation.

While there is an evolving neurological problem, immunisation should be deferred.

Risk of severe reaction   Controversy persists over the risk of permanent brain damage after pertussis vaccination. In a 3-year case-finding study (the National Childhood Encephalopathy Study (NCES), 1976–79), only a small number of cases were found suggesting a temporal relationship between pertussis vaccine and neurological illness; there was insufficient evidence to prove any causative association.

It is incontrovertibly true that the incidence of neurological complications after whooping cough (~1 in 1000 cases) is greater that the risk of a neurological reaction to vaccine (estimated at 1 in 110 000 immunizations, with the majority being transient). The Committee on Safety of Medicines and the Joint Committee on Vaccinations and Immunizations therefore conclude, "the benefits of vaccination outweigh the very small risk of serious neurological reactions which may arise in relation to pertussis vaccination".

Diphtheria   Diphtheria toxoid provokes antitoxin production which provides immunity to the effects of the toxin. It is very effective. Diphtheria immunization was introduced in 1940 when there were 46 281 cases in the UK. Between 1986 and 1991 there were only 13 cases with no deaths.

Diphtheria antitoxin should be given simultaneously with the vaccine in suspected cases. Contacts should be given a full course or a booster as indicated. The Schick test is used to assess immunity to diphtheria. Contacts should also be given a prophylactic course of erythromycin.

Note: low-dose vaccine must be used for anyone aged over 10 years.

Tetanus   Tetanus spores are present in soil and usually infect through deep puncture wounds but any injury, including burns, may become infected. Tetanus neonatorum (due to infection of the umbilical stump) is still an important cause of death in developing countries.

The vaccine is given routinely as a component of the triple vaccine, see p. 68. Children who have received full primary immunization with school entry booster should be considered immune until the age of 15 years. Too frequent administration of booster doses results in severe local reactions. Patients with tetanus-prone wounds whose last reinforcing dose was >10 years previously should receive human tetanus immunoglobulin and a booster dose of adsorbed vaccine, together with thorough wound cleaning.

Polio   Inactivated polio vaccine (IPV) was introduced in 1956 and replaced in 1962 by attenuated live oral vaccine (OPV). Notifications of paralytic polio in 1955 reached nearly 4000; from 1985 to 1991, 20 cases were reported.

Live attenuated OPV contains virus types 1, 2 and 3 and is always given by mouth. The virus simulates antibody formation in the intestine and in the blood, providing protection locally against subsequent infection with wild polio viruses.

One dose of 3 drops is given directly into the mouth or on a lump of sugar. (It tastes very bitter and teeth can always be brushed!)

Vaccine strain virus may be excreted for up to 6 weeks after OPV. Parents must be advised that faecal virus excretion may lead to infection and care must be taken to wash hands after nappy changing. Any non-immune parent or sibling should be immunized at the same time.

Note:

— HIV-positive children may excrete the virus for much longer
— IPV, not OPV, is used for the immunization of immunosuppressed children and their siblings

Adverse reactions   Vaccine-associated poliomyelitis rarely may affect OPV recipients, or their contacts. The risk is of the order of 1 case per million doses.

MMR   This vaccine was introduced in 1988 with the aim of eliminating rubella, congenital rubella syndrome, measles and mumps. Uptake of at least 90% must be attained in order for this to be achieved. In practical terms this means all eligible children (i.e. those without a valid contraindication) must be immunized; by May 1992 the overall uptake was 92%.

For maximal effect the vaccine must be given before the age of 5 years. The current DoH recommendations state that the vaccine should be given to:

(a) Children of both sexes (unlike the previous policy of vaccinating girls only) preferably between the ages of 12 and 15 months.
(b) Non-immune children of both sexes aged 4–5 years. (This will only continue until the present infants reach school age.) MMR should be given at the same time as the pre-school booster of diphtheria, tetanus and polio, which should be given in the other arm and *after* the MMR as the latter is usually less painful.

Note: single antigen rubella vaccine will still be given to girls aged 10–14 years (unless they have received MMR) and non-immune women.

Contraindications   (a) General, see p. 68.
(b) Documented evidence of MMR vaccination (but single antigen measles vaccination is not a contraindication).
(c) Serological evidence of immunity to measles, mumps and rubella.
(d) Any child with a history of anaphylaxis due to any cause.

Children with a history of febrile fits cannot receive immunoglobulin as previously used with measles vaccine, as it may inhibit the immune response to rubella and mumps. Parents should be advised about antipyretic measures, including administration of paracetamol.

Adverse reactions   — fever, malaise, rash appearing about 1 week after vaccination and lasting 2–3 days
— parotid swelling 2–3 weeks after vaccination (1%)
— vaccine-associated mumps meningoencephalitis; incidence up to 1 in 11 000 immunised children from Urabe strain of mumps vaccine (Pluserix-MMR, Immravax) withdrawn in 1992. Lower incidence after Jeryl Lynn mumps vaccine (MMRH, Wellcome), which is the only type now available.

Children with post-vaccination symptoms are not thought to

be infectious, although isolated cases of vaccine-associated disease in contacts have been reported.

Haemophilus influenza

Haemophilus influenza type B (Hib) is the most common cause of serious infections such as meningitis, epiglottitis, cellulitis and septic arthritis in young children.

In the US, vaccination against Hib has been licensed since 1985, consisting of purified Hib capsular polyribosylribitol phosphate (PRP). It is poorly immunogenic in children <2 years however, so several conjugate vaccines have now been developed, which have enhanced immunogenicity due to linkage of PRP to a carrier protein, e.g. diphtheria toxoid PRP-D) or tetanus toxoid (PRP-T).

Routine immunization was implemented in the UK in October 1992. With 95% uptake in the primary schedule, immunization has the potential to prevent 90% of *H. influenzae* type B infections in young children.

Adverse reactions
— *local* reactions in up to 10% of recipients
— *systemic* reactions (crying, fever) in 10–15% but no excess over rates in placebo groups

Tuberculosis

Intradermal BCG (Bacillus Calmette-Guerin) vaccine contains live attenuated bacteria derived from *Mycobacterium bovis*. Protection should last at least 15 years. It is about 70% effective when given in adolescence, but less so when administered in neonates. It is given by intradermal injection on the upper arm (usually left).

Groups for which vaccination is *recommended*:
— contacts of cases
— children of immigrants in whose communities there is a high prevalence of TB
— school children aged 10-13 years
— infants who will be travelling to, or who live in, areas of high risk
— health service staff

Adverse effects
Usually due to faulty injection technique:

— large ulcers and abscesses
— adenitis, occasionally with suppuration

Note: if isoniazid is to be administered prophylactically following contact with a known case, isoniazid-resistant BCG vaccine should be used.

Hepatitis B

Hepatitis B vaccine (HBVac) antigen is produced by yeast cells using a recombinant DNA technique (Engerix B).

— about 90% effective (response best in the under 40s)
— duration of immunity ~ 5 years
— Post-vaccination serology to confirm immunity should be checked at 2–4 months

Indications   Recent WHO recommendations are that all children receive hepatitis B vaccination. In the UK current guidelines recommend vaccination of the following groups:

— infants at risk should receive active/passive immunization within 48 h of birth (see p. 46)
— after exposure to infected blood, e.g. needlestick injury
— susceptible groups, e.g. patients with chronic renal disease awaiting dialysis or transplantation, health care staff, active homosexuals, intravenous drug users

Immunoglobulins

Normal immunoglobulin   Human normal immunoglobulin (HNIG) confers passive immunity to a number of infections, including measles, chickenpox, hepatitis and other viruses. It is obtained by pooling plasma from blood donors negative to hepatitis B and HIV and prepared by processes which kill all viruses.

HNIG interferes with the immune response to live vaccines, which should therefore be given at least 3 weeks before or 3 months after HNIG.

Uses of HNIG:

(a) For prophylaxis in children at special risk of contracting measles, e.g. after exposure in children with immunosuppression, or recent serious illness for whom measles could be dangerous.

(b) HNIG does not prevent rubella infection after exposure but reduces the likelihood of clinical symptoms. It should be given as soon as possible after maternal exposure where a termination of pregnancy would not be acceptable to the patient.

(c) Can be used for protection against hepatitis A for travellers to all countries except those in Europe, the USA, Australia and New Zealand. It is also used to control outbreaks in institutions.

Specific immunoglobulins   Available for:

— tetanus
— chickenpox
— rabies
— hepatitis B

1. *Antitetanus immunoglobulin (Humotet)*. Can be used for the immediate treatment of wounds at high risk of tetanus infection in patients who are not immunised or need an immediate booster dose.

2. *Antivaricella/zoster immunoglobulin (ZIG)*. Recommended for:

— contacts of chickenpox or herpes zoster who are:
  • immunosuppressed
  • suffering from severe concurrent illness

- neonates whose mothers have no antibodies to chickenpox (i.e. mothers with no history of the disease or who develop it after delivery)
- pregnant
— babies born before 30 weeks' gestation or with a birth weight of <1 kg whose mothers have been in contact with the disease, even if they themselves are immune, as antibody may not have crossed the placenta

3. *Rabies-specific immunoglobulin (HRIG)*. Provides effective post-exposure protection. Administered simultaneously with the first of six injections of human diploid-cell rabies vaccine given over 90 days.

4. *Hepatitis B immunoglobulin (HBIG)*. Confers immediate post-exposure protection. Combined with simultaneous injection of hepatitis B vaccine at different site.

Advice for travelling

Polio
: Infants and children must be fully immunized before visiting countries where polio is endemic; if necessary, an accelerated programme of immunization at monthly intervals is used.

Cholera
: Vaccine offers only limited protection, lasting only 3–6 months.

— risk to tourists is very small even in endemic areas
— best protection is by scrupulous hygiene
— not to be given to children under 1 year

Typhoid
: Monovalent vaccine (vaccine no longer available against parathyphoid A and B (TAB)).

— one injection gives 70–80% protection for 1 year
— two injections 1 month apart confer 3 years' protection
— not recommended for children under 1 year

Oral typhoid vaccine (live attenuated) now available; duration of protection may be less.

Smallpox
: Global eradication of smallpox declared in December 1979. No vaccination required.

Yellow fever
: Acute arbovirus infection occurring in tropical Africa and South America. Spread by mosquito bite, therefore protection by insect repellants and covering nets.

Prophylaxis: live attenuated vaccine available only from designated centres.

— single dose gives 100% immunity lasting about 10 years
— not recommended for infants <9 months
— (may be given with HNIG to travellers needing protection against hepatitis A)

Meningococcal infection
: Vaccine effective against serotypes A and C. (There is no vaccine against Group B, the commonest strain in the UK).

Recommended for travellers to the 'Meningitis Belt' across Africa, New Delhi, Nepal and Mecca (where epidemic Group A infection occurs).

Children from 2 months should be vaccinated, although immune response is poor in the very young, especially to Group C polysaccharide.

General   — use sterilizing tablets in all drinking water
— use sterilized water to wash fruit and vegetables
— no swimming in rivers or ponds
— use mosquito repellants and nets; malaria chemo-prophylaxis for endemic areas, see p. 156
— encourage children to wear clothes which minimize areas of exposed skin. Shoes should be worn at all times
— travel with some oral rehydration mixture and simple medications

Dental health

Dentition   There are 20 deciduous or 'milk' teeth which erupt from the age of about 6 months onwards. The first permanent teeth are the 6-year molars. The permanent teeth total 32 (including four wisdom teeth which usually erupt during the late teens).

Calcification of the milk teeth begins at about 28 weeks' gestation and continues until age 3 years. Calcification of the permanent teeth starts around term and continues until age 14 years, hence the need to avoid tetracyclines which stain enamel as it is being laid down. Similarly, severe nutritional problems or systemic illness may lead to defects in the enamel. Resistance to dental caries can be increased by the administration of fluoride drops from birth onwards.

Dental caries   Dental decay results from the action of bacteria in the mouth on refined carbohydrates, leading to the formation of acids, which demineralize the enamel surface of the tooth, thus causing cavities. These are most likely to occur in the molar and premolar teeth, due to the pits and fissures in the tooth surface which trap food debris. In children there is rapid progression of decay, so prevention is the most effective method of control. In addition, prolonged infection in the peri-apical area of primary teeth may affect the development of erupting permanent teeth. The severity of dental caries has decreased markedly over the last 20 years due to fluoride (see below) in preventive dentistry.

Preventive measures   (a) Avoid dummies and bottles of sweetened fruit juices which can cause rapid decay of the upper incisors.
(b) The first visit to the dentist should be before the age of 3 years. This allows early diagnosis of potential problems and familiarizes the child with the surgery environment.
(c) A dental check up every 4 months provides a good

opportunity for continuing dental health education as well as identification and treatment of caries and gum disease.

(d) *Tooth brushing*. Children should have their own tooth-brush and be encouraged to start brushing from about 2 years. Children do not have the hand–eye coordination to clean the teeth properly until 8–10 years, so parents should re-brush the teeth and gums at least once daily.

(e) *Fluoride* strengthens enamel making it more resistant to decay. Children living in areas where the water is fluoridated (1 part per million) have at least 50% fewer fillings. Fluoride can be administered in various ways if the local water supply has low levels:

— fluoride drops from the age of 6 months to 16 years
— topical fluorides
  • tooth gels which are brushed onto the teeth after cleaning
  • more concentrated pastes can be applied by the dentist
  • mouth washes
  • fluoride toothpastes (most common method)

(f) *Fissure sealants*. These are plastics used to seal the permanent molar and premolar teeth to minimize the risk of caries starting in the occlusal surfaces. Best applied at 6–7 years, soon after the teeth have erupted

(g) *Dietary advice* to minimize the frequency of eating sweets. A once a week 'sweets day' is best, encouraging fresh fruit snacks at other times.

Dental problems   1. *Teething*. Teething pains may occur at any age but are most common in the first 2 years of life. Teething does not cause pyrexia.

2. *Eruption cysts*. These may occur around an erupting tooth and are occasionally haemorrhagic. The tooth then appears to be black. They should be left alone as incision may introduce infection and most resolve before the tooth breaks through the gum.

3. *Trauma*:

(a) a sharp blow to the tooth may cause damage to the periodontal ligament, resulting in bleeding around the gum margin. Antibiotics, e.g. amoxycillin, prevent possible infection.

(b) teeth which subsequently darken due to nerve damage should be assessed regularly for abscess formation, which may occur after a latent period of up to 2 years.

(c) complete avulsion of an incisor tooth is not uncommon in young children following falls:

— rinse the tooth in clean water and push it back into the socket, as far as it will go

— if this is not possible, store the tooth in a small amount of milk, making sure that it is completely covered and refer to dentist immediately
— the dentist will hold the tooth in position with an acrylic splint. Ideally the tooth should be replaced within 30 min (maximum 2 h). 95% of avulsed teeth survive if replaced in this way

4. *Malocclusion.* May follow thumb sucking. Refer for orthodontic assessment.

Accident prevention   In Britain two children die every day in accidents. They are the single largest cause of death in children between the ages of 1 and 14 years. In addition, one in five children attend an A & E department each year.

The DTI Home Accident Surveillance System collates statistics from 20 A & E departments nationwide. The Child Accident Prevention Trust is concerned with establishing the causes and patterns of accidents and methods of reducing their number and severity.

Falls   The commonest accidents at all ages.

Prevention   — stair gates, highchairs, playpens, harnesses
— window locks
— good lighting
— tidiness
— well designed playgrounds with slides set into banks of earth and wood chippings, rubber or grass instead of tarmac
— protective wear for limbs and head when cycling or skateboarding

Burns   These cause about 14% of childhood trauma deaths, and terrible morbidity. Toddlers are most at risk of scalds and older children of starting more serious fires.

Prevention   — turn saucepan handles inwards on the cooker
— keep cups, teapots, etc. away from the edges of tables
— keep flexes short on kettles and irons and never leave them on floors
— maintain the temperature of domestic hot water at <54°C
— fireguards and cooker guards
— run baths with cold water first and always supervise children in baths and showers

House fires:
— installation of smoke alarms with regular testing and family fire drills
— fire-retardant materials should be used as much as possible for furniture and clothes, particularly night gowns

— storage of matches out of reach of children
— fire-guards and -extinguishers

Emergency treatment Advise parents about first-aid measures:

(a) Plunge the affected part into cold water immediately for *at least* 10 minutes.
(b) If the child's clothing is soaked in scalding liquid, lift it away from the skin whilst running to the cold tap.
(c) Remove belts or tight clothing in case of swelling.
(d) Cover area with a clean sheet and seek medical advice.

Further management (a) Take detailed history to find out what caused the burn.

(b) Assess the extent and depth of the burn.
(c) For *minor* scalds:

— clean if necessary with topical antiseptics
— cover with a clean dressing and leave for 7–10 days
— if dressing needs changing, try to leave the adherent bottom layer untouched
— tetanus immunization if non-immune
— may need systemic antibiotics if wound dirty

(d) Refer if:

— burn exceeds 5% of total body surface (palm of hand is 1.25%)
— full thickness burns
— burns of hands, face, joints or flexor surfaces; circumferential burns
— chemical burns
— electrical burns (these may cause unseen damage below the skin as well as cardiac arrhythmias)
— suspected smoke inhalation: risk of acute pulmonary insufficiency, pulmonary oedema and bronchopneumonia

(e) Management of *severe* burns:

— assess and maintain airway
— assess circulation and extent of burns. Replace fluid losses:

$$\frac{\% \text{ burn} \times \text{wt (kg)}}{2} = \text{ml to be given in first 4 h}$$

Monitor urine output and fluid balance carefully.

(f) If *inhalational* burn:

— high concentrations of oxygen
— assess blood carboxyhaemoglobin levels
— bronchodilators
— antibiotics and steroids may be indicated
— gastric protection, e.g. ranitidine, sucralfate

(g) Analgesia

(h) Plastic surgery referral

(i) Tetanus toxoid booster

Choking
Causes over 100 child deaths each year. Young babies and toddlers are most at risk as they instinctively explore objects by putting them in their mouths.

Management
(a) Place the child face down and apply several blows to the back between the shoulder blades. (The older child should be laid down and the heel of one hand placed in the midline between the umbilicus and the rib cage. The other hand is placed on top of the first exerting pressure upwards and inwards.)

(b) If this fails, an emergency airway can be established by cricothyrotomy using a 14 G cannula.

(c) Direct laryngoscopy under anaesthetic as soon as possible.

Swallowed objects
These are usually passed without any problem but watch for:

— hearing-aid type batteries (used in all small computer games). These may leak heavy metals

— sharp or long, thin objects which may impact and cause obstruction. These should usually be removed

Road accidents
Although >60% of childhood accidents occur in the home and <5% on the roads, 400 children are killed every year in road traffic accidents, with the child victim a pedestrian in 50% of cases. Boys between 5 and 8 years are at maximum risk. Accidents to cyclists are most common in older children.

Prevention
— Use of proper restraints for children travelling in cars:
  • newborn to 9 months: a rear-facing baby car seat
  • toddler to 4 years: second stage front-facing car seat
  • 4–10 years: booster seat

— teach children road safety from a young age

— ensure child cyclists pass the cycling proficiency test before allowing them on the road

— encourage the use of proper cycle safety helmets

— improve visibility at night by wearing reflective clothing

— separation of pedestrian areas from traffic and reduction of traffic speed, particularly near schools and play areas

Accidental poisoning
Every year about 40 000 children present to A & E departments in England and Wales with accidental poisoning. Most escape without serious problems but there are some fatalities, and ingestion of toxic substances remains a common reason for admission to hospital.

Toddlers from the age of about 18 months can undo screw tops. Older children are at risk of inadvertant poisoning if chemicals are transferred into soft drinks bottles.

The poisons which are most frequently accidentally ingested have changed with alterations in prescribing habits, wider use of child-resistant packaging for some drugs and adoption of other preventive measures. Before 1970, salicyclates were the most commonly fatal poison. Paracetamol is now the most frequently accidentally ingested drug. Tricyclic antidepressants are the commonest cause of death due to poisoning.

Prevention   — store medicines and household products carefully
— fit child-proof catches on cupboards
— never transfer chemicals to drinks bottles
— advise parents to insist on child-resistant packaging for prescriptions, including blister packs, strip packs and child-resistant tops

Emergency treatment   (a) Identify ingested substance.
(b) Induce emesis *unless* child unconcious or has ingested corrosives or hydrocarbons. Give syrup of ipecacuanha
    10 ml if <18 months
    15 ml if >18 months
    Note: salt-induced emesis is dangerous; mechanically induced emesis is ineffective.
(c) Gastric lavage may be indicated up to 10–12 hours (24 hours for aspirin) after ingestion of toxic substances such as tricyclics, salicylates and 'slow-release' preparations, with activated charcoal slurry ('Medicoal') left in the stomach after washout.
(d) Admit unless ingested substance known to be of low toxicity (e.g. most antibiotics, oral contraceptives, some plants and household products) and no adverse social factors.

Specific poisons   1. *Tricyclic antidepressants* (e.g. imipramine). Effects of ingestion of >10 mg/kg

— neurological disturbances
— respiratory depression
— arrythmias

Management:

— gastric lavage + activated charcoal
— ECG monitoring on ITU
— anticonvulsants, respiratory support, antiarrythmics as necessary

   2. *Salicylates.* Effects of ingestion of >150–200 mg/kg

— respiratory then metabolic acidosis
— hyperglycaemia, ketosis
— fever
— dehydration

— coagulopathy
— nausea and vomiting, haematemesis

Management:

— emesis or gastric lavage
— confirm diagnosis with urine ferric chloride test (Phenistix). Purple reaction = positive
— 4-hour serum salicylate level:
  <40 mg/100 ml (2.9 mmol/l) — rarely symptomatic
  >120 mg/100 ml (8.8 mmol/l) — usually lethal
— fluid and electrolyte treatment: correct dehydration, acidosis, hypoglycaemia. Maintain urine output 5–6 ml/kg/h and urine pH >7.5.
— vitamin K and FFP for hypoprothrombinaemia and clotting disturbances
— dialysis or exchange transfusion may be necessary

3. *Paracetamol.* Life-threatening hepatotoxicity, which may not become evident for several days, may follow ingestion but is fortunately rare in children.
Other effects of ingestion of >150 mg/kg:

— vomiting, gastrointestinal haemorrhage
— disturbance of carbohydrate metabolism
— renal tubule damage
— cerebral oedema

Management:

— emesis or lavage
— 4-hour blood paracetamol level. Interpret using nomogram. Hepatotoxicity likely if 4-h level >200 μg/ml
— if presents within 10 h treat with oral methionine; if between 12–15 h treat with i.v. acetylcysteine
— monitor liver function and coagulation profile

4. *Iron.* Effects of ingestion of >30 mg elemental iron/kg:

— vomiting and haematemesis
— shock
— liver failure
— convulsions and coma

Management:

— gastric lavage (intubate first if unconcious)
— desferrioxamine i.m. stat and leave 2 g in solution in stomach after lavage
— continue desferrioxamine i.m. 4–8 hourly or by s.c./i.v. infusion (max. rate 15 mg/kg/h)
— supportive treatment, particularly fluid balance

5. *Lead.* Rare. Usually chronic. Seen in infants and young children who live in old homes where original paintwork

contains lead. Rarely it may be due to pica (compulsive dirt eating), which is seen most commonly in socioeconomically or emotionally deprived children, and also in the mentally retarded.

Other sources include:

— lead pipes
— lead painted toys
— cosmetics, e.g. kohl, surma
— exhaust fumes
— contaminated water

Presentations:

— recurrent abdominal pain, vomiting, anorexia, constipation
— anaemia, with basophilic stippling
— encephalopathy presenting gradually with irritability, ataxia and developmental retardation or acutely with convulsions and coma

Diagnosis. Suggested by:

— anaemia with red cell basophilic stippling
— dense metaphyseal line on X-rays of long bones
— radiological opacities in GI tract

Confirmed by:

— blood lead levels
— serum-free erythrocyte protoporphyrin and urine coproporphyrins are also raised

Treatment
— mild cases: D-penicillamine orally
— severe: chelation therapy with sodium calcium edetate. Supportive treatment for cerebral oedema, etc.
— remove source of lead

5. Growth and development

Growth A healthy child grows at a normal rate. Prenatal growth is the most rapid and during this time the brain is especially susceptible to damage as a result of nutritional deprivation.

The measure of growth as an indicator of health begins antenatally, using serial US measurements. The first indication of slow growth is a reduction in abdominal circumference and, if very severe, head growth also slows. Variations in fetal growth are influenced by fetal, maternal and environmental factors (see p. 6).

After birth serial measurements of head circumference and weight are the best indicators of growth, as length measurements at this time are often inaccurate. There is rapid general growth in the first 2 years, during which time the child's growth pattern may correct for prenatal influences. Babies who suffered prolonged intrauterine growth retardation (IUGR), starting in the second trimester of pregnancy, may never fully 'catch up' their lost growth.

From 2 years, growth continues steadily until puberty, when there is a sudden increase in growth velocity. Timing of the onset of puberty is very variable (see p. 89).

The brain grows to 90% of the adult weight by age 5 years and 95% by age 10 years.

Centile charts The normal distribution of most biological variables follows a Gaussian curve. A standard centile chart gives a range of growth curves with limits of 2 SD from the mean. These correspond to the 3rd and 97th centiles. By definition these limits will encompass about 94% of the population, but it must be remembered 6% of *normal* children are outside the limits. Serial measurements are far more valuable than single measurements to assess the pattern of the child's growth.

When monitoring height and predicting final adult height, adjustment should be made for parental height. The height of the parents should be plotted as if aged 19 years (the end of the scale), with 12.5 cm added to mother's height before plotting a boy's chart and 12.5 cm deducted from father's height when plotting a girl's chart. The midpoint between the two parental heights is the mid-parental height centile and the child's height should be within 8.5 cm (±2 SD) of this centile.

Measurement
(a) in babies, weight, length and head circumference should approximate to the same centile. Disproportionate measurements should be monitored closely.

(b) the first sign of hydrocephalus or megalencephaly may be head circumference measurements accelerating across centiles. Early referral is imperative.

(c) a growth-retarded baby with a height and weight consistently below the 3rd centile but a head circumference around the 50th centile shows preservation of neural growth and is likely to do well, although small stature may persist.

(d) accurate and reproducible measurements are essential, therefore always:

— reduce observer error by having the same person take all readings.
— calibrate scales before each weighing
— weigh without clothes
— measure length using an infant measuring table or similar device with fixed head plate and adjustable foot plate
— use a non-stretching tape measure for head circumference
— in older children, measure height using a stadiometer (this has a flat surface applied to the head). Gentle traction should be applied to the mastoids to correct postural slumping. Check that feet are flat on the ground and that the outer canthus of eye is at the same level as the external auditory meatus.

Growth velocity
The rate of growth (growth velocity, GV) is a far more valuable guide to health than a single measurement of either height or weight. Regular measurements of height and weight should be made on all children as a routine part of primary care:

(a) At least five readings should be taken in the 1st year, three in the 2nd, and then annually or every time the child is seen in the surgery if less frequent. The values should be plotted on a centile chart.

(b) The GV is calculated as an annual GV rate and plotted at the age midpoint between the two measurements.

(c) Children found to have a GV below the 25th centile or above the 75th should be referred, even if the actual height values are within the norm. Do not wait until the height is below the 3rd centile before referring.

Abnormal growth
Deciding whether growth is abnormal in an individual child requires:

— estimation of growth velocity
— reference to standard growth charts and familiarity with normal and abnormal growth patterns
— consideration of genetic and environmental contributory

factors, e.g. parental height, ethnic group, nutrition, emotional status, general physical health

If the above indicate that growth may be abnormal and the cause is not obvious from the history and examination, the following may help to determine the cause:

— weight, skinfold thickness
— sitting height
— occipito-frontal circumference
— pubertal staging
— investigations:
  • FBC, ESR
  • U & E, creatinine, calcium, phosphate, alkaline phosphatase, iron
  • skull X-ray
  • bone age for skeletal maturity
  • thyroid function tests
  • basal gonadotrophins
  • karyotype in all short girls
  • ± jejunal biopsy
  • screening tests for suspected growth hormone deficiency (see below)

Causes of short stature

1. Short with currently normal GV:

— constitutional
— previous growth-delaying problem, now resolved

2. Short with slow GV

— with increased skinfold thickness — endocrine: hypopituitarism, GH deficiency, hypothyroidism, Cushing
— disproportionate, e.g. dyschondroplasia, mucopolysaccharidoses, metatrophic dwarfism
— chronic illness, e.g. asthma, coeliac disease, congenital heart disease, renal disease
— psychosocial deprivation

Growth hormone (GH) deficiency

Causes:

— hereditary: due to GH gene deletion
— psychosocial deprivation
— secondary to: infection, head injury, cranial irradiation
— idiopathic GnRH deficiency
— hypothalamo-pituitary tumour
— developmental abnormalities, e.g. pituitary hypoplasia, midline brain anomalies

Diagnosis

(a) Screening tests for suspected GH deficiency include plasma GH on sample collected:

— post-prandial
— post-exercise
— during sleep

Serum GH >15 mu/l excludes GH deficiency. If serum GH <15 mu/l, formal provocation GH testing is required, and is usually performed at a regional growth centre.

(b) Formal provocation tests for diagnosis of GH deficiency include:

— insulin tolerance test (ITT)
— intravenous arginine test (may be combined with ITT)
— oral clonidine test
— intramuscular glucagon test

The insulin hypoglycaemia test has been the most widely used but it is potentially hazardous and should no longer be used when only the GH reserve needs to be tested. If both GH and ACTH function are to be assessed, a closely supervised ITT may be performed in a paediatric endocrinology unit. It may be combined with other provocation tests, e.g. TRH, LH–RH.

Partial GH deficiency   Patients with subnormal growth and peak serum GH between 7 and 15 mu/1 in two formal tests are eligible for GH treatment.

Severe GH deficiency   Children with peak serum GH <7 mU/1 in a formal test. Incidence 1 in 5000. Clinical features may include cherubic facies, high pitched voice, tendency to obesity and sexual underdevelopment in boys.

Treatment: Daily subcutaneous GH injections. Optimal dose disputed but for example 15 U/m^2 week. Dose tailored individually according to height velocity.

Pituitary human GH withdrawn in 1985, replaced by biosynthetic human GH produced by recombinant DNA technology.

Other indications for GH treatment include some children with chronic renal failure and also Turner syndrome, where growth is improved especially if used in combination with anabolic steroids, e.g. oxandrolone. It is important to start therapy as soon as indication for treatment is established, as lost growth may never be made up. Treatment is continued until epiphyseal closure takes place.

The treatment of normal small children with GH may help them attain their final adult height at an earlier age and thereby avoid some of the psychological problems associated with short stature; this approach is under evaluation.

Syndromes featuring
disorders of growth

Short stature   1. *Turner syndrome* (XO syndrome)

— must always be considered in girls of short stature

— look for associated features:
- webbed neck
- low posterior hairline
- short 4th metacarpal and/or metatarsal, cubitus valgus
- pigmented naevi
- congenital lymphoedema
- aortic coarctation
- ovarian dysgenesis with absence of secondary sex characteristics

2. *Ulrich–Noonan syndrome*
— Turner-like syndrome but normal karyotype
— more likely to have mental retardation and congenital heart disease, particularly pulmonary stenosis, or ASD
— short stature
— secondary sex characteristics may be normal or absent
— can occur in males and females

3. *Prader–Willi syndrome.* Usually sporadic. Associated with a deletion on chromosome 15.

— short stature
— usually history of low birth weight
— obesity presenting after 1st year
— small genitalia
— small hands and feet
— hypotonia

4. *Silver–Russell syndrome.* Cause unknown, usually sporadic.

— short stature of prenatal onset
— skeletal asymmetry
— small triangular facies
— short and incurved little fingers (clinodactyly)

5. *Achondroplasia.* Incidence 1 in 25 000. Autosomal dominant inheritance. 80% of cases are new mutations.

— disproportionate short stature with shortening of limbs (predominantly proximal), often apparent at birth
— large head with frontal bossing
— flat nasal bridge
— hydrocephalus due to small foramen magnum

6. *Mucopolysaccharidoses.* See p. 285.

Tall stature   1. *Cerebral giantism* (Sotos syndrome)

— usually sporadic: occasional familial cases inherited as autosomal dominant
— prenatal onset of large size with birth weight and length usually above 90th centile
— rapid growth in first few years to >97th centile
— large head with down-slanting palpebral fissures and hypertelorism.

— large hands and feet
— mental retardation with clumsiness and learning difficulties
— growth hormone levels normal

2. *Marfan syndrome*

— autosomal dominant with variable expression
— connective tissue disorder
— limbs long with fingers long and tapered (arachnodactyly)
— lax ligaments producing hyperextensibility of joints, flat feet
— upward lenticular subluxation
— severe myopia
— retinal detachment
— dilatation of the aorta with or without dissecting aneurysm and secondary aortic regurgitation
— mitral valve disease

3. *Homocystinuria.* See also p. 283. Resembles Marfan syndrome but other features include:

— osteoporosis
— mental retardation
— malar flush
— downward lenticular subluxation
— thrombo-embolic phenomena

4. *Klinefelter syndrome* Incidence 1 in 1000. Usually XXY chromosomes, some mosaics.

— mental retardation
— antisocial behaviour
— tall, slim with long legs
— relative androgen deficiency, delayed puberty, infertility (azoospermia), gynaecomastia, hypogenitalism

Treatment: Testosterone replacement from age 11–12 years.

Causes of small and large heads	Small	Large
	Normal variation, often familial	Normal variation, often familial
	Small baby	Large baby
	Microcephaly	Hydrocephalus
	Craniostenosis	Cerebral tumour
	Cerebral atrophy	Megalencephaly
		Hydranencephaly
		Subdural effusion
		Cerebral gigantism
		Gangliosidoses

Fontanelles   Posterior fontanelle usually closes by 6 weeks and anterior by 18 months.

Causes of delayed closure:

— hydrocephaly
— rickets
— raised intracranial pressure
— syndromes, e.g. Down's, Zellweger, etc.

Abnormal closure of sutures   Premature closure of the sutures (craniosynostosis) results in abnormal head shapes and may cause damage to the growing brain.

Puberty   Puberty is a series of physical and psychological changes by which a child matures into an adult capable of reproduction. The essential changes are:

— a growth spurt
— an alteration in body proportion
— the development of secondary sex organs and characteristics

The newborn has high levels of gonadotrophins but low levels of testosterone and oestradiol due to positive feedback. The trigger for normal puberty is unknown; it follows an elevation of the threshold for feedback. The first endocrine event of puberty is an increase in adrenal androgens occurring from 5–8 years in both sexes. Pre-pubertally the pituitary responds to GnRH by producing more FSH than LH. After puberty the LH response is greater than that of FSH.

When puberty begins, GH levels rise. GH and sex steroids act synergistically to promote the pubertal growth spurt.

Girls have an earlier puberty than boys (onset between 9 and 13 years in 95%). 80% start with breast formation, 20% with pubic hair growth. Average age of menarche is 13 years. Menarche corresponds with bone age.

Boys have a longer growth spurt. Early in puberty the increase in GH production results in longer legs. Later, an increased testosterone level causes increasing spinal growth.

Normal staging   1. *Boys: genital development*

Stage 1   Preadolescent; the testes, scrotum and penis are the same size and proportions as in early childhood

Stage 2   The scrotum and testes grow, and the skin of the scrotum reddens and changes in texture

Stage 3   The penis begins to grow longer

Stage 4   Growth continues; the penis broadens and the glans develops, the testes and scrotum enlarge and the scrotal skin darkens

Stage 5   The genitalia are adult in size and shape

2 *Girls: breast development*

Stage 1   Preadolescent; only the papillae are raised

Stage 2   Formation of the breast bud; the breast and papilla become elevated into a small mound, and the areola enlarges

Stage 3   Further enlargement and elevation of breast and areola

Stage 4   The areola and papilla project to form a secondary mound above the level of the breast

Stage 5   Mature stage, only the papilla projects, the areola recedes to the general contour of the breast

3. *Both sexes: pubic hair*

Stage 1   Preadolescent; no pubic hair

Stage 2   Sparse growth of long pigmented downy hair, sometimes curly, at the base of the penis or along the labia

Stage 3   Hair spreads sparsely over the junction of the pubes and is coarser, darker and more curled

Stage 4   Hair is now adult in type, but has not spread to the medial surface of the thighs

Stage 5   Hair is adult in type and in distribution, having spread to the medial surface of the thighs. Spread up the linea alba occurs much later

Precocious puberty   Onset of sexual maturation before 8 years in a girl and 9 years in a boy. More common in girls.

Causes   1. *Constitutional.*
2. *Central*:

— idiopathic (more common in girls)
— secondary to
   • hypothalmic or pituitary tumours (particularly haematoma, craniopharyngioma–more common in boys)
   • injury — post traumatic, post infection, hydrocephalus, cranial irradiation
   • tuberose sclerosis
   • primary hypothyroidism

3. *Gonadotrophin-independent* precocious puberty (familial testotoxicosis).
4. *Gonadal disorders*:

— Gonadal tumour
— McCune–Albright syndrome

5. *Ectopic gonadotrophic production*, e.g. hepatoblastoma.
6. *Adrenal disorders*:

— CAH
— Cushing
— adrenal tumour

Investigation   The presenting clinical feature will determine which specific tests are indicated but these may include:

— plasma dihydroepiandrosterone sulphate, 17 hydroxy-progesterone, sex hormones, gonadotrophins, LH and FSH, corticotrophin, response to GnRH
— thyroid function tests
— bone age
— X-ray skull and long bones
— pelvic US
— CT brain scan

Premature thelarche Usually affects under 2-year olds and is often cyclical. Distinguishing features from central precocious puberty include:

— no other concomitant signs of sexual development
— normal GV
— skeletal maturation appropriate for age

May be caused by isolated ovarian follicular cysts. Usually resolves after a few years.

Delayed puberty In contrast to precocious puberty, delayed puberty is more common in boys than girls. Investigation should be undertaken if there are no signs of puberty by 14 years.

Causes 1. *Constitutional.*
2. *Central* (low gonadotrophins):

— isolated gonadotrophin deficiency or with GH deficiency
— GnRH deficiency
— panhypopituitarism
— post-cranial irradiation
— tumour, e.g. craniopharyngioma, prolactinoma
— any chronic systemic illness
— malnutrition, anorexia nervosa
— syndromes, e.g. Prader-Willi, Laurence–Moon–Biedl

3. *Gonadal* (high gonadotrophins):

— gonadal dysgenesis, e.g. Turner syndrome
— sex-steroid deficiency due to anorchia/hypoplastic testes
4. *Adrenal*: enzyme defects in steroidal biosynthesis.
5. *Hypothyroidism.*

Investigation Depending on clinical features, may include:

— lateral skull X-ray, bone age and skeletal survey
— thyroid function tests
— serum gonadotrophins, serum prolactin
— chromosomes in short girls
— pelvic US
— high resolution cranial CT scan

Gynaecomastia Common in adolescence. Usually · mild and transitory. Differential diagnosis includes:

— obesity
— Klinefelter syndrome
— oestrogen-producing tumour
— hyperprolactinaemia

6. The child with a handicap

The handicapped child must be seen as an individual. There are often associated problems which complicate management and require close cooperation between health, education and social services.

The team approach is used to define and provide for each individual child's special needs although parents need to have access to someone who will coordinate care. The GP, Consultant Community Paediatrician or Head Teacher are probably the best choices.

The effect of a severely disabled child on family life is tremendous. Sympathetic listening and practical help are essential. Parents need the chance to discuss how the problem affects family members, the financial implications and the prognosis for the future.

Early diagnosis

The aim is to prevent handicap as far as possible. Early diagnosis and intervention are essential to maximize potential. Handicap may be suspected in the following ways:

— antenatal diagnosis, e.g. microcephaly, Down's syndrome
— examination after birth
— parents may notice the child not developing like other children
— concern may be raised by health care workers e.g. health visitor, nursery nurse, GP, teacher

Assessment

If handicap is suspected by anyone, immediate referral to a paediatrician should be arranged. The Consultant Community Paediatrician is usually the best person to organize assessment, ideally in the Child Development Centre, with access to the full multidisciplinary team.

The *medical examination* includes:

(a) general background history, including details of birth, development to date, medical problems, family and social history, etc.
(b) discussion of presenting concerns
(c) general physical examination, looking for clues to aetiology of problem
(d) a full developmental assessment is performed by combining information from the parents with observation of

the child's behaviour. Areas of development are examined separately to assess individual need in each:
- posture and gross motor
- vision and fine motor
- hearing and speech
- social and emotional

(e) investigations if indicated

The other professionals involved in assessment include:

1. The *physiotherapist* assesses motor function and defines likely problems for the future.

2. The *occupational therapist* assesses how much the child can do for himself with regard to the activities of daily living.

3. The *educational psychologist* estimates how the handicap may affect intellectual development and prognosis for independent living. The IQ cannot be accurately assessed in children under 2 years but will affect not only the speed at which the child can learn but also the choice of necessary communication aids.

4. The *speech therapist* will assess communication skills. Hearing must always be tested at an early stage in the handicapped child, as the prognosis with early intervention is very much better.

Subsequent management

(a) Define areas of disability.

(b) Identify which professional will coordinate and oversee care. This is important for parents who will want to discuss day-to-day problems with someone who knows their child well.

(c) Devise a structured treatment programme with the help of relevant specialists: physiotherapists, occupational therapists, educational psychologists, speech therapists and specialist teachers for the deaf and visually handicapped. Pre-school advisory teachers can visit children at home.

(d) Prepare a Statement of Special Educational Needs if necessary (see p. 95).

(e) Assess which communication aids, including sign language, are indicated.

(f) Emphasis should be placed upon teaching social and self-help skills. Competence in activities of daily living is essential for independence.

(g) Management of behavioural difficulties. Emotional and behavioural disturbances are common in children with disabilities. In some instances these responses may cause more problems than the underlying handicap. These may either be due to mental retardation or be a complication of the brain damage responsible for the handicap. These may present simply with a child who is easily angered and frustrated or in other ways, e.g.:

— poor concentration span
— self-centred behaviour
— repetitive mannerisms
— self mutilation
— autistic features

Behaviour modification techniques, involving positive and negative reinforcement, are often helpful.

(h) Counselling and support for the family. The needs of the family must be considered and practical help given. Prolonged counselling may be required as parents come to terms with their child's handicap. Lack of information is the most frequent complaint of these parents. They must be involved at every stage.

Sympathetic listening is vital. Many parents will express anger at involved professionals as part of the grief reaction for the loss of their normal child. They may be helped by contact with self-help groups who offer support from parents with similarly affected children and also provide additional information about aids, respite care, new therapies, e.g. MENCAP, Spastic Society.

Discuss possibilities for respite care, e.g. to a purpose-run unit or to family or friends.

Advise about allowances, local charitable funds, etc.

Refer for genetic counselling if appropriate.

Plan for the future by discussing school leaving and subsequent care. Provide information about adult training centres, sheltered employment, day centres, etc.

The Statement of Special Educational Need (SSEN)

As a result of the Enquiry into the Education of Handicapped Children and Young People (The Warnock Report), the Education Act of 1981 (Section 10) requires a Health Authority to notify the Local Education Authority (LEA) when they become aware of a child who may have special educational needs. The LEA has a statutory duty to identify such children between the ages of 2 and 16 years and to refer them for an assessment. Parents may request an assessment if a child is under 2 years. The assessment will result in the preparation of a Statement (with a copy to the parents) of special educational needs and how they are to be met.

(a) The statement must include recommendations for schooling, i.e. whether or not the child can be educated in a normal school with or without additional resources from the Local Education Department or needs to attend a special school.

(b) The statement must be reviewed annually. Schools must provide information about how a child is coping with the new arrangements and the views of the parents and professionals involved.

(c) The child must be fully reassessed at the age of 14 years (if the statement is made before 11 years).

(d) The Act allows for withdrawal of special educational provision if the child's needs have been met.

(e) Parents can appeal if they disagree with the decisions made.

Placement   This depends on:

— degree of handicap
— learning ability /IQ
— personality of the child
— whether or not school can provide special educational resources
— wishes of parents, including practical aspects of getting to and from school, wheelchair access, etc.

Where possible, children with handicaps should be placed in ordinary schools. This gives them the opportunity to mix with normal children and benefits both handicapped and non-handicapped children.

If the handicap is severe the child may need to attend a special school (day or residential). In extreme cases, home tuition or education in hospital or other centres may be needed.

Benefits and allowances   1. *Child benefit*: payable weekly until the child is 16 years (or 18 years if in full-time education).

2. *Attendance allowance*: payable for any child over the age of 2 years who requires either frequent attention or continual supervision as a result of severe physical or mental handicap. There is a different rate for day and night attendance.

3. *Mobility allowance*: payable for any child over 5 years of age who is unable or virtually unable to walk.

4. *Invalid care allowance*: paid to carer of person receiving an attendance allowance.

5. *Severe disablement allowance*: paid to the severely handicapped who are incapable of working (after 16th birthday).

Other sources of financial help:

1. Family Fund: a government fund independently administered by the Rowntree Memorial Trust. It provides for purchase of expensive items directly related to needs posed by caring for a handicapped child at home.

2. Local charities.

3. Local businesses or companies manufacturing aids.

Visual handicap

Prevalence

Defect	Prevalence (per 1000 children)
Squint	30
Refractive error	50
Registered blind	0.25
Registered partially sighted	0.3

Causes of severe visual handicap

— myopia
— optic atropy, e.g. genetic, secondary to perinatal insult
— cataract, e.g. genetic, metabolic, rubella, drugs
— ocular malformations, e.g. anophthalamia, aniridia
— glaucoma
— severe refractive error
— retinoblastoma
— retinopathy of prematurity
— inherited choroido-retinal degeneration
— trauma

Commonly associated with other handicaps, e.g.:

— cerebral palsy
— severe mental retardation
— deafness

Screening for visual defects

1. *History,* especially of abnormal eye movements, lack of fixation, photophobia. Selective screening of high-risk infants, e.g. with history of familial visual defects, intrauterine infection, prematurity, etc.

2. *Examination* of eyes for red reflex, exclude cataract, coloboma, microphthalmia, etc.

3. *Vision screening in developmental assessment.* Tests of visual acuity (VA) are difficult and inaccurate in children under 3 years. STYCAR assessments (Sheridan Tests for Young Children and Retardates) are used but are not very sensitive and may only detect severe impairment.

— 6 weeks. Elicit social smile. Observe following face or bright light
— 8 months
   • rolling graded balls at 3 m
   • 'hundreds and thousands' test for near vision
   • mounted balls test for peripheral vision
— 2 years. Matches miniature toys
— 3 years. STYCAR 5 letter test
— 6 years. STYCAR 9 letter test
— 7 years+. Snellen chart. Each eye tested separately. Repeat every 3 years (or more often if strong family history of myopia). Used at distance of 6 m. VA for distant vision expressed as pseudo-fraction, e.g. 6/60 means the child can see at 6 m a letter visible to a normal person at 60 m, i.e. very poor vision.
   Normal VA at 6 months = 6/18

At 18 months = 6/12
From 3 years onwards = 6/6
Partially sighted = 6/24 in better eye
Registered blind = <3/60

— test for *squint* (incidence 3–7% of children):
  • corneal reflections from bright torch at 30 cm
  • look for head tilt
  • cover tests
— tests for *colour blindness*. Should be done at school entry using modified Ishihara plates. Incidence: boys 8%, girls 0.5%, therefore boys screened again at secondary school entry

4. *Specialized techniques*:

— electrophysiology: electroretinogram, visual evoked responses
— CT scan

Management of impaired vision

(a) Refer to Ophthalmologist and Child Development Centre. Refractive errors must be corrected and the child's special needs assessed.

(b) Education. Many children with visual handicaps can go to normal schools with classroom aids, e.g. large type books, magnifiers, Braille books, talking books.

(c) Refer to the Royal National Institute for the Blind (RNIB) for social and family support and information regarding talking books, benefits, peripatetic teachers, etc.

(d) Refer for genetic counselling.

Deafness

Prevalence

1 in 1000 — severe (more than 70 dB loss); need hearing aid and special schooling.
2 in 1000 — moderate (50–70 dB loss); need hearing aid.

Diagnosis

Early diagnosis is vital as early habilitation improves all aspects of development, especially language.

A moderate hearing loss of 50 dB will cause delay in language development; with loss >70 dB, acquisition of speech is very difficult.

Causes

1. *Inherited*:

— autosomal recessive, e.g. Pendred's syndrome (deafness with goitre), Usher's syndrome (deafness with retinitis pigmentosa)
— autosomal dominant, e.g. Waardenburg syndrome (deafness with white forelock)
— X-linked

2. *Inner ear and facial malformations*, e.g. Treacher–Collins syndrome.

3. *Congenital rubella syndrome* (CRS).

4. *Perinatal*:

— asphyxia
— kernicterus
— ototoxic drugs
— meningitis

5. *Acquired*:

— chronic secretory otitis media
— head injury
— meningitis

Screening   1. *Neonatal screening* of infants at increased risk of hearing loss:

— family history of deafness
— congenital infection (rubella, CMV, toxoplasmosis, herpes and syphilis)
— low birth weight
— severe jaundice
— birth asphyxia
— external ear malformation or cleft palate

Methods:

— brain stem auditory evoked responses
— acoustic cradle
— click evoked otoacoustic emissions

2. *Developmental surveillance checks* (see Chapter 4).
3. *Older children*:

— sweep test for all school entrants (pure tone audiogram at fixed intensity, usually 20–25 dB)
— all children with other handicap, e.g. cerebal palsy, Down's syndrome
— language disorder or delay
— secretory otitis media (glue ear). This is the commonest cause of deafness. Can cause language delay if persistent, but generally resolves with time and/or grommets.

Management of the   (a) Diagnosis and investigation. Refer to audiologist.
deaf child   (b) General assessment:

— physical examination
— visual assessment
— speech therapy
— educational psychology; non-verbal intelligence tests

(c) Education and support:

— peripatetic teacher of the deaf (employed by Local Education Authority)
— family counselling and support
— Royal National Institute for the Deaf (RNID)

— 50% of hearing impaired children taught in normal schools. Others attend partially hearing units attached to normal schools, or schools for the deaf
— aids and language training. Wide variety of aids available, usually selected by audiologist. Used with ear mould which must fit well and will need replacing as child grows. Most can be used with 'loop' wiring systems in schools which transmit the teacher's voice and bypass background noise

Methods of education remain controversial. 'Total communication' combines oral methods (amplification, lip reading and touch) and non-verbal methods, such as sign language (e.g. British Sign Language (BSL), Makaton, Paget–Gorman) and is probably the best approach, especially for children with associated mental or visual handicap.

Language delay

Prevalence   1 in 1000 (severe delay).

Causes   — constitutional
— socio-emotional deprivation
— mental retardation
— deafness
— abnormalities of speech apparatus:
  • neurological, e.g. cerebral palsy
  • physical, e.g. cleft palate
  • lip and tongue dyspraxias
— specific language disorders
— autism

Diagnosis   Speech therapist assesses whether comprehension or expressive language delay, or both (e.g. Reynell developmental language scale). Isolated expressive delay is more common, has a good prognosis and is often managed by speech therapist alone. More complex or severe delay requires multidisciplinary assessment, including general neurodevelopmental examination, audiometry and psychometry.

Management   Depends on cause:
1. *Constitutional speech delay* — regular speech therapy. Most will catch up anyway. Increased incidence of reading and writing difficulties at school.
2. *Deafness* — refer to audiologist.
3. *Articulation problems*; plastic surgery and orthodontist for malformations. Speech training when child is old enough to understand. Augmented communication methods in cerebral palsy, see p. 103.
4. *Specific language disorders* — speech therapy. If severe may need daily language programmes and communication aids in special schools.

Learning disabilities Referral to educational psychologist or paediatrician may be made because of difficulties keeping up with school work.

— boys affected more commonly than girls
— prevalence ~5%
— various theories as to pathogenesis, including disorders of laterality, minimal brain dysfunction (characterized by poor attention span and motor coordination) and difficulties in the coding and sequencing of information in the brain

Causes Include poor teaching, frequent school absence, mild mental handicap, vision and hearing defects, petit mal epilepsy, anticonvulsant drugs, neurodegenerative disorders and space-occupying intracranial lesions.

Reading difficulties Commonest learning disability. Increased incidence in lower socioeconomic groups but all are affected. Correlation with:

— developmental delay
— intrauterine growth retardation
— speech problems
— IQ
— positive family history

The term 'specific reading retardation' refers to children with reading age below the expected for IQ and chronological age after adequate schooling.

'Dyslexia' is a more generalized abnormality of language skills, involving not only reading failure but also difficulties with mathematics, sequences (e.g. time tables), writing, left–right confusion and spelling.

Management (a) Psychologist's assessment.
(b) Consider underlying disorders, check vision and hearing.
(c) Remedial teaching, e.g. phonetic drills, tracking exercises, spelling packs.

Physical handicap

Cerebral palsy

Definition A permanent but not necessarily static disorder of movement and posture caused by non-progressive brain damage sustained prenatally or in childhood.

Prevalence 2.5 in 1000. Commonest physical handicap.

Associated disabilities
— visual   25%
— language   90%
— hearing loss   25%
— mental handicap up to 50%

Causes

Prenatal	Perinatal	Postnatal
Cerebral malformation	Hypoxic–ischaemic injury	CNS infection
Intrauterine infection	Complications of extreme prematurity, e.g. PVH, see p. 33	Trauma
Metabolic defect	Metabolic, e.g. kernicterus, hypoglycaemia	Hypoxia
Obstetric complications Chronic anaemia	Neonatal meningitis	

Types

— spastic • hemiplegia (arm more affected than leg)
          • diplegia (leg more affected than arm)
— ataxic
— choreo-athetoid
— mixed

Diagnosis

Early diagnosis with intervention reduces subsequent disability. History of risk factors in pregnancy, at delivery or postnatally necessitates increased surveillance.

The diagnosis of cerebral palsy under the age of 6 months may be difficult unless it is severe. Some children with neurological abnormalities appear to develop normally in the early months. Warning signs in the first few months include:

— feeding difficulties (poor sucking/swallowing/late chewing)
— decreased spontaneous movements, hands kept tightly closed
— small head/excessive head lag
— exaggerated tendon reflexes, sustained clonus
— persistence of immature reflexes, e.g. Moro, grasp and ATNR beyond 3 months
— failure to develop protective reflexes, e.g. parachute
— hearing loss
— squint
— fits
— involuntary movements (do not usually appear until after the age of 1 year)

Management

The aim is to allow children to reach their full potential in all areas. It is important to control abnormalities of movement and posture, so avoiding deformities which would ultimately restrict mobility. About 75% of children with cerebral palsy will eventually learn to walk.

1. *Physiotherapy* is the mainstay of treatment. Methods include Voojta, Kabat, Bobath, Doman-Delcato and *conductive education*, which is practised in the Peto Institute in Hungary. Carried out by 'conductors' who have been trained in the many disciplines required by the physically handicapped child and are therefore physiotherapist, occupational

therapist, speech therapist and behavioural therapist all rolled into one.

Children are residential and stay with the same conductor throughout. They are encouraged to become mobile however they can, even if this involves abnormal patterns of movement. Artifical aids are not encouraged.

Parents are involved at every stage and taught to recognize abnormal persisting primitive reflexes and dystonic movements and how to inhibit these reactions. In addition, the importance of preventing deformities by repeated correction of seating position and passive stretching of the limbs is emphasized.

The physiotherapist supervises the use of *physical aids* to enable children to sit upright and to increase mobility at a time when they are naturally curious about their environment, and this allows them to develop other skills. Physical aids include simple devices such as:

— sticky mats and heavy dishes to prevent spills
— high-sided potties for reassurance in toilet training
— prone boards and rollators as crawling supports
— standing supports, e.g. flexistand, tripods
— child seats, e.g. Chailey adapta seat, Cloudesley chair, bath seats
— firm boots may be recommended to aid independent walking
— pushchairs or wheelchairs may be individually designed

All physical aids can be supplied through the Disablement Services Authority if available on the NHS. Various charitable institutions donate money for single item purchases.

2. *Occupational therapy.* Home visits may be needed to assess necessary alterations, e.g. stair rails/lifts, bath rails or hoists, ramps and wheelchair access. These are the responsibility of the local social services department.

3. *Speech therapy.* An individual language programme is developed for each child. Sign language may be used if the child has good IQ but difficulty with the mechanics of speech, e.g.:

— Makaton: simple hand signs
— British Sign Language: needs good function of both hands
— Paget–Gorman: involves precise and complex signalling, therefore mostly used for children with speech impairment only
— BLISS symbols: pictograms instead of words. Laborious to use but does not require precise motor skills
— POSSUM: typewriters or computer operated by single movements. Supplied on NHS after assessment by DHS

4. Assessment by *educational psychologist* to give an idea of IQ. Special tests are available for children with vision, hearing and speech problems.

5. *A Statement of Special Educational Needs* is likely to be made for all children suffering from cerebral palsy. The aim is full-time education in an ordinary school wherever possible.

Social and self-help skills are taught early, e.g. toilet training, washing, dressing, eating, cooking. These skills may be taught in special sessions within the school day for the less severely handicapped, or may involve attending a school designed and equipped for the physically handicapped.

6. *Counselling and support* for the family (see p. 95).

Spina bifida

Early management See p. 23.

Long-term management This should be home-based wherever possible with family interaction encouraged throughout. The level of the neurological lesion and associated anomalies governs the range of problems experienced and therapy required.

Involved professionals will usually include:

— neurosurgeon, orthopaedic surgeon, urologist
— physiotherapist, occupational and speech therapist
— paediatrician, clinical medical officer, GP
— educational psychologist

Problems and management 1. *Hydrocephalus.* After early detection of a spinal defect, shunt insertion may be necessary. Often need lengthening as child grows. Shunt complications usually present with evidence of raised intracranial pressure, e.g. headache, vomiting, drowsiness.

— blockage occurs in > 50%
— infection of shunt in 10%. Most common organism is *Staph. albus.* May develop shunt nephritis
— subdural haematoma

If shunt is inserted in time to prevent damaging compression, the prognosis for intellectual development is good. Untreated hydrocephalus causes irreversible brain destruction.

2. *Orthopaedic.* Kyphosis, scoliosis, contractures, foot deformities. Spine and hip surgery may be necessary. Soft tissue release, callipers and walking aids may improve positioning and mobility.

3. *Bladder and bowel.* May have:

— flaccid paralysed bladder with overflow incontinence, constant dribbling and reflux
— spastic bladder with reflex emptying. Outlet obstruction may lead to ureteric reflux

— UTIs are a consequence of urine stagnation and reflux. May lead to chronic pyelonephritis and renal failure

Bladder emptying may be achieved using expression or catheterization. Urinary diversion procedures occasionally necessary. Early bowel training with regular enemas and laxatives facilitates the achievement of a degree of control by most children.

4. *Cerebral*:

— damage secondary to raised ICP
— cerebral palsy
— epilepsy
— mental retardation
— optic atrophy

5. *Psychological.* Stress, anxiety and depression may be associated with medical problems, repeated hospitalization, limitations on activity and worry about the future. Play therapy, group activities to foster peer-group interaction and coping strategies for families are important in assisting adjustment.

ASBAH (Association for Spina Bifida and Hydrocephalus) provides local support, disabled living advice and independence training programmes.

Psychological testing and early vocational guidance help in planning educational programmes, use of leisure time and training and work opportunities.

Sexual counselling in adolescence and advice about accommodation options outside the home help the young person become self-confident and achieve as much independence as possible.

Mental handicap

Definition A global delay in development of cognitive learning.

— severe mental retardation, IQ usually <50. Will remain dependent
— mild or moderate retardation, IQ usually 50–70. Can usually learn to live independently

Causes About 3% of the population has an IQ <70, with about 0.04% <50.

1. *Idiopathic.*
2. *Chromosomal.*
3. *Embryopathy*:

— infection
— drugs, alcohol
— metabolic
— radiation

4. *Perinatal*:

— hypoxia, birth trauma
— prematurity-associated problems
— metabolic: hypoglycaemia, hyperbilirubinaemia

5. *Genetic*:

— biochemical: amino acid/carbohydrate/lipid/organic acid metabolism
— endocrine, e.g. hypothyroidism
— syndromes, e.g. Apert, Sotos, Laurence–Moon–Biedl, Smith–Lemli–Opitz, etc.

6. *Postnatally acquired*:

— environmental including subcultural, psychosocial deprivation, restrictive child rearing practices, nutritional deprivation
— trauma
— post-meningitis, septicaemia, encephalitis
— hypernatraemic dehydration
— hypoxia: cardiac arrest, near drowning, status epilepticus, etc.
— hypoglycaemic coma
— lead poisoning

Management (a) Initial referral should be made to the local Child Development Centre or District Handicap Team for assessment once developmental delay is suspected.

(b) Assessment includes:

— history: • full perinatal history
            • history of illness, hospital admissions
            • developmental milestones
            • family history
            • social circumstances
— medical examination.
— investigation. The extent of investigation will be determined in each case by the results of careful history and examination of the child, as there are a very large number of comparatively rare causes of mental retardation and it would be impossible to exclude every condition in each child.

If dysmorphism is present, useful reference may be made to a 'dymorphologist' (a geneticist with wide experience of syndrome recognition and access to genetic computer databases).

The yield of positive laboratory results is often low, but it is worthwhile testing for the following in case of unexplained non-progressive mental subnormality:

• *blood*:   fasting calcium, phosphate and alkaline phosphatase

thyroid function
amino acid chromatography
blood lead ± zinc
liver function
± chromosome analysis ± search for fragile X sites
± blood ammonia
± blood vacuolated lymphocytes
± blood B12 and folate
± creatine phosphokinase in boys
± serology for syphilis and for toxoplasma, rubella, CMV in <3 years

- *urine*: note ? unusual odour, e.g. MSUD — sweet maltlike smell; isovaleric acidaemia — 'sweaty feet'
amino acid chromatography
reducing substances
ferric chloride test (positive in PKU, MSUD, tyrosinaemia)
cyanide nitroprusside test for sulphydryl groups (positive in homocystinuria, cystinuria, Fanconi syndrome, Wilson's disease)
2, 4-dinitrophenylhydrazine test for keto-acids (positive in PKU, MSUD, ketosis)
± glycosaminoglycans
± CMV

- *radiology*: skull, spine X-rays
± wrist for bone age
± CT brain
± NMRI

- *other*: EEG
Wood's light
(in some cases) psychometry, audiology assessment, ophthalmological opinion

(c) An honest but compassionate approach is needed to help parents accept diagnosis and foster bonding. Optimize learning opportunities from an early age. Developmental stimulation programmes such as the Portage system involve parents working with therapists in helping retarded children to acquire skills. Educational placement will depend upon assessment of behaviour and abilities.

(d) Practical and financial assistance including respite care, organized holidays and residential placement.

(e) For adolescents, consider family planning services, sheltered workshops and supervized group homes.

Down's syndrome   Commonest single cause of severe mental retardation, accounting for 1 in 4 of all children with severe learning difficulties. Affects 1 in 660 births on average. Incidence rises with maternal age to 1 in 100 at age 37 years and 1 in 40 at age 40 years.

Four types:

— 90% trisomy 21 (non-disjunction during meiosis; maternal-age related)
— 6% double trisomy (XXY + trisomy 21)
— 3.5% translocation trisomy (some, but not all, have a balanced translocation carrier parent)
— 1% mosaics

Recurrence risk:
— trisomy 21   1%
— mosaic   <1%
— translocation trisomy:
        parents not carriers   <1%
        mother carrier   10–20% (depending on type D/G, G/G)
        father carrier   1–2%

Antenatal screening   See p. 7.

Features   1. *Mental retardation.* IQ range 20–75. Development may progress quite well over first few years but retardation becomes more evident from 3–4 years onwards.

2. *General appearance*:

— brachycephaly with flattened occiput. Mild microcephaly
— eyes: upslanting, epicanthic folds, Brushfield's spots, cataracts
— small nose with low bridge
— small mouth with protruding tongue
— hands: spade-like with Simian crease (45%), clinodactyly, distal palmar axial triradius
— feet: wide gap and plantar crease between 1st and 2nd toe
— skin: dry, mottled
— hair: soft, sparse
— general hypotonia, joint laxity

3. *Cardiac.* Anomaly in 40%, particularly atrioventricular septal defects and patent ductus arteriosus.

Also increased incidence of duodenal atresia, thyroid disorders, leukaemia.

Management   (a) Both parents should be told diagnosis together, and the likely development of their child discussed.
(b) Introduction to the Down's Children's Association and information about developmental programmes to stimulate early progress may help parents to adopt a positive approach.
(c) Practical help and support.
(d) Genetic counselling when appropriate.

7. Behaviour disorders and child psychiatry

Helping disturbed children requires an understanding of the normal process of socio-emotional development from infant to adult and the ability to recognize the variety of ways in which psychological problems may present, including developmental, emotional, behaviour and psychophysiological disorders.

Disturbed behaviour in a child must be assessed in relation to:

— stage of development
— family life cycle
— socio-cultural background
— physical problems

Normal child and family development

All aspects of a child's biological, psychological and social development are interdependent and are influenced by both hereditary and environmental factors. Most children grow up within a family unit of some sort. Families vary greatly in their composition and character, from the single parent to very large extended families. An understanding of family dynamics is essential in assessing a child's developmental problems.

Personality development

Personality refers to the distinguishing behavioural qualities of an individual which are displayed persistently in a variety of situations. It is the unique result of interaction between the individual's genetic constitution and his environment and in childhood it has potential for change as a result of adverse events, therapeutic intervention, etc.

Many interesting theories of child development have been advanced, including:

(a) The psychoanalytic theory developed by Sigmund Freud concerned essentially with emotional psychosexual development
(b) Social learning theories based on premise that behaviour is modified by experience
(c) Causal theory and studies of intellectual development by Jean Piaget in the 1950s

Milestones in socio-emotional and cognitive development

Age	Developmental milestone	Common related behaviour problems
2–3 months	Selective social smiling	Feeding and sleeping problems
3+ months	Attachment behaviour	
6–8 months	Anxiety in presence of strangers	
9–12 months	Separation anxiety	
1–2 years	Main advances are in motor development enabling exploratory behaviour Learns to distinguished self and non-self Satisfaction from achievement and exerting his own will Anxiety from disapproval of others	Temper tantrums Refusal to leave mother Constipation
3–5 years	Egocentricity Sexual curiosity Conscience formation Increased complexity of language Establishment of defence mechanisms Increasing socialization	Encopresis Nightmares and fears Speech delay Clinginess
6–10 years	Concrete operational logic prevails Cultural affiliation Learning at school and peer group relationships Striving for conformity	Learning difficulties
10–12 years +	Abstract thinking develops Social and sexual roles established Separation from parents	Rebelliousness Delinquency

Family influences   Children's experiences of family life have a major effect on their development and behaviour. Important family characteristics include:

1. *Child rearing practices.* Over protectiveness with prolongation of infantile care and excessive constraint may result in overinhibited anxious children. Factors contributing to this pattern include:

— history of miscarriages/infertility
— death of other children
— chronic illness in the child
— deprivation of love or protection in the mother's own childhood
— submissive father
— sexual maladjustment between parents
— neurotic parent

Parents with obsessional traits may develop rigid depersonalized patterns of care which frequently lead to emotional problems for the child, e.g. phobias, feeding disorders, delayed bowel/bladder control.

2. *Family size and ordinal position.* Children from large families tend to have lower intelligence with slower attainment of verbal and reading skills. Suggested explanations include the possibility that such children receive less intensive interaction and infant care, less encouragement with schooling and less material resources. They are more likely to develop conduct disorders.

First-born children tend to have higher levels of scholastic achievement but are also at greater risk of emotional disorder than later born children.

3. *Parental problems:*

(a) Chronic or recurrent mental disorder in parents leads to substantially greater risk of psychiatric disorder in the child.

(b) Intergenerational cycles:

— family discord or disruption is associated with increased incidence of delinquency, teenage pregnancy and unmarried motherhood in children of such families

— up to one-third of battering parents were themselves subject to serious abuse in childhood

(c) Parental criminality is associated with delinquency in children.

4. *Separation and family relationships.* Bowlby and others have argued that separation experiences play a crucial role in the genesis of anxiety and hence in the development of a range of psychiatric disorders occurring in childhood.

Acute reactions to separation have been most studied in children admitted to hospital. Emotional distress is most marked in those aged between 6 months and 4 years; many children show an immediate reaction of acute distress and crying (period of protest) followed by misery and apathy (phase of despair) and finally a stage where the child appears more contented and to lose interest in the parents ('detachment'). When returned to the parents the child may at first ignore them and subsequently remain bad-tempered and demanding for several weeks. Parents may need help to understand a child's difficult behaviour after a separation and to learn gradually to introduce the child to happy separations with a familiar adult whilst the parent is away, in preparation for nursery and school attendance.

Single separations less than a week rarely have long-term sequelae. Recurrent stressful separations (e.g. multiple hospital admissions) are associated with increased risk of psychiatric disorder, particularly if there are other family problems.

Socio-cultural influences

As children grow older they are exposed to a wider range of influences and attitudes at school and in their neighbourhood. The peer group exercises an important influence on children's behaviour.

1. *Geographical area and delinquency.* Crime and delinquency are often concentrated in particular areas such as inner city slums or new housing estates. Delinquency is associated with family conflict, poor housing and low income. It is likely to be a behaviour learned through interaction with other delinquent individuals: it is strongly associated with delinquency in siblings and criminal parents, though the higher proportion of delinquents from poor homes may stem in part from differences in the way police treat people from differing social backgrounds. It is usually a transient phase which in some areas is so common that it may be regarded as normal behaviour in the child's subculture. Recidivist delinquency, however, is a more serious indicator of maladjustment and of likely adult disturbance than is the presence of neurotic symptoms.

In general, psychiatric referral rates are higher in families living in high density city areas of low social status. Various stresses of inner city life may contribute to this including:

— lack of community facilities
— overcrowded households
— anonymity and lack of community involvement
— school factors • high turnover
              • inadequate facilities
              • rigid streaming systems
              • teaching styles

2. *Immigrant families.* Difficulties with adaptation to change in socio-political structure, language and climate are particularly experienced by immigrants without an established community in the UK, e.g. Vietnamese boat people.

Parental insecurity may result in altered behaviour, including marital difficulty and increased anxiety about children, which in turn causes the children to feel anxious and insecure. Trans-cultural problems in reconciling the differences between the behaviour expected at school and that required at home may be difficult for children. Parental restrictions on social life are a frequent source of conflict, particularly for Asian girls who are often expected to enter into arranged marriages. Poor school progress due to linguistic difficulties or to unhappiness may be compounded by considerable parental pressure to succeed, particularly in those groups who came to Britain with high financial expectations.

Several studies have found that West Indian children have

higher rates of behavioural disorders at school, but not necessarily at home. In contrast they are less likely to have emotional disturbances or difficulties with peer group relationships.

There are many variations in family structure, child rearing practices and discipline as well as wider socio-cultural influences which must be considered when assessing the causes of behavioural disturbance in children of ethnic minority families.

Development and habit disorders

Feeding problems

Poor appetite may be a symptom of physical illness, such as acute infection, etc., but by far the commonest cause of persistent food refusal is poor training and food forcing. Questioning will often reveal other evidence of mother–child disharmony or excessive maternal anxiety about the child's nutrition and weight.

Management

(a) Allay maternal anxiety by demonstrating that child is growing normally for age, explain that children often eat less in the 2nd half of their 1st year and that there is great variation in the range of 'normal appetite'.
(b) Listen to mother's concerns and discuss any background anxieties which are exacerbating the situation.
(c) Explain that this is a common problem which can be overcome.
(d) Discuss feeding tactics to be employed and stress the importance of firm and consistent handling by all those involved with care of the child.
(e) In severe cases, if the child is not thriving, it is helpful for someone such as the health visitor to visit the family at home to observe feeding practices and suggest possible improvements. Rarely, in difficult cases, mother and child are admitted to hospital to exclude underlying illnesses and check that the child gains weight when adequate calorific intake is ensured.

Sleep disorders

Duration of sleep usually about 10–12 h/day at 6 months and 8–10 h/day at 2 years.

Sleep problems:

— difficulty settling to sleep
— failure to sleep through the night
— night terrors (commonest at 4–7 years)
— nightmares (commonest at 8–10 years)
— sleep walking (commonest at 11–14 years)

Aetiological factors include:

— perinatal complications

— variations in temperament
— anxiety related to separation or parent–child interactions

Management (a) Exclude physical illness or underfeeding.
(b) Take full history to investigate for underlying anxieties.
(c) Explain normal variations in sleeping patterns and reassure.
(d) Occasionally, sedation for a brief period (e.g. a week) is useful to break the pattern of night terrors.
(e) If the disorder is persistent or the symptom hazardous, e.g. sleep walking, specialist psychiatric therapy may be needed.

Habit disorders — rocking
— headbanging
— nailbiting
— thumbsucking
— masturbation
— tics

These are generally not of pathological significance and are usually outgrown by the 4th birthday. They can, however, be manifestations of tension or emotional disorder when they are often persistent and associated with other symptoms.

Manifestations of stress Infants — excessive crying
— disturbed sleep
— poor feeding
— vomiting
Toddlers — persistent thumbsucking
— frequent open masturbation
— overactivity
— separation anxiety
— night terrors
— withholding faeces
— asthma
Children — impaired concentration
— excessive fears
— night terrors
— tics, e.g. shrugging, blinking
— speech hesitancy
— recurrent abdominal pain or headache
— enuresis
— encopresis

Enuresis Inappropriate voiding of urine after the age at which bladder control should have been achieved. Most children are dry by day at 2–3 years and at night by 3–4 years.

Prevalence Approximately 10% of children are enuretic at 5 years, 5% at 10 years and 1–2% of teenagers.

— falls with age

— boys more often affected
— commoner in intellectually retarded children
— often familial: 70% have first-degree relative with history of enuresis
— associated with delayed speech development

Aetiology   May be associated with:

— neurophysiological maturational delay
— faulty training (delay in social learning response)
— emotional disturbance leading to regression
— organic causes:
  • UTI (6% of enuretic girls have UTI *cf*. 1.5% of non-enuretic girls)
  • diabetes mellitus
  • diabetes insipidus
  • Neurological disorders affecting bladder control, e.g. myelomeningocele, sacral agenesis, diastematomyelia, lipoma of cauda equina, epilepsy
— Genitourinary abnormalities:
  • bladder outflow obstruction, e.g. posterior urethral valves
  • ureterocele, ectopic ureter
  • urethrovaginal fistula
  • epispadias
  • bladder exstrophy

Investigations   Should be kept to a minimum unless history is suggestive of physical problem, e.g. persistent dribbling, neurological symptoms. Urinalysis for sugar, albumin, microscopy and culture in all cases. Consider renal US, IVU, MCU if organic cause suspected.

Management   (a) Full history of child and family, plus examination of child.
(b) Explain to child that this problem is shared by many other children. Reassure parents that the problem, though inconvenient, is not serious and is likely to be outgrown.
(c) Explain that punitive methods serve only to increase anxiety and may make matters worse.
(d) Conditioning methods:

— reward systems
— pad and buzzer alarm; requires careful initial demonstration and regular follow-up, but if used properly the success rate is up to 70%.

(e) Medication:

— imipramine may help, but high relapse rate
— desmopressin (DDAVP) 20 µg intranasal at bedtime. Improvement in up to 80% within days but only 12–40% completely dry. Best response in children >9 years. High relapse rate

Encopresis   Passage of faeces into the clothes by day or night. Children usually achieve faecal continence by 3 years. Soiling after 4 years is abnormal.

Four types:

1. *Primary or continuous* soiling — may be due to lack of, or inconsistent, training.

2. *Stress (regressive)* soiling — symptom of anxiety.

3. *Aggressive* soiling — usually reflects disturbed child–parent relationship in children who feel oppressed by parental demands to be clean. Parents of such children sometimes have obsessive personalities and employ rigid coercive toilet training practices.

4. *Retentive* soiling — may be emotional in origin or may have physical cause, including anal fissure or Hirschsprung disease.

Management   (a) Establish if there is retention with soiling due to overflow incontinence by abdominal and rectal examination. May require abdominal X-ray, barium enema.

(b) If there is severe retention, disimpaction with laxatives or enema is needed and admission to hospital is occasionally necessary.

(c) Alleviate causes of any anxiety if possible. Individual psychotherapy may be needed.

(d) Consistent patient retraining, preferably at home.

(e) Family therapy or counselling.

Breath-holding attacks   Occur between 6 months and 5 years. Child when thwarted or hurt cries, then holds his breath in expiration, turns blue and after 10–15 seconds goes limp. He may lose consciousness and usually when this happens a normal breathing pattern is resumed and a pink colour returns.

If the breath-holding continues for a further 10–15 seconds a convulsion may ensue. This may be differentiated from an epileptic convulsion in which the cry is synchronous with the tonic phase and cyanosis occurs late.

Management   (a) Take a full history and examine the child to establish diagnosis.

(b) Discuss mother's anxieties about diagnosis, management and outcome.

(c) Discuss setting limits of allowable behaviour and the importance of firm and consistent handling if limits are exceeded.

(d) Reassure mother that child will outgrow the habit by 4–5 years at the latest.

Hyperactivity (attention deficit disorder)   Term applied to children who are unusually overactive with accompanying lack of concentration, short attention span, impulsiveness and emotional immaturity. Diagnosed more frequently in the USA (5–10% of primary schoolchildren). In the UK held to be uncommon in isolation but perhaps occurring more frequently in association with conduct disorders or mental retardation. Five times more common in boys.

Causes
— normal variation
— maturational delay — particularly in mentally handi-capped or associated with specific learning difficulties
— neurogenic • birth asphyxia
         • cerebral palsy
         • TLE
— autism
— psychosocial • parent–child conflict
         • abnormal fears
         • excessive restraint
         • parental alcoholism
— lead poisoning
— drugs — Phenobarbitone, phenytoin, theophylline
— foods, e.g.: additives • tartrazine   E102
            • sunset yellow   E110
            • carmiosine   E122
            • amaranth   E123
      other — cow's milk, wheat in some children

Management   1. *Behavioural*:

— psychosocial assessment. Counselling parents, teaching simple behaviour modification techniques. Structured environment, regular quiet routines, consistent manage-ment. Day care, respite care
— educational psychology assessment. Special help with specific difficulties

2. *Pharmacological*. Methylphenidate used in the USA. Neuroleptics, e.g. haloperidol, may be effective in more severe cases associated with brain damage or mental retardation.

3. *Dietary*. Exclusion diets, e.g. Feingold diet (avoiding additives and colourings), should be supervised by dietician to avoid nutritional inadequacy. May benefit certain sub-groups of hyperactive children but trial results are equivocal.

School absence   Causes of repeated or prolonged absence from school include:

— chronic physical illness
— school or family problems
— truancy
— school refusal

School refusers are often younger than those children who play truant. They tend to be quiet, concientious children who have no obvious problems at school but are reluctant to attend, becoming panicky as school-time approaches. Problem usually stems from separating from mother and home. May present with physical symptoms, e.g. headache. abdominal pain.

Contrasting features of school refusal and truancy

	School refusers	Truants
Age (years)	5–11	>8
Previous school attendance	Good	Poor
Family	Conventional cohesive family	Unaware or unconcerned
	Collude over non-attendance	
	Small family	Large family
	Social class I, II, III	Social class IV, V
Personality	Concientious, conforming	Rebellious
Achievement	Good with high goals	Nonacademic, only practical goals
Psychosomatic features	Common	Rare
Triggers	Accidents	Domestic crisis
	Illness	Change of school
	Bereavement	

Management
(a) Examination to enable confident exclusion of physical causes. Avoid prolonged investigation.
(b) Discussion with parents about nature of problem.
(c) Set date for early return to school and thereafter firm insistence that child attends every day.
(d) Involve school staff: meet child at gate and reinforce and reward positive behaviour for few weeks to help child readjust.
(e) In some cases it is appropriate and necessary to involve the Educational Welfare Officer or the Child and Family Psychiatry team.

Problems of adolescence

Anorexia nervosa
Increasing problem in Western society. Predominantly females aged 12–18 years, though sometimes seen in boys.

Incidence
1 in 250 girls aged 15–18 years.

Features
— persistent refusal to eat
— may be bouts of overeating followed by self-induced vomiting
— may use laxatives or diuretics to try and reduce weight
— disturbed perception of body image — sees and portrays herself as fat even when emaciated
— intense fear of gaining weight or becoming fat
— endocrine disturbance — secondary hypothalamic dysfunction often first manifest by amenorrhoea

— family tend to be overprotective, restrictive or un-adaptable. May be family history of obesity
— premorbid personality — often emotionally immature, obsessional traits, ambivalent mother–child relationship
— physical • very thin
         • weak and lethargic
         • reduced basal metabolic rate, hypothermia, bradycardia
         • acrocyanosis
         • lanugo
— biochemical
    • LH, FSH, oestrogen low
    • electrolyte disturbances, particularly hypokalaemia in those who vomit or purge
    • neurochemical abnormalities — associated changes in noradrenaline, serotonergic and opioid systems
— Psychopathological
    • conflict associated with fear of growing up and assuming adult sexual role
    • pressure in Western society for women to be slim

Management
(a) Establish rapport with patient and family.
(b) Mild cases: outpatient psychotherapy.
(c) Admission to hospital necessary for more severe cases.
(d) Structured environment, set contracts with privileges as reward for achievement of target weight gains.
(e) Individual psychotherapy.
(f) Family therapy.
(g) Drug treatment with, e.g. anxiolytics and anti-depressants, helpful in some cases.

Prognosis
Half these patients remain underweight with social and sexual difficulties. Mortality rates are up to 8% from inanition.

Alcohol, drug and solvent usage
The extent to which a child experiments with such substances varies from place to place and time to time, depending on fashion and availability.

In the UK, 0.5–1% of the secondary school population abuse solvents regularly and deaths in the UK have increased from 2 in 1971 to over 100 each year since 1985. The Ontario child health study in 1983 found that solvents were used by 8–9% of those aged 12–14 years, with marijuana and hard drugs more commonly used by those aged 14–16 years. Amongst the latter group, 15% of boys and 25% of girls smoked tobacco regularly.

Factors associated with drug use include:

— low self esteem
— social isolation
— depression

— family conflicts
— other conduct disorders

Drugs and solvents used in the UK

Substance	Active constituent	Route
Model airplane glue	Toluene, benzene, acetone, xylene	Sniffed
Petrol	Hydrocarbons, tetraethyl lead	'Huffed' — cloth over face or from plastic bag
Cleaning fluids	Trichloroethylene, carbon tetrachloride, toluene	
Aerosols, lighter refills	Fluorocarbons, butane	Sprayed direct into mouth
Paints, varnishes, lacquers	Trichloroethylene, methylene chloride, toluene	Sniffed
Nail varnish remover	Acetone, amyl nitrate	
Cocaine		Inhaled 'snorting'
Crack	Cocaine separated from its hydrochloride salt: 'free base cocaine' More rapid effect, higher blood levels than cocaine hydrochloride	Smoked in cigarette or freebase pipe
Amphetamine: 'speed'		Oral, i.v.
Hallucinogens: LSD, 'acid', mescaline, phencyclidine		Oral
PCP, 'angel dust'		
Tranquillisers: benzodiazepines		Oral
Narcotics: heroin, morphine, codeine, methadone		Oral, i.v.

Detection   Presentations suggestive of substance use include:

— altered behaviour: mood swings, violent excitement, loss of self control, truancy, theft, deterioration in schoolwork
— 'sniffer's rash': inflammation and ulceration around mouth and nose
— injection sites
— chronic upper respiratory tract inflammation
— irregular pulse

— signs of glue on skin or clothes

— acute intoxication ± ataxia, coma, respiratory depression and cardiac arrhythmias

Effects of solvent abuse

(a) Initial euphoria; subsequent confusion, perceptual distortion, hallucinations and delusions.

(b) Large doses can cause CNS depression with ataxia, nystagmus, dysarthria, coma and convulsions. Toluene inhalation can cause encephalopathy. Chronic abuse can cause hepatic and renal damage.

(c) Sudden death may result from anoxia, vagal inhibition, respiratory depression, cardiac arrhythmias or trauma.

(d) Solvent use in pregnancy may result in neonatal depression and there may be teratogenic effects.

Management

(a) 95% of children who experiment with solvents only do it a few times and can be dealt with by the GP or adolescent unit, sometimes enlisting help from other involved professionals such as a social worker or probation officer. Obtain consent to deal with school-year heads, probation officer or youth leaders. Activity based self-help groups in many areas.

(b) Emergency treatment for acute presentations in A & E. If diagnosis uncertain measure blood toluene, acetone or drug levels.

(c) Subsequent referral to:

— child guidance clinic

— psychotherapy with casework by social worker

— voluntary organizations (contactable via Health Education Council, e.g. Re-Solv, National Campaign vs Solvent Abuse)

— child and family psychiatry team

— drug dependancy unit

GPs have a legal obligation to notify addicts to the Home Office whether prescribing treatment or not. GPs may prescribe controlled drugs to registered addicts on a blue FP10 form.

Prevention

(a) Education in public health.

(b) Restrictions on sale of solvents to children <18 years (Intoxicating Substances Act 1985), though solvent abuse is not illegal.

Major affective disorders

These disorders involve a persistent and pervasive disturbance of mood. Mania is rare before puberty. Depressive symptoms may be seen in association with:

— adverse life events

— constitutional factors

— physical disease, e.g. diabetes, asthma, viral illness

— medication, e.g. steroids, some anticonvulsants

— severe sociocultural deprivation
— other psychiatric disorders

Symptoms vary with age and may include:

— direct expression of depressed mood:
  • ± loss of energy and of interest in friends, hobbies
  • feelings of worthlessness and self reproach
  • psychomotor retardation
— vegetative symptoms:
  • disturbance of sleep or appetite
  • regression — enuresis, soiling
— indirect:
  • vandalism
  • drug use
— suicidal behaviour

Treatment   Look for emotional stresses to alieviate when possible and help child to cope with stress by means of:

— individual psychotherapy
— milieu therapy offering supportive environment
— behaviour therapy

Antidepressant drugs may be helpful in severe cases in initial stages.

Suicide   Rare before puberty. Incidence increasing in adolescents in most Western countries. Slightly more common in males though sex difference less than in previous decades.

Mean annual rate (1980–1986) is 1.3 per million population aged 10–14 years in England and Wales. Suicide *attempts* are much commoner with a 7:1 female preponderance. Must always be taken seriously with a full psychosocial assessment and work with child and family to try to relieve conflicts and improve relationships.

Childhood psychosis   This group of disorders is characterized by severely disturbed, bizarre and unpredictable behaviour resulting from a disturbed perception of reality.

Many psychotic children function at a regressed level, whilst the mentally handicapped are at more risk of developing psychosis than normal children. It is important to consider organic causes for such behaviour.

1. *Acute confusional states*:

— systemic infections
— chemical intoxication, including drug reactions
— metabolic disturbances, e.g. hypoglycaemia, hyper-ammonaemia
— TLE
— acute brain injury or infection

2. *Chronic organic causes* of disintegrative psychoses:

— lead encephalopathy
— cerebral lipidosis
— infection: SSPE, HIV encephalopathy

3. Psychoses of *mixed aetiology*:

— infantile psychosis or autism
— late onset psychosis or schizophrenia in childhood

Autism   'Pervasive developmental disorder of infancy'. Autism means to be withdrawn into one's self. It is not an all-or-none phenomenon; autistic features may coexist with other pathology, e.g. mental handicap, deafness. Male:female ratio 3:1. Onset before 30 months.

Incidence   4 in 10 000 in Britain.

Features   1. *Failure to establish social relationships*:

— avoids physical and eye contact
— forms attachments to objects rather than people

2. *Impaired language development*:

— delay or absence of speech
— echolalia

3. *Ritualistic and compulsive phenomena*:

— obsessive desire for sameness
— stereotypical behaviour patterns
— catastrophic reactions to changes in routine

Aetiology   Unknown. Possible associated factors:
1. *Genetic*. Higher concordance rate in monozygotic than dizygotic twins. Increased incidence of autism and learning disorders in siblings.
2. *Family dynamics*. Parental coldness, aloofness and mechanistic methods have been blamed but these theories are discounted because of lack of evidence.
3. *Brain damage*. Associated with focal neurological defects, abnormal EEG and subsequent development of epilepsy in up to 28%, often around puberty.
4. *Biochemical*. Elevated blood serotonin levels have been found in up to a third of autistic children. This led to trials of treatment with fenfluramine, but results so far are inconclusive.

Treatment   Various approaches have been tried; none has been proven to affect long-term outcome.
(a) Educational and behaviour modification treatment with positive re-inforcement and one-to-one teaching helps some children. Forced holding therapy: good results are

claimed by exponents in Germany; efficacy controversial and emotionally exhausting for parents.

(b) Parents need practical advice and guidance. Day-care centres are useful sources of support, as are associations of parents of autistic children, e.g. The National Autistic Society.

(c) Drugs such as tranquillizers may be necessary to control panic attacks and sleep disorders. Haloperidol may reduce stereotypies.

(d) Residential placement is avoided but is necessary in severe cases if families are unable to cope with their autistic child.

Prognosis   Poor. 60% need long-term hospital or special institutional care.

Late onset psychoses   Affected children have a period of normal development before the onset of the disorder which may be sudden or insidious. Such conditions are much rarer than infantile autism until puberty, when schizophrenia occurs more frequently.

Most children with late-onset psychoses have symptoms similar to those of adult schizophrenics, as described by Schneider. Others not fitting this clinical picture are categorized as atypical or undifferentiated late-onset psychoses.

Schizophrenia in childhood is very rare before the age of 5 years; most cases present after 7 years. A useful set of diagnostic criteria was proposed by Schneider, the 'First Rank Symptoms' of schizophrenia:

— auditory hallucinations
— thought withdrawal and insertion
— thought broadcasting
— somatic passivity phenomenon
— delusions
— feelings and volitional acts experienced by patient as influence of others

Four types:

— simple
— hebephrenic ('hebe', Greek: puberty)
— catatonic
— paranoid

Simple and hebephrenic types have worse prognosis, particularly if onset before 20 years or positive family history.

Treatment   (a) Antipsychotic drugs, principally long-acting phenothiazines and butyrophenones.

(b) Social rehabilitation and long-term family support. Voluntary associations, e.g. National Schizophrenia Fellowship, offer advice and support.

(c) Institutional care becomes necessary for some patients.

Role of the family doctor   The GP will often be the first doctor the parents consult if a child has behaviour problems or physical symptoms. It is important to be aware of the different ways children may react to stress and to consider emotional problems when looking for the cause of somatic disorders.

A classic study of 9–11-year olds on the Isle of Wight in the 1960s found a 6.8% incidence of psychiatric illness. Only 1 in 10 were receiving treatment. Considerable overlap was found between psychiatric illness and other handicaps such as educational retardation and physical disorders. Subsequent epidemiological studies in inner London showed much higher rates of educational retardation and psychiatric disorders than the Isle of Wight survey. A study of children attending GPs in Manchester in 1986 found mental health problems as the main reason for presentation in 2% but psychiatric disturbance was identified as background to somatic disorder in 23%.

The GP is known and trusted by the family, and often may have a knowledge of the family's structure and problems which places him in a unique position to understand their needs.

Many behavioural disorders in children can be managed with the family, either by the GP alone or jointly with other agencies, e.g. schools, paediatricians, voluntary organizations or psychiatrists. Even if specialist help is needed, the GP acts to coordinate available resources and offer essential supportive care, providing explanations and reassurance and helping to restore parents' confidence in their ability to cope.

8. Child abuse

— physical
— sexual
— emotional
— neglect

Epidemiology
Notification of child abuse has increased more than 20 times in the last decade. This may indicate a true increase in incidence but certainly reflects increasing awareness of the problem.

Exact prevalence unknown but about 4–10 in 1000 children are physically abused each year in the UK. The majority are <4 years old; 1 in 1000 children in this age group suffers severe abuse every year (e.g. cerebral haemorrhage or life-threatening internal injuries). Mortality estimated to be 2–4 children per week in the UK.

Aetiology
Certain common factors may be helpful in anticipating the likelihood of abuse:

1. *Parents*:

— often from broken homes, lack personal experience of good parenting skills and family support. Abuse is 20 times more likely if parent was abused in childhood
— may have personality disorders or psychiatric illness
— may have unreasonable expectations of the child

2. *Child*:

— result of unwanted pregnancy
— neonatal problems, such as prematurity (three times greater risk) or birth defect
— wrong sex
— difficult child, e.g. chronic illness, feeding or sleeping problems

3. *Social background*:

— family crises, e.g. marital strife, unemployment, eviction, bereavement
— drug/alcohol dependence
— poor housing, debt, social isolation
— frequent pregnancies, maternal exhaustion or depression
— change in family structure; step children at increased risk
— 'abusive society'. Children often victims of ideological

and political conflicts which expose them to risk of both physical and emotional injury. In South Africa the black infant mortality rate is 6 times that for white infants; in Northern Ireland nearly 200 children under 14 years have been victims of the violent struggle over the last 20 years

Recognition Clues which should raise the suspicion of abuse include:

— delay in presentation
— inadequate or inconsistent explanation of symptoms or lesions
— parents expressed fear of damaging child or inability to cope
— parental attitude, e.g. abnormal interaction with child, aggression, reluctance to allow full examination, derogatory comments about child
— multiple consultations about minor symptoms
— child's appearance
  • unkempt, frightened, withdrawn
  • 'frozen watchfulness'
  • failure to thrive
  • developmental retardation
  • physical injuries

± history of possible contributory aetiological factors in family or social background as above.

Patterns of injury in physical abuse

1. *Superficial injuries*:

— bruises: suspicious if child <9 months or on face, upper arms (finger and thumb grip marks), around wrists or ankles, ears. Fade from purple through brown through green to yellow, each change taking 3–7 days
— bite marks
— black eyes, particularly bilateral
— torn frenulum (force feeding, blows)
— hair loss
— lacerations, wheals, ligature marks
— petechiae
— burns and scalds: seen in 10–15% of physically abused children. May be deliberately inflicted as punishment or result from negligence:
  • contact burns; brand marks, sharp demarcation
  • cigarette burns: deep, small, circular, may be multiple
  • forced immersion scalds: particularly buttocks, glove and stocking distribution
  • hot feed scalds

2. *Bone injuries*. Over 90% of non-accidental fractures are inflicted on children <3 years old. In this age group, at least a quarter of all fractures are probably non-accidental.

Suspicious fractures:

— multiple fractures at different stages of healing
— epiphyseal or metaphyseal avulsion fractures (corner and bucket handle)
— unusual sites: posterior ribs, lateral clavicle, scapula, sternum
— unpresented fractures

If radiology of a tender site is negative, a repeat film in 10–14 days may reveal periosteal new bone formation or callus around an undisplaced epiphyseal separation.

3. *Head injuries.* Commonest cause of death in abused children. 95% of serious intracranial injuries in infants are due to abuse.

(a) *Skull fractures.* Accidental fractures tend to be single, linear, narrow and parietal. Associated intracranial injury is uncommon except after severe trauma, e.g falls >3 m.

Suspicious skull fractures:

— multiple or complex
— crossing suture lines
— depressed
— bilateral
— occipital
— wide (>3 mm) and 'growing'
— associated intracranial injury

(b) *Subdural haemorrhage.* Coexistent fracture in <50%. Due to direct trauma or shaking causing rupture of bridging veins between cerebral cortex and venous sinuses. Look for retinal haemorrhages, grip marks or other bruising.

(c) *Intracerebral haemorrhage.*

(d) *Cerebral oedema and contusions.*

(e) *Subgaleal haematoma.*

Long-term sequelae of head injuries include mental retardation, hydrocephalus, blindness and epilepsy.

4. *Ocular damage*:

— acute hyphaema, may lead to secondary glaucoma
— dislocated lens
— retinal haemorrhage or detachment.

Approximately half those with serious head injury sustain permanent visual impairment.

5. *Visceral injuries.* Remember to look for these, as are important cause of morbidity and there may be little external evidence.

— rupture spleen/liver
— intestinal perforation, torn mesentery

6. *Poisoning*. Deliberate poisoning is more often seen in children <2 years old *cf*. accidental poisoning commonest in 2–4 year olds.

— drugs: hypnotics; laxatives, emetics; methadone, cannabis; insulin
— salt
— alcohol

7. *Suffocation*. Signs of smothering:

— petechiae, particularly face
— bruising, fingermarks
— bleeding from mouth/nose

8. *Drowning*.

Emotional Abuse

All forms of child abuse involve some emotional injury. The fact that only 2.5% of children on NSPCC registers are under the category of emotional abuse does not mean that it is less common than other forms of abuse, but rather reflects the fact that emotional abuse is a diffuse concept which can be difficult to define and to prove. It often accompanies and underlies failure to thrive.

Modes of presentation

Infants

— developmental delay, particularly social and psychomotor skills
— absent/abnormal attachment behaviour to parents
— failure to thrive
— Characteristic appearance — pale, apathetic, paucity subcutaneous fat, thin face, prominent ribs, sparse dry hair, spindly limbs, napkin rash, acrocyanosis
— decreased spontaneous movement, watchful 'radar gaze'

Children

— behaviour problems: limited attention span, hyperactivity, aggression, indiscriminate friendliness, enuresis, encopresis
— learning difficulties
— withdrawal, difficulty with peer group relationships
— failure to thrive, 'psychosocial dwarfism'
— reversible growth hormone deficiency

Child sexual abuse (CSA)

Definition

CSA is the involvement of children in activities for the sexual gratification of adults.

Prevalence

Estimated frequency varies depending on case definition, type of study and population sample.

From the NSPCC's statistics for 1986 an annual incidence rate of 0.57 cases per 1000 children under 17 years old has been estimated. The number of reported cases has increased over the last 2 years due to heightened awareness and recognition of the problem, but available figures are probably an underestimate.

Perpetrator	%
Father	30
Older brother	10
Step-father/male cohabitee	9.5
Baby-sitter	7
Uncle	5
Mother	4
Grandfather	4

CSA may occur in all types of family and to children of any age and either sex. Certain factors lead to increased vulnerability to CSA:

— parental sexual abuse
— socioeconomic risk factors
— maternal depression/illness
— child deprived of affection

All doctors who work with children must be familiar with the principles of dealing with CSA. *Requirements for medical assessment* include:
(a) Awareness of possible forms of presentation of CSA.
(b) Ability to discriminate normal cultural and familial variations in lifestyle from abusive practices.
(c) Familiarity with normal pre-pubertal genital appearance.
(d) Knowledge about STD, incidence and significance in the pre-pubertal child.
(e) Legal aptitude about documentation.

Presentation   In some cases the child makes a verbal allegation but often the suspicion may arise from a combination of physical or behavioural factors.

1. *General*:

— superficial injuries–bruises, bites, scratches
— difficulty walking or sitting
— torn/stained clothes
— teenage pregnancy, especially if concealed/unidentified father
— recurrent UTI
— recurrent abdominal pain/headaches/fainting

2. *Genital ± rectal*

— soreness/itchiness

— persistent vaginal discharge
— vaginal bleeding
— dysuria
— faecal soiling/retention/rectal bleeding
— signs of STD, e.g. warts, discharge
— foreign body

3. *Behavioural*

— sexualized: child with detailed knowledge of, or pre-occupation with, sexual behaviour in conversation, play or drawings. May act in a sexually provocative manner towards adults
— regression
— depression, guilt, loss of self esteem, withdrawal
— fearfulness
— disruptive, attention-seeking behaviour
— sleep disturbance
— bedwetting
— inappropriate displays of affection
— daughter adopting maternal role within a family
— school: poor peer group relationships, deteriorating academic performance, avoidance of school medical, truancy
— alcohol/solvent/drug dependence
— suicide attempts

In investigation of suspected CSA it is essential for all involved agencies to cooperate fully, sharing information and resources, with the aims of protecting the child and minimizing the trauma of investigation for the child and family.

(a) Concern regarding CSA may be aroused by a verbal allegation or suggestive behaviour and brought to the attention of a doctor not specially trained in child abuse work. To avoid the need for repeated examinations it is often best to defer detailed examination until arrangements are made for it to be conducted by a doctor with training in this area. The case should be discussed promptly with another professional working in child abuse, so that assessment of urgency and type of response required can be made.

(b) If it is agreed that there are serious grounds for concern, a planning discussion or strategy meeting will be held with other professionals in local child abuse services, including senior members of social services, hospital and community paediatricians, police and others as appropriate. The strategy meeting will decide who should see the child and where.

(c) Interviewing is kept to the minimum. Special interview techniques are used to help children relate their experiences, including the use of drawings, anatomically complete dolls and video-recording; these 'disclosure techniques' should be employed only after careful consideration by professionals trained in their use. Full interviews, where necessary, are usually done by social workers in collaboration with a paediatrician and a member of the police child protection team. Consent should be obtained from the parent before the interview and the child offered the opportunity to have a trusted adult present.

(d) Medical examination should be performed only with the consent of parent and child. (If parents refuse and examination is deemed essential, a court order is sought).

Children must be carefully prepared for the examination which should be performed in a comfortable private environment by an experienced doctor trained in child abuse work, together with a medical forensic examiner who collates forensic evidence using a specially designed kit, and provides a second opinion so that repeated examinations should not be necessary.

The medical examination

(a) The doctor should have a clear history of the child's previous health, development and behaviour as well as of the alleged incident.

(b) The child should be put at ease as much as possible.

(c) Full general examination should precede examination of the genitalia.

(d) Examination of the genitalia should be performed:

— with the child relaxed
— in a good light
— magnifying lens and measuring card may be helpful
— special microbiological and forensic swabs, plates and containers should be readily to hand if required
— clinical photography is useful in some cases

Interpretation of physical findings

The DHSS guidelines for doctors (1988) stress the important point that 'No physical sign can at the present time be regarded as uniquely diagnostic of CSA'. Any signs must be interpreted in the knowledge of the full clinical picture; the attribution of undue importance to any single sign in isolation must be avoided.

Findings which *may* indicate abuse:

— clothing: torn, stained, inside out or back to front, smell
— superficial signs of a struggle: scratches, bruises, broken finger nails (NB scrapings from underneath nails)
— burns, particularly cigarette burns (may be associated with sado-masochistic abuse)
— ligature marks: neck, wrists, ankles
— oropharynx : bruising, petechiae, ulcers
— abdomen; bruises, pressure marks, tenderness, masses
— genitalia
  • erythema, oedema, bruising, lacerations on vulva/labia

- dystrophic skin changes
- pubic hairs or lubricants
- tears/scars of posterior fourchette (may also follow accidental straddle injuries)
- vaginal discharge or bleeding
- perineal warts
- tears or scars of hymen

(But note *normal variations* in size and shape. The hymen is rarely imperforate; usually has a central orifice <0.5 cm in diameter, of varying shape. There may be several openings (septate, cribriform). Bumps on the hymeneal ring may be residual after healed tears or previous genital infection. Tears are usually in the posterior half. The horizontal vaginal introitus normally measures up to 0.75 cm in pre-pubertal girls.)

— buttocks and anus:
- bruises, scratches on buttocks, inner thighs
- erythema, swelling, venous dilatation around anal ring
- perianal warts
- fissures, skin tags, scars
- anal dilatation: with the child in the left lateral position, buttocks are gently separated. In a positive test, the anal sphincter relaxes (within up to 30 seconds) so that the interior of the anal canal is seen, with the dilatation persisting at least 2–3 seconds. This may indicate stretching or injury to the internal anal sphincter and should raise the level of suspicion of possible abuse, but the sphincter may be relaxed physiologically by faeces in the lower rectum, and the presence of anal dilatation is *not* pathognomic of abuse

It is essential to make a detailed record, including clear drawings and authenticated photographs when appropriate of the findings at examination. If further action is necessary, this must be explained to the child and parents; if not, they should be reassured.

Differential diagnoses   1. *Bruises*

— bleeding diatheses; haemophilia, leukaemia, ITP
— Mongolian blue pigmentation

2. *Fractures*

— osteogenesis imperfecta
— osteoporosis
— bone cysts
— neoplasia
— rickets
— osteopetrosis
— Caffey's disease
— copper deficiency

3. *Periosteal reaction*

— syphilis
— scurvy
— copper deficiency
— physiological (1–10 months, diaphyses only)

4. *Multiple scars*

— previous surgery
— Ehlers–Danlos
— ceremonial scars, Moharran scars (Schia Moslem adolescents in Islam New Year)

5. *Intracerebral haemorrhage*

— birth injury
— meningitis
— bleeding diatheses, e.g. HDN, thrombocytopenia
— deccelerative force, e.g. RTA

6. *Self injury.*
7. *Sickle cell disease*

— hand–foot syndrome

8. *Genital lesions*

— infective vulvo-vaginitis
— contact dermatitis
— lichen sclerosis et atrophicus
— vitiligo
— threadworm infestation

9. *Anal*:

— constipation
— neurogenic patulous anus
— Crohn disease

Prevention
Parents should teach children how to respond to advances from strangers and encourage them to tell parents of any advances or behaviour which has frightened them or made them uncomfortable, even from people they know. This may be re-inforced in schools by teachers and counsellors; structured video-interactive classroom prevention programs have been shown to increase children's awareness of self-protection and assertiveness.

Investigation of suspected child abuse
(a) Full history and examination.
(b) Consider:

— haematology: FBC, platelets, film; clotting profile
— biochemistry: serum calcium, phosphate, alkaline phosphatase; copper, caeruloplasmin if fractures in infant

— radiology: skeletal survey
— Sexual abuse
- if within 72 h: forensic kit, spermatozoa (neg. after 24–48 hours), blood group, acid phosphatase, saliva (secretor status)
- throat and rectal swabs for gonococcus
- MSU
- vulval swabs: C&S, gonococcus, chlamydia, viruses
- syphilis, HIV serology
- pregnancy test

(c) Discuss with health visitor, GP, SMO, other involved professionals.
(d) Check previous attendances A&E/known to social services/on Child Protection Register?
(e) Social work investigation.
(f) Police investigation.
(g) Psychiatric opinion about parents is sometimes valuable.
(h) Share information at case conference.

Role of the GP

- Any doctor involved in suspected child abuse has a responsibility to care for the acute needs of the child and to share his concern with other professionals to formulate a plan to safeguard the child. (This does *not* always necessitate the removal of the child from his family, though this step may need to be considered if return home may expose the child to further danger).
- In most cases of suspected abuse the child is referred to hospital for the opinion of a doctor skilled in child abuse work and for investigation of alternative diagnoses or treatment if required. It is advisable to telephone ahead so as to ensure that the child is seen by an experienced doctor in a suitable environment, and to facilitate exchange of information.
- The GP must keep detailed written records, be prepared to submit a formal medical report and attend case conferences or care proceedings if requested.
- The GP will often have a unique knowledge of the family background and dynamics and can play a valuable role in developing a therapeutic relationship between the family and other professionals at a time when the family may feel very threatened.
- The family doctor should also be involved in monitoring the progress of children who remain at home and in supporting the family through a stressful period.
- To ensure that management follows recommended procedures, all doctors, including family doctors, should be familiar with their local Area Child Protection Committee policy and with the District Health Authority handbook.

Following the Butler-Sloss report of the inquiry into child abuse in Cleveland 1987, the DHSS responded with several publications, including *Child Abuse — Working Together* and *Child Sexual Abuse: Guidance for Doctors*, which lay down principles of management and clear guidelines for their implementation.

Case conference   Part of child abuse procedure since 1974.

Composition
— chairman: senior officer from Social Services
— social worker and team leader
— health visitor, school nurse, nurse manager
— GP
— paediatrician
— child psychiatrist if involved
— police child protection team
— solicitor from local authority
— NSPCC, education welfare officer, nursery or school teacher, as appropriate

The Butler-Sloss report recommends that parents should be invited to attend all or part of the conference unless the Chairman feels that their presence will preclude proper consideration of the child's interests.

Purposes
(a) To share all relevant information and review evidence of abuse, causative factors and likelihood of recurrence.
(b) To consider safety of child(ren) in family and to decide whether legal action is needed to protect the child(ren).
(c) To decide whether the child's name should be placed on the Child Protection Register.
(d) To formulate a plan for future work with the child and family, including assessment of needs of family and help available locally, nomination of a key worker and recommendations for follow-up and case review.

Apart from the decision about registration, the case conference acts in an advisory capacity only; decisions are the responsibility of directors of social services who will take the recommendations of the case conference into account.

Child Care Legislation   Subject of much recent revision. Legal procedures to protect children previously included the Children and Young Person's Act (1969) and the Child Care Act (1980); legislation reformed by the new Children Act (1989), implemented in 1991.

1. Based on the principle that the welfare of the child is always the paramount consideration.

2. Range of new Court Orders emphasizing parental responsibility rather than parental rights. Encourages parent participation in decision making with statutory authorities.

(a) Replaces the Place-of-Safety Order (28 days) with the *Emergency Protection Order* (EPO) lasting 8 days, renewable for 7 days. Parental responsibility transferred to applicant for order; parents can challenge in court after 72 h.

(b) *Child Assessment Order*; to facilitate investigation if there is a lack of cooperation and need for more evidence, e.g. medical examination. Parental responsibility retained. Maximum duration 7 days.

(c) *Police Protection Provision*: police have power to remove a child, without a warrant, into police protection for a maximum of 72 h during which an EPO may be sought.

(d) Changes in *Care Proceedings*:

— *Care Order*: simplified grounds. Court must be satisfied that the child has suffered, *or is likely to suffer*, significant harm attributable either to standard of care given to the child (being below that which it is reasonable to expect) or that the child is beyond parental control
  • *Interim Care Orders*: duration limited to 8 weeks, with renewals to maximum of 4 weeks
  • *Full Care Order*
— *Supervision Orders* : place child under supervision of local authority. Time limit 3 years

(e) Power of assumption of parental rights removed. Under the Child Care Act the local authority had the power in certain circumstances to take over the parental rights of a child already in voluntary care without resource to court.

(f) New rules about appointment and role of Guardian *ad litem*, appointed by Court to act independently on behalf of child.

(g) Changes in Wardship. High Courts no longer able to make care or supervision order in wardship proceedings, which will be used less often and more selectively.

The majority of children on whom child protection procedures are invoked do not become the subject of legal proceedings and are not removed from home. In many cases where children are removed, the long-term aim is to re-unite them with their parents.

It is therefore important to work with parents so that they or their representatives are involved participants during investigation and subsequent plans for the care and protection of their children.

— keep parents informed and involve them in decision-making
— encourage them to draw on their extended family support

— ensure they are aware of other available sources of
  support:
  • individual psychotherapy, family therapy
  • family centres (local authority or voluntary)
  • Family Rights Group, established 1974 and DHS-
    funded
  • 'Parentline — OPUS' (Organizations for Parents Under
    Stress) self-help groups for parents, telephone help-
    line, etc.

9. Children and the law

Employment
(a) It is an offence to employ a pupil without notifying the Education Welfare Service.
(b) No child is allowed to work under the age of 13 years. After then they may work part time and *out* of school hours.
(c) A work permit will be issued by the Education Welfare Service on application from an employer if the conditions are correct.
(d) Parental consent is necessary together with confirmation from GP that work will not have any deleterious effect on the child or his education. (Head teacher is informed when work permit is issued.)
(e) Some types of work are never approved, e.g. factories with machinery, betting shops, cooking food.
(f) Baby sitting is not included in work regulations.
(g) Acting and entertainment come under different regulations.
(h) On Sundays and in mornings before school only newspaper or milk delivery is permitted. After school 2 h daily maximum; Saturdays 4 h maximum (<15 years), 8 h (>15 years).

Road Traffic Act
The use of seat belts and other restraints dramatically reduces the risk of death and injury to children in cars.
(a) It is the driver's responsibility to ensure that children under 14 years wear the restraints that are available and appropriate for age and weight. Infants must be strapped into a safety rear-facing car seat. Booster seats and seat belts for older children.
(b) Children of any age may ride in the front seat of the car but must wear a seat belt or suitable restraint at all times.

Adoption

Definition
A permanent and irreversible transfer of legal rights of natural parents to adopters. The child assumes the adopters' surname and full inheritance rights.
(a) Applicants to adopt must be over 21 years old.
(b) All adoptions must be through agencies recognized by the British Agencies for Adoption and Fostering (BAAF).
(c) Applications for adoption are made through the court. The consent of the natural parent (only the mother if

the child is illegitimate) is essential (unless there is a history of neglect or child abuse).

(d) Recognized agencies all have an adoption panel, including:

— social worker
— medical advisers
— manager
— at least two independent advisers (often an adoptive parent or legal adviser)

Role of the medical adviser   The medical adviser carries out a full medical examination of the child, the aim of which is to ascertain whether the child has any short- or long-term medical problems or special needs. Information is obtained regarding antenatal, intrapartum and neonatal difficulties and a full physical and developmental assessment is made.

Newborn babies who are to be adopted are usually examined at birth, 6 weeks and again at about 3 months (or within 1 month of final adoption order).

Fostering   Children generally do better in good foster care than in children's homes. 18% of all children in care are with a parent, guardian or nominated family friend.

1. *Short-term*:

— babies awaiting adoption
— young children whose parents cannot look after them temporarily due to illness
— whilst child abuse proceedings take place

2. *Long-term*:

— foster parents paid allowance of up to £250 a week
— children have 6-monthly medical examination

Disadvantages   (a) Disorganized medical care: increased risk of missing immunizations and routine developmental examinations.
(b) Interrupted schooling with risk of subsequent learning difficulties or behavioural problems.
(c) Psychological/psychiatric disorders due to insecurity.

GP has a very important role in coordinating services and ensuring continuing medical care.

Child care   Local authorities must:

— identify children in need
— provide appropriate services to meet these needs
— promote care by the family
— publish information about services
— keep register of disabled children
— make assessment of need with regard to education

Child protection   See Chapter 8.

10. Infectious diseases

Infections are the commonest reason for children attending their GP (on average 4 times per year), with respiratory viruses being the most frequent infective agents.

Notifiable infections

Anthrax
Acute encephalitis
AIDS
Cholera
Diphtheria
Dysentery
Erysipelas*
Food poisoning
Hepatitis B
Legionella*
Leprosy
Leptospirosis
Malaria
Measles
Meningitis
Meningococcal infection
Ophthalmia neonatorum
(gonococcal and chlamydia)

Mumps
Paratyphoid fever
Pertussis
Plague
Poliomyelitis
Rabies
Relapsing fever
Rubella
Scarlet fever
Tetanus
Tuberculosis
Typhoid
Typhus
Varicella
Yellow fever

*Scotland only

Incubation and school exclusion periods

Infection	Mode of transmission	Incubation (days–range)	School exclusion period
Measles	Resp. droplet	7–14	4 days from onset of rash
Rubella	Resp. droplet	14–21	4 days from onset of rash
Chickenpox	Direct contact, droplet or airborne	10–24	6 days from onset of rash provided all lesions crusted
Mumps	Droplet or saliva	12–31	7 days after swelling subsides
Scarlet fever	Droplet	2–5	2 days after treatment with penicillin started
Roseola	Unknown	9–15	Until rash gone (about 2 days)
Glandular fever	Saliva	30–50	Not required
Hepatitis A	Faecal–oral	15–50	At least 7 days from onset of jaundice

Measles Acute viral infection with highest incidence in the pre-school child. Caused by RNA virus of the paramyxovirus family.

Prodromal catarrhal phase for 3–4 days before rash, with fever, runny nose, dry cough and conjuntivitis. Koplik's spots visible 2–3 days before eruption of rash (tiny white lesions on buccal mucosa). Typical maculopapular rash, 3 or 4 days after first symptoms, starts behind the ears and spreads to face, then body, becoming confluent over upper trunk.

Complications Important cause of morbidity and mortality in immuno-suppressed patients and in malnourished children in developing countries.

— otitis media
— respiratory (4%): croup, bronchopneumonia, giant cell pneumonia
— convulsions
— encephalitis: 7–14 days after onset in up to 1 in 1000 cases. High morbidity and mortality (15%)
— Guillain-Barré syndrome (see p. 262)
— Subacute sclerosing panencephalitis (SSPE). Thought to be a late reactivation of the measles virus 5–10 years after initial infection, affecting about 1 in 100 000 cases. M:F ratio is 4:1. Presents with deteriorating school performance, memory loss, behavioural problems, then progresses to choreoathetosis, myoclonus, and dementia. Fatal in 50% of cases

Prevention See p. 71.

Rubella (German measles) Mild infectious viral disease affecting mainly 6–12 year olds.
(a) Fine macular rash on face is usually first sign, can coalesce and spreads to trunk. Transient, 1–3 days.
(b) Lymphadenopathy, especially post-auricular and occipital.
(c) Mild fever.

Differential diagnosis — scarlet fever
— adenovirus
— echovirus
— coxsackie virus
— drug allergy

Complications Rare:

— arthritis (usually older children and adults)
— encephalitis and myelitis
— thrombocytopenia

Congentital rubella syndrome See p. 44.

Chickenpox (varicella) Highly infectious disease, commonest in children between 2 and 10 years. Caused by Herpes varicella-zoster primary infection.

May be mild coryzal prodrome. Usually presents with vesicular rash, mainly on trunk. Spreads to all areas, but centripetal. Vesicles become pustular over 3–4 days, then crusted. Itchy; can scar if severe scratching or secondary infection occurs. Evolution of rash in series of crops means different stages seen together.

Mucous membranes often affected; very irritating, can cause anorexia.

Complications — secondary infection of lesions; may lead to pneumonia, osteomyelitis and septic arthritis
— haemorrhagic chickenpox
— Encephalitis (1 in 1000), often mild cerebellitis with ataxia. Generally good prognosis
— pneumonitis
— shingles (zoster). Due to reactivation of latent infection in sensory nerve root ganglia
— Reye's syndrome has been reported after chickenpox. Possible link with ingestion of aspirin which should now be avoided in febrile children

Treatment (a) Symptomatic, with calamine lotion or oral histamine for itching.
(b) Acyclovir is effective against varicella-zoster infections and is indicated for immunocompromized children and for serious complications.

Mumps Acute infection with *Myxovirus parotidis*. Highest incidence is in school-age children. Low infectivity so significant proportion of population is not immune.

Characteristic painful parotid swelling (unilateral in 25% of cases), with fever. Submandibular and sublingual salivary glands are occasionally involved. Sub-clinical infection occurs in about one-third of cases.

Complications — aseptic meningitis: may precede or develop 3–7 days after parotitis
— post-infectious encephalitis or myelitis
— sensorineural deafness (may be bilateral and permanent)
— orchitis: rare before puberty. Impairs fertility in 13%
— pancreatitis
— facial palsy, usually transient

Treatment Symptomatic. (Passive immunization with mumps gamma-globulin is not effective in preventing mumps or its complications.)

Scarlet fever Caused by erythrogenic-toxin producing strains of Group A beta haemolytic streptococci.

Presents with tonsillitis plus high fever, headache and malaise. After 1 day, fine macular rash on trunk and limbs.

Facial rash with circumoral pallor. Followed by desquamation, especially of the extremities. Tongue coated white with inflammed papillae (strawberry tongue).

Complications (All preventable by adequate antibiotic therapy.)
   1. *Local*:

— cervical adenitis
— otitis media
— retropharyngeal abscess

   2. *Later, toxic*:

— rheumatic fever
— glomerulonephritis
— erythema nodosum

Treatment Penicillin for 10 days (or erythromycin if definite history of allergy).

Erythema infectiosum (Fifth disease) Parvovirus B19 infection: usually affects children under 10 years of age. Incubation period 4–14 days.

Presents with general malaise and characteristic rash on one or both cheeks ('slapped cheek disease') with later spread to limbs. Usually resolves within a week without sequelae. (Patients with hereditary anaemias may develop aplastic crises after B19 human parvovirus infection.)

Roseola infantum (Sixth disease/Exanthem subitum) Common infectious disease of infancy, probably due to human herpes virus 6.

Presents with high fever for 3–4 days which subsides as a fine maculopapular rash appears, first on the trunk then widespread. Resolves in 2–3 days.

Other than febrile convulsions, no associated complications.

Glandular fever (Infectious mononucleosis) Infection caused by Epstein-Barr virus (EBV), which is a herpes virus, and affects young children and adolescents. It has low infectivity and is spread by direct contact with saliva ('kissing disease'). The incubation period is variable, usually <4 weeks.

Clinical course: prodromal phase of general malaise, headache and fever followed by sore throat in over 50%, with grey-white exudate covering tonsils (anginose variety) and petechiae on palate. Generalized lymphadenopathy and splenomegaly is seen in the majority sometimes with jaundice. A rash present in 10%. Seen frequently after inappropriate treatment of this infection with ampicillin.

Diagnosis (a) large atypical mononuclear cells in peripheral blood.
(b) heterophile antibody tests (Paul Bunnel, 'Monospot'): may take several weeks to become positive. Many children do not produce these antibodies at all.
(c) mildly abnormal LFTs in over 50% of cases.
(d) specific EBV IgM antibodies.

Complications — airway obstruction in severe anginose variety
— thrombocytopenic purpura
— splenic rupture
— neurological: aseptic meningitis, transverse myelitis, Guillain-Barré syndrome

Treatment Usually symptomatic only. Corticosteroids for severe airway oedema, hepatitis or neurological complications.

Herpes simplex virus (HSV)

HSV 1 Primary infection in childhood may be asymptomatic, or cause serious infection necessitating hospital admission.
1. *Acute hepatic gingivo-stomatitis.* This is the commonest presentation. There is fever, severe inflammation and ulceration of the mouth and gums, with general systemic upset and lymphadenopathy. The child is often unable to eat or drink. Hospital admission may be necessary to ensure adequate hydration. Usually resolves within 2 weeks. Treatment is supportive, with the addition of acyclovir in severe infections or immunocompromized children.
2. *Keratoconjunctivitis.*
3. *Meningo-encephalitis* with prediliction for temporal lobes; mortality 50%.
4. *Eczema herpeticum* (Kaposi's varicelliform eruption).

HSV 2 Causes genital infection. May be seen in cases of child sexual abuse or as acquired intrapartum infection of the newborn, see p. 45.

Recurrent herpes simplex Provoked by acute illness, emotional stress, over-exposure to sunlight. Clusters of small vesicles usually around nose or mouth (but can be anywhere).
Topical treatment with acyclovir is only effective in the very early stages of cutaneous infection. In recurrent herpetic eye infection 5-iodo-2-deoxy-uridine (IDU) may be helpful

Hand, foot and mouth disease

Caused by Coxsackie virus A 16. Presents with a typical rash on hands, soles of feet and inside mouth. The spots have a target-like appearance, white in the centre with a red halo.
Usually there is no systemic upset, although ulcers in the mouth may cause reluctance to feed.

Adenovirus infections

Usually cause pharyngitis with or without:
— keratoconjunctivitis
— rubelliform rash
— diarrhoea
— flu-like symptoms
— pneumonia
— encephalitis

Hepatitis   Causes of viral hepatitis:

— hepatitis viruses A, B and C
— Epstein-Barr virus
— cytomegalovirus

Hepatitis A (infectious hepatitis)   Hepatitis A virus (HAV) infection is commonly found in areas with poor living conditions, overcrowding and poor sanitation. In these areas most children are HAV antibody +ve by late childhood.

Presents with acute onset of fever, anorexia, nausea, vomiting, general malaise and mild hepatosplenomegaly. Young children often have mild infection and may be anicteric. Jaundice, when present, usually clears in about 2 weeks. Very rarely complicated by acute hepatic failure or progression to chronic hepatitis.

Diagnosis   (a) Virus isolation.
(b) Serology: specific anti-HAV IgM indicates recent infection.
(c) LFTs.

Treatment   (a) Rest.
(b) Decrease dietary fat if very nauseated.
(c) Hospital admission rarely necessary.

Prevention   (a) Passive immunization of contacts with human normal immunoglobulin (HNIG).
(b) Water sterilization.
(c) Careful washing of hands, foods, etc.

Hepatitis B   Hepatitis B virus is usually transmitted directly by infected carrier mothers (see p. 45), or transfusion of blood products. The incubation period is 50–180 days and the child should be kept off school only while unwell (carrier status should be notified).

Presents with similar symptoms to hepatitis A with anicteric infection common, but illness tends to be more severe and prolonged. About 10% develop chronic liver diseases, such as chronic active hepatitis or primary liver carcinoma.

Treatment   As for hepatitis A.

Prevention   (a) Vaccination, see p. 72.
(b) Screening blood donors for HBs antigenaemia (positive in ~1 in 500).

Polio   Highly infectious enteroviral illness now rare in the UK but endemic in many developing countries.

There are three strains: types 1, 2 and 3. Type 1 has caused the most severe epidemics.

Spread by oral-faecal route with an incubation period of 1–3 weeks. Virus multiplies in tonsils and intestinal wall, spreads to regional lymph nodes and thence into the blood-stream. May attack anterior horn cells of the spinal cord or cause a more extensive invasion of CNS with encephalitis involving motor cells in the brainstem and cerebral cortex.

Presentation Ranges from subclinical to paralytic form.

Initially minor illness with fever, sore throat and 'flu-like' symptoms. Resolves in a few days. May then recover completely or develop major illness due to viraemia and invasion of the CNS manifested by headache, vomiting, neck stiffness, bulging fontanelle. Some cases then recover, but others develop paralysis. This is usually patchy and asymmetrical with legs more often affected than arms. Respiratory muscles may be involved leading to respiratory failure. Bulbar palsy presents with dysphagia, cranial nerve palsies and cardio-respiratory distress, which may lead to fatal circulatory collapse.

Complications of paralytic poliomyelitis include permanent paralysis with severe muscle atrophy.

Diagnosis (a) Virus isolation from throat swab or faeces.
(b) Serology

Treatment Supportive: bed rest in acute phase, ventilation, NG feeding, etc.

Prevention Immunization, see p. 70.

HIV infection Increasing numbers of children worldwide are infected with human immunodeficiency virus type 1 (HIV-1). It is therefore important for family doctors to develop a high degree of awareness of the spectra of medical and social problems associated with HIV and of the need for coordinated family-oriented services to care for patients with this infection.

Epidemiology WHO statistics in June 1989 recorded nearly 160 000 cases of AIDS. Almost 2000 cases are reported in children <13 years. These figures are certainly a gross underestimate due to inadequate diagnosis and underreporting. WHO forecasts 5–6 million cases by the year 2000.

70–80% of new cases in children are due to perinatal infection so the number of infected children is expected to rise in line with the increasing numbers of women of childbearing age with AIDS.

The vertical transmission rate in Europe is estimated at 13–25% (whereas it seems to be much higher in Africa). Clinical symptoms in pregnancy are thought to increase the risk of disease in children.

Up to 1991, about 200 children born to HIV-positive mothers have been reported to the Centre for Disease Surveillance and Control (CDSC), London, of whom 36 have developed AIDS or died. 178 children with haemophilia in the UK have been infected; there have been no new cases since the introduction of heat-treated factor VIII in 1985.

Immunopathogenesis The virus attaches itself to a receptor molecule, CD4, found mainly on T4 lymphocytes but also on monocytes, macrophages and dendritic cells. (During normal immune response, the CD4 molecule is the receptor for major histocompatibility complex molecules.) Having entered the cell, the virus destroys it by interfering with its DNA synthesis. Infection also causes functional impairment of B cells, causing global immunosuppression and increasing susceptibility to fatal infections and neoplasms.

Diagnosis All children born to HIV positive mothers are HIV positive due to high levels of passively transferred maternal antibody, which may persist for up to 18 months (median 10 months). In the UK, only about 15–30% of these children are actually infected. Present criteria for diagnosis of infection include:

— persistence of HIV antibody after 18 months of age
— clinical and/or immunological manifestations (e.g. hyper-gammaglobulinaemia, low T4:T8 ratio) of HIV infection
— culture of virus from blood (can predict 45% of children with HIV infection at birth if specialized techniques are used)

Alternative methods being developed to detect infection earlier include:

— detection in serum of the P-24 antigen fragment of the virus. Indicates poor prognosis
— polymerase chain reaction (PCR) for detection of proviral gene sequences in infected lymphocytes
— Western blot antibody patterns, e.g. anti-HIV IgA

Clinical manifestations   1. *Non-specific* — weight loss or failure to thrive
— recurrent unexplained fever
— persistent or recurrent diarrhoea
— generalized lymphadenopathy
— splenomegaly, hepatomegaly
— parotitis
— oropharyngeal candidiasis
— repeated common infections

2. *Respiratory*:
(a) *Lymphoid intersititial pneumonitis (LIP)*. Chronic lung disease, often asymptomatic in children in early stages but chest X-ray shows bilateral fluffy nodular infiltrates and hilar lymphadenopathy. In later stages, progressive tachypnoea, hypoxia and clubbing develop. Occurs in 20-40% of vertically-infected children. Treat with oxygen; antiretroviral drugs, e.g. azidothymidine, cause symptomatic improvement and the role of steroids is also under study.

(b) *Pneumocystis carinii pneumonitis (PCP)*. Often the first clinical sign; most commonly diagnosed between 3 and 6 months of age. Much more acute onset than LIP. Carries poor prognosis with mortality rate of about 60%.

Treatment with cotrimoxazole or pentamidine (i.v. or nebulized) and oxygen. Some centres also treat with steroids for the first few days.

Indications for PCP prophylaxis (Atlanta Center For Disease Control 1991):

— CD4 cell count below lower limit for age
— CD4 cell count <20% total lymphocytes regardless of absolute count
— any child who has had an episode of PCP

3. *Neurological*:
HIV encephalopathy due to HIV infection of brain. Progressive with poor prognosis. Features include acquired microcephaly, loss of developmental milestones and progressive motor deficits. CT scan shows cerebral atrophy and calcification in basal ganglia and periventricular white matter. P-24 antigen or virus may be isolated from CSF.

4. *Gastrointestinal*:

— candidiasis
— diarrhoea
— malabsorption, may be non-specific villous atrophy

5. *Severe recurrent bacterial infections*:

— septicaemia
— meningitis
— septic arthritis, osteomyelitis, cellulitis, abcesses

6. *Opportunistic infections*. PCP, candidiasis and CMV are the commonest in children. Others, e.g. toxoplasmosis, histoplasmosis, cryptococcosis and TB, occur but less commonly in children than in adults with HIV infection.

7. *Rare manifestations in children*:

— Burkitt lymphoma
— Kaposi sarcoma
— cardiomyopathy, arteriopathy
— chronic hepatitis
— nephropathy
— 'fetal AIDS' syndrome reported in the USA, but it is as yet uncertain whether dysmorphic features are associated with HIV infection

Management (a) Immunize as per schedule, except with BCG, which is not recommended in the UK.

— (in countries with high prevalence of TB, BCG should be given to newborn but not to older children with HIV infection)

— immune globulin should be given if infected children are exposed to measles or chickenpox
— inactivated polio vaccine should be used
— in infected children, Pneumovax should be considered

(b) Monitor growth and development.
(c) Nutritional support.
(d) Treat bacterial and opportunistic infections promptly.
(e) Intravenous gammaglobulin is given every 3 weeks prophylactically in some centres for children with recurrent infections.
(f) Antiretroviral drugs. Azidothymidine (AZT), a reverse transcriptase inhibitor, slows progression of the disease and lengthens survival in adults. Early studies of AZT and newer analogues such as dideoxyinosine (ddI) in children are promosing, suggesting an increase in growth and well-being and an improvement in HIV encephalopathy. Several trials are in progress to determine when and in what dosage these drugs may be indicated in children.
(g) Psychosocial support. Parents and siblings of an infected child may themselves be fatally ill and comprehensive medical care must be combined with effective social, psychological and developmental services for all family members. Specialized counselling and support groups can help families to deal with the denial, guilt, anger and repeated losses caused by AIDS. Education is needed to prevent isolation and stigmatization occurring through fear of contamination. Depressive symptomatology is not uncommon and may respond well to anti-depressants, but close monitoring of use of any psycho-therapeutic drugs is essential.

WHO estimates during the 1990s more than 10 million children uninfected with HIV will be orphaned by AIDS; urgent international efforts are needed to care for these children, particularly in sub-Saharan African countries where health services are already severely overstretched.

Confidentiality and HIV testing

The BMA has stated that children can be tested without parental consent if it is essential to the child's care, but parental consent should be obtained wherever possible.

The GP should always be informed because of the importance of early treatment of infections. Notification of others depends on circumstances; the Department of Education and Science has stated that there is no need for school staff to be informed of the HIV status of infected children who are clinically well; where the child is symptomatic, specific educational needs are assessed in the usual way and infection control guidelines are provided by Departmental booklets and the school health team.

Antenatal testing   The Royal College of Obstetricians and Gynaecologists recommends that the antibody status of pregnant women with risk factors should be determined if informed consent is given. Women found to be seropositive should be counselled and given the option of termination of pregnancy.

Transmission of HIV in breast milk   There is some evidence that HIV can be transmitted via breast milk, but the risk is thought to be very small. WHO recommends that in countries where safe alternatives to breast feeding are available (such as in the UK), breast feeding is not recommended for infants of HIV-positive mothers, but in developing countries where safe alternatives are not available, all mothers should be encouraged to breast feed, since the risks of malnutrition, diarrhoea and death in bottle-fed babies far outweigh any risk of breast-milk transmission of HIV.

Kawasaki syndrome   An acute febrile mucocutaneous syndrome with lymphoid involvement and desquamation, first described in Japan in 1967 and since recognized worldwide.

Incidence   0.6 in 100 000 children. 80% of cases are under 5 years old.

Cause   Obscure. Tendency to clustering of cases and several outbreaks of epidemic proportions suggest an infectious agent and many have been postulated, e.g. dust mites, rickettsiae and retroviruses, which may trigger an abnormal immunological reaction.

Clinical features   — fever for at least 5 days, up to several weeks
— generalized urticarial or morbilliform rash
— conjunctivitis
— cervical adenitis
— prominent tongue papillae, pharyngitis, fissuring of lips
— swollen hands and feet, red palms and soles, progressing to periungual desquamation after 2–3 weeks
— thrombocytosis with increased platelet aggregation due to increased synthesis of thromboxane A_2
— cardiac involvement in at least 30%:
  • heart block, arrhythmias, pericardial effusion
  • coronary artery aneurysms
  • risk of sudden death due to myocarditis or coronary thrombosis in early stages, or coronary artery aneurysms and stenosis leading to ischaemic heart disease later. Occurs in about 10% of patients with aneurysms (1–2% of all patients with the disease)
— arthralgia and arthritis
— aseptic meningitis
— urethritis
— hepatitis
— hydrops of gall bladder

Diagnosis   Clinical, requiring prolonged fever and four of the first five features listed above.

Investigations   Non-specific:

— ESR raised
— leucocytosis, mild normochromic, normocytic anaemia and thrombocytosis
— CRP elevated
— serum α_2 globulins elevated
— serum bilirubin and transaminases may be abnormal
— mild CSF lymphocytosis
— ECG: prolonged PR and QT_c intervals; flattening T waves and depression of ST segment
— serial cross-sectional echocardiography from 2–3 weeks
— if symptoms or ECG evidence of ischaemia, selective coronary angiography or thallium myocardial imaging

Treatment   (a) Antiplatelet therapy: aspirin, dipyridamole
(b) Intravenous immunoglobulin (IVIG) reduces the frequency of development of coronary artery abnormalities.

Tuberculosis   Infection with *Mycobacterium tuberculosis* is usually acquired from infected close family contacts. Primary infection is usually by inhalation through the lung with enlarged hilar nodes, and less commonly by ingestion or skin trauma.

Probability of infection varies with dose, virulence and host resistance. The younger, poorly nourished child is more likely to become infected. Overcrowding and deprivation predispose to spread of the disease.

Presentation   — cough
— failure to thrive
— fever
— weight loss
— general debility with or without respiratory symptoms
— lymphadenopathy
— hepatosplenomegaly

Many have no symptoms and are detected as a result of screening contacts. There may be a mild, non-specific illness at the time of tuberculin conversion. Hypersensitivity phenomena, e.g. erythema nodosum, phlyctenular conjunctivitis may be seen at this stage. Rarely, disseminated disease is the first presentation. Complications may develop, usually 6 months to 2 years after primary infection, e.g.:

— progressive pulmonary disease
— infection of bones, joints, kidneys, CNS
— miliary disease

Diagnosis   (a) chest X-ray showing primary complex plus enlarged regional hilar lymph nodes

      (b) acid-alcohol fast bacillus (AAFB) present in sputum, nasopharyngeal aspirates or gastric washings

      (c) Mantoux test: single intradermal injection of 0.1 ml of purified protein derivative (PPD) of tuberculin:

      0.1 ml 1:10 000 (if suspected)

      0.1 ml 1:1000 (for routine use to exclude diagnosis)

      results read at 72 h

      positive result = induration of 6 mm or more

Treatment Antituberculous drugs in double or triple combinations, e.g. Isonazid and rifampicin for 6 months + pyrazinamide with or without streptomycin for first 2 months. (Ethambutol is not used in children under 6 years because of difficulty in monitoring for its major toxic effect, optic neuritis.) Complicated cases require longer courses.

Prevention (a) neonatal BCG vaccination of at risk infants: except in babies of HIV +ve mothers (UK only).

      (b) Heaf testing of all school children at 13 years followed by vaccination if Heaf test negative.

      (c) BCG vaccination of at risk adults.

Imported infections Protozoa — malaria
           — amoebiasis
           — giardiasis
           — leishmaniasis

Malaria Infection is caused by:

— Plasmodium falciparum
— Plasmodium vivax
— Plasmodium malariae
— Plasmodium ovale

Transmitted man to man via bite of Anopheles mosquito. The incubation period is 1–40 weeks (varies with species).

    Classical malaria is uncommon in children, and very rare in infants <6 months due to maternal antibody (if in endemic areas). In endemic areas children usually develop natural immunity by 5 years of age with little in the way of clinical symptoms. In the UK, international travelling is causing increasing numbers of imported cases from the Indian subcontinent (Pl. vivax) and Africa (Pl. falciparum).

Presentation 1. *Symptoms*: Fever, general malaise, drowsiness, vomiting, diarrhoea. May also have cough, abdominal pain and headache.

    2. *Clinical signs*:

— fever/rigors
— anaemia
— tender hepatosplenomegaly
— metabolic acidosis

— dehydration
— albuminuria

Complications Cerebral malaria: due to Pl. falciparum malaria and is frequently fatal. Presents with pyrexia, convulsions and altered level of conciousness with few focal signs. Retinal haemorrhage often seen. CSF normal in most cases.

Diagnosis A thick Field's stained blood film will demonstrate the parasite under the microscope. The film is best taken when the patient is febrile.

Treatment Treatment should be started if the diagnosis is suspected (with or without a confirmatory blood film). The choice of drug (e.g. chloroquine, quinine) depends on the patterns of resistance in the area where infection was acquired, so specialist advice is essential.

Prophylaxis (a) Prevention is best 'treatment' if travelling to endemic areas
(b) antimalarials should be started a week before travel, continued throughout the stay and continued 4 weeks after returning home
(c) avoid mosquito bites by:

— applying insect repellants to skin
— minimizing areas of exposed skin after sunset
— staying indoors at dusk, especially if near water
— insect screens on windows and doors should be closed at all times

Amoebiasis Infection with the protozoon Entamoeba histolytica. Transmitted through food and water. Cysts remain viable in chlorinated water but are destroyed by boiling, drying or antiseptic. After ingestion trophozooites migrate to large intestine, producing mucosal ulcers. Haematogenous spread leads to abscess formation in liver, lungs, spleen, kidneys and brain.

Presentation Depends on general health and nutritional status of host. Mild cases have only vague symptoms and irregular bowel habit, with relapsing diarrhoea. Severe cases present with dysentery, which may be complicated by perforation and peritonitis. Hepatic abscess formation occurs even in mild infection.

Diagnosis (a) Examination of fresh stool.
(b) Direct sigmoidoscopy — ulcerated mucosa.

Treatment Metronidazole.

Giardiasis Caused by the flagellate protozoon, Giardia lamblia. Transmission via food and water containing cysts which can remain viable for months outside host.

Presentation — *acute* with anorexia, vomiting and diarrhoea

— *chronic* with prolonged diarrhoea and malabsorption causing failure to thrive

Diagnosis (a) Fresh stool microscopy for cysts — several specimens may be needed as excretion is intermittent

(b) Examination of duodenal juice aspirates for trophozoites

Treatment Metronidazole.

Leishmaniasis Protozoon infection, conveyed to man by sandflies. Three species:

— Leishmania donovani (visceral leishmaniasis, Kala-Azar)
— Leishmania tropica (cutaneous leishmaniasis)
— Leishmania braziliensis (muco-cutaneous leishmaniasis).

Presentations 1. *Kala-azar*. Commonest in infants and young children. Incubation period 2–6 months. Acute illness with recurrent fevers, weight loss, hepatosplenomegaly, lymphoedema, pancytopaenia and diarrhoea. Secondary infection is common.

2. *Cutaneous leishmaniasis*. Single or multiple nodules which ulcerate and leave depressed scar. Satellite nodules may develop. No systemic upset.

Diagnosis Microscopy and culture of tissue fluid from ulcer. In visceral form, serology may be helpful; bone marrow aspiration and culture is method of choice.

Treatment (a) Pentamidine.
(b) Allopurinol.
(c) Blood transfusion.
(d) Antibiotics for secondary infection.

Salmonella infections There are more than 1000 salmonella serotypes. Most cause a relatively mild gastroenteritis and rarely invade systemically.

Typhoid fever Systemic infection caused by S. typhi. Spread is by direct contact with infected faeces or urine, usually via contaminated food and water. This is therefore a disease seen predominantly in countries with poor sanitation. In the UK it is an imported disease with most cases acquired on the Indian subcontinent. The incubation period is 7–21 days.

Presentation Usually acute onset:

— diarrhoea and vomiting; liquid stools with mucus and blood
— headache and meningism in some cases
— high fever and abdominal pain
— rose spots crop on trunk and limbs (<20% of cases)
— hepatosplenomegaly usually in second week
— weight loss
— anaemia
— dehydration

Symptoms generally last 3–4 weeks. May resolve spontaneously if untreated. Chronic carriage ensues in about 2% of cases.

Complications — small bowel perforation, GI bleeding
— meningo-encephalitis
— UTI
— arthritis and osteitis

Diagnosis Culture of blood, faeces or urine.

Treatment (a) Chloramphenicol or ampicillin.
(b) Supportive treatment, including intravenous hydration, electrolyte balance and bed rest.

Salmonella food poisoning — commonly acquired from eggs, poultry and salad
— short incubation period 5–24 h
— usually only GI symptoms of diarrhoea, vomiting and abdominal pain, without systemic upset. Dehydration may develop, especially in younger children

Management (a) Supportive only. Antibiotics are not indicated as they do not shorten the illness and may prolong carriage.
(b) Notify environmental health officer.
(c) Child should be excluded from school until there have been three consecutive clear stool cultures.

**Shigella infections
(Bacillary dysentery)** Four clinically important species, listed in order of severity of illness produced:

— Sh. dysenteriae
— Sh. flexneri
— Sh. boydii
— Sh. sonnei

Sh. dysenteriae and Sh. flexneri cause tropical epidemics. Sh. sonnei is dominant in the UK.
   Present with fever, abdominal pain and diarrhoea with mucus and blood.

Treatment (a) Restoration of fluid and electrolyte balance.
(b) Occasional use of antibiotics, e.g. co-trimoxazole, if systemically ill.
(c) Careful hygiene to avoid cross-infection.

Worm infections — roundworm
— tapeworm
— threadworm
— whipworm
— hookworm

Ascariasis Infection with the roundworm, Ascaris lumbricoides, is transmitted hand to mouth by eggs picked up from soil. The eggs hatch in the intestine into larvae which penetrate the intestinal wall into the bloodstream which carries them to the liver, heart and lungs. In the lung they pass up the trachea, are reswallowed and complete their development into adult worms (about 8″ long) in the small intestine. Worms and eggs can survive for up to 2 years. In the UK, most infection is acquired from family pets.

Presentation
— a healthy child on a normal diet may have few symptoms
— commonly the first sign of infection is the passage of a single adult worm in the stool or vomit
— lung infection may present with peristent cough and haemoptysis
— heavy worm loads may cause malabsorption and occasionally intestinal obstruction or intussusception

Diagnosis
(a) Stool microscopy to confirm the presence of eggs.
(b) Eosinophilia on blood film.

Treatment
(a) Piperazine or mebendazole.
(b) Ascariasis is the commonest worm infestation worldwide. Prevention relies primarily on stopping the use of human faeces as fertilizer and preventing contamination of drinking water.
(c) Periodic deworming is useful in areas with high prevalence

Tapeworms
Species of these flat worms which affect man include:
1. Taenia saginata (beef tapeworm).
2. Taenia solium (pork tapeworm).
Occur worldwide, especially Middle East, Africa and India. Ova hatch in small intestine and hook firmly onto wall where they may remain for 25 years or more.

Symptoms
Often none. May be weight loss, abdominal pain with eosinophilia. Occasionally larvae migrate into the blood and lodge in muscle and brain leading to palpable subcutaneous cysts ± epilepsy (cysticercosis).
3. Echinococcus granulosis — Dog tapeworm (Hydatid disease). Ova hatch in small intestine and embryos migrate through intestinal wall into portal circulation and thence to liver, lungs, brain and bone. They develop into hydatid cysts which gradually enlarge, particularly in lungs and liver.

Presentation
Related to site and shape of cyst.

— pulmonary: chronic cough, wheeze, haemoptysis
— liver: abdominal pain, hepatomegaly
— cerebral: signs of raised ICP, epilepsy, etc.

Treatment
Surgical excision of cyst without spillage.

Threadworm (Enterobius vermicularis)
Commonest worm infestation in the Western world. Inhabit caecum and adjacent intestine. Females migrate to anus at night to lay eggs and then die.

Presentation   Perianal or vulvovaginal pruritis usually at night. Often asymptomatic.

Diagnosis   (a) worms may be visible in the stool.
(b) sellotape test. A small strip of sellotape is pressed against the anus in the morning before bathing, then stuck on a glass slide. Examination of the tape under a microscope will usually reveal the ova.

Treatment   Mebendazole. The whole family must be treated. May need multiple courses.

Whipworm (Trichuris trichiura)   Commoner in hot damp climates. Ingested eggs hatch in small intestine and migrate into large bowel.

Presentation   Symptoms related to worm load:
— abdominal pain
— growth retardation
— chronic diarrhoea
— clubbing
— rectal prolapse
— iron deficiency anaemia (due to GI bleeding)

Treatment   Mebendazole, thiabendazole or pyrantel.

Hookworm (Acyclostoma duodenale and Necator americanus)   Occur in tropical areas. One of the commonest causes of anaemia worldwide. Larvae penetrate skin at the site of contact (usually bare feet), causing a papulovesicular rash ('ground itch'). They enter lymphatics, travel to the lungs, migrate up the trachea and are swallowed, then attach to the duodenum.

Presentation   — iron deficiency anaemia
— respiratory symptoms — cough
— anorexia, diarrhoea, marasmus in severe cases

Treatment   Thiabendazole, bephenium or pyrantel.

Schistosomiasis (Bilharziasis)   Affects 200 million people worldwide. Due to parasitic flat worms (trematodes). Three species infect man:

— Shistosoma haematobium (Africa and Middle East)
— Shistosoma japonicum (Far East)
— Shistosoma mansoni (Africa and Americas)

S. japonicum and mansoni affect the large bowel and liver; S. haematobium affects the urinary tract.
Infection is via infected water where the larvae live in the intermediate host, the water snail, which excretes cercariae. These enter through unbroken skin or mucous membranes. They are carried by lymphatics to the liver, then migrate to lay eggs elsewhere. Eggs cause intense inflammatory reaction.
In S. haematobium infection eggs are deposited in the

bladder wall, prostate, urethra, cervix and vagina. In S. mansoni and japonicum infection, eggs are laid in the colon, liver, small intestine, pancreas and spleen.

Diagnosis — detection of ova in urine, faeces or rectal biopsy
— eosinophilia

Complications — renal: pyelonephritis, calculi, bladder calcification and renal failure
— GI: granulomatous tumours and fibrosis
— liver: fibrosis, portal hypertension, ascites, splenomegaly
— respiratory: chronic cough, wheeze, Cor pulmonale

Treatment Niridazole, antimonials, praziquantel.

11. Respiratory problems

Causes of wheeze
— asthma
— acute bronchiolitis
— sensitivity to cow's milk protein, drugs, food additives
— foreign body
— inhalation of smoke, milk
— cystic fibrosis
— uncommon causes:
  • non-specific suppurative bronchitis and bronchiectasis
  • α1-antitrypsin deficiency
  • obstructive lesions of trachea or bronchus:
    tracheomalacia, bronchomalacia
    vascular ring
    tracheal webs, stenosis, tumour
    tuberculous and mediastinal lymphadenopathy
    mediastinal cysts and tumours.

Asthma   Characterized by cough, breathlessness and wheezing due to reversible airway narrowing caused by bronchial smooth muscle spasm, mucosal oedema and increased secretions.

Prevalence   Wide geographical variation in reported prevalence due in part to difference in survey methodology and in definition. Cumulative prevalence in school children in western Europe is 7–10%. Apparently increasing over last 20 years. Possible contributory factors:

— increased awareness
— pollution
— changing infant feeding patterns

Morbidity and mortality   1. *School absence.* Causes one-fifth of all school absences. One-third of asthmatics miss >3 weeks of school/year.

2. *Hospital admissions.* Up to 4% of known asthmatics require admission each year. Since 1980 asthma has been the reason for admission in 20% of 0–4 and 12% of 5–14-year olds.

3. Mortality. Causes ~50 deaths/year. Most are teenagers with chronic severe asthma.

Pathogenesis   In infancy a genetic predisposition is usually expressed when induced by environmental factors, particularly viral respiratory infections. In childhood an atopic tendency (manifested by personal or first-degree family history of asthma, eczema or hayfever) is the commonest associated factor.

Common triggers for asthma attacks include:

— exercise
— climatic change
— passive smoking
— psychosomatic
— gastro-oesophageal reflux

The central feature is bronchial hyperreactivity to such stimuli. Different mechanisms causing bronchial hyperresponsiveness may coexist in individual children.

Bronchial narrowing may result from mucosal oedema, increased mucus secretion and smooth muscle contraction. The bronchial smooth muscle tone is under the influence of parasympathetic cholinergic fibres in the vagus nerve tending to cause bronchoconstriction; this is counteracted by the bronchodilator effects of circulating catecholamines on $\beta2$-adrenergic receptors. In addition there is a third non-adrenergic, non-cholinergic (NANC) inhibitory pathway, stimulation of which produces bronchodilation. The intracellular mediators of the adrenergic and cholinergic pathways are believed to be cyclic 3,5-adenosine monophosphate (cAMP), which is increased after adrenoceptor stimulation and causes bronchodilation, and cyclic guanidine monophosphate (cGMP), a cholinergic mediator causing bronchoconstriction. These cyclic nucleotides act by altering calcium flux across the smooth muscle cell membranes.

As well as these neural influences, there are a range of chemical mediators released from mast cells, neutrophils and other inflammatory cells which play an important role in determining airway diameter in asthmatic children. >90% of children with asthma have evidence of type 1 allergic reactions, i.e. develop IgE antibodies to common environmental allergens, e.g. house dust mite, pollens and mold spores. These IgE antibodies then become attached to mast cells. An environmental allergen will interact with the IgE causing disruption of the mast cells and release of mediators. The principle mediators are histamine and SRS-A; others include leukotrienes, prostaglandins, thromboxanes and eosinophil and neutrophil chemotactic factors. These mediators cause airway narrowing by stimulating mucus secretion and causing mucosal oedema and smooth muscle spasm.

Pathology   Bronchi may be plugged with mucus, inflammatory exudate and shed epithelial cells. The basement membrane is thickened. Bronchial muscle and bronchial mucus glands are hypertrophied. There may be contributory abnormalities in mucociliary clearance.

Natural history   During childhood

— 40% asthmatic children become symptom free

— 34% improve considerably
— 24% remain unchanged
— 1% deteriorate
— 0.5% die

Persistent asthma is more likely if the following factors are present

— onset <2 years
— frequent attacks in the 1st year of life
— strong personal or family history of atopy
— infantile eczema
— severe asthma at onset of puberty

Management
(a) Explain diagnosis to child and family.
(b) Discuss plan of treatment and allay anxiety about effects of medication. Stress that the aim of treatment is for the child to have a normal lifestyle with no exercise limitation.
(c) Ensure parents understand purpose of treatment and have adequate instruction about selected mode of drug delivery. If the regimen includes more than one drug, written guidelines for reference may be helpful.
(d) Give clear advice about when to seek medical help.
(e) Try to identify trigger factors:

— history
— coexistence of other atopic features
— skin prick tests
— serial exclusion diet (under dietician's supervision). Dietary precipitants more common in Asian children, particularly orange squash, milk, cola, ice, nuts, oily food.
— avoidance tactics: house dust mite elimination; consider sending pets on holiday for a few weeks
— treatment of gastro-oesophageal reflux

6. Regular review of:

— response to treatment: daily symptom score record card; home peak flow monitoring
— delivery system still most appropriate for child's age and abilities? Check technique with inhalers, etc.
— growth
— frequency of GP/A&E attendances/admissions
— emotional and educational impact of asthma on child and effects on family life

Most children with asthma can be dealt with in the community with management coordinated by GP and involving health visitor, teacher and school medical officer. Parents may obtain useful information and support from self-help groups, such as the National Asthma Campaign which runs a junior asthma club with activity holidays and provides literature in several languages.

Children with persistent symptoms despite treatment or who have severe acute attacks will need hospital referral.

Management of acute exacerbations

Some acute attacks can be managed at home. Treatment may include:

— bronchodilator given via home/surgery nebulizer or GP's portable nebulizer
— short course oral prednisolone

provided parents understand the signs of possible deterioration and have the means to get the child to hospital quickly if necessary. Give written instructions of danger signs to watch for.

Children should be referred urgently to hospital if

— deteriorating despite 2 doses of bronchodilator 3–4 h apart
— too breathless to talk
— using accessory muscles
— cyanosed

Management in hospital:

(a) Assessment, including:

— BP; paradoxical swings of >25 mmHg difference in systolic pressure between inspiration and expiration suggest severe airway obstruction
— arterial gases in any child who is cyanosed or deteriorating

(b) Oxygen.

(c) Nebulized bronchodilators with O_2.

(d) i.v. hydrocortisone bolus 4 mg/kg stat, then 1 mg/kg/h (or 4 mg/kg 6 hourly) (aiming to produce a plasma cortisol level at least that obtainable by maximal stimulation of adrenal cortex, i.e. in excess of 100 µg/ml). *Note*: i.v. route — response within 6–8 h.

(e) i.v. aminophylline: bolus 6–8 mg/kg over 20 min (providing not on maintenance oral theophylline), then 1 mg/kg/h.

(f) CXR to exclude pneumothorax, pneumonia, etc.

(g) Antibiotics if suspected bacterial infection.

(h) Monitor O_2 saturation, blood gases, PEFR if child able to cooperate.

(i) Transfer to ITU if progressive signs of respiratory failure, including $PaCO_2$ >8.0 kPa

Drugs used in childhood asthma

Drug	Mode of action	Adverse effects	Route of admin.
β2-adrenergic agonists	Intracellular cAMP Relaxation of smooth muscle	Tremor, tachycardia	Oral, inc. SR preparations, inhaled: metered dose aerosol (MDA) ± spacers, e.g. nebuhaler; dry powder, e.g.rotacaps, rotadiscs, nebulized i.v.
Theophyllines	Inhibit phosphodiesterase which catalyses breakdown of cAMP Possible effect on NANC nerves Central resp. stimulant	Nausea, vomiting Abdominal pain Sleep disturbance	Oral, inc. SR preparations i.v.
Anticholinergic (e.g. ipratropium bromide)	Competitive blockade of cholinergic nerves	None	Inhaled: MDA nebulized
Sodium chromoglycate	Inhibits release of mediators from mast cells	None	Inhaled: MDA, spincaps, nebulised
Corticosteroids	Sensitise β2-receptors to sympathomimetics Anti-inflammatory effect Reduced production of mediators from mast cells by inhibition of enzyme phospholipase A2	Growth suppression Adrenal suppression Oral candidiasis	Oral Inhaled i.v.

Modes of delivery appropriate at different ages

Allowance must obviously be made for individual variation in cooperation and coordination!

Age	Formulation	Examples
Infants and toddlers	Oral syrups Capsules containing SR granules which can be opened and sprinkled on food Spacer devices — MDA + plastic coffee cup — MDA + open proximal half of a nebuhaler — MDA + nebuhaler + soft face mask Home nebulizer + soft face mask	Salbutamol, terbutaline, theophylline Theophylline SR capsules
>3 years as above +	Spacer devices + MDA	Nebuhaler, volumatic
>3.5 years as above +	Turbohaler	
>4–5 years as above +	MDA alone Dry powder systems	Spincaps, rotacaps, disc systems
Older children as above +	SR tablets	Salbutamol spandets, terbutaline SR

MDA = Metered dose aerosol; SR = slow release

Seasonal allergic rhinitis (Hayfever)

Prevalence   Like asthma, the prevalence of this allergic respiratory disorder appears to be increasing, affecting about 4–9% of children in the UK. More common in boys and first-born children. Occurs in 75% of children with asthma. Often starts around 4–6 years and may persist through adolescence to adult life.

Pathogenesis   Sufferers are genetically predisposed to atopy, i.e. the ability to produce high concentrations of IgE against common allergens, which may be inherited as an autosomal dominant with variable penetrance, carried on chromosome 11.

Environmental factors contributing to sensitization of atopic children include:

— viral RTI
— parental smoking
— damp housing
— industrial environmental pollution

Clinical features   — intense nasal irritation, congestion and sneezing, mucoid nasal discharge and postnasal drip
— conjunctival injection and lacrimation
— 20% of affected children have hearing loss which may lead to speech delay and learning difficulties
— ±allergic 'shiners':bluish infra-orbital swellings due to venous stasis secondary to mucosal oedema
— chronic cases may develop nasal polyps
— FBC may show eosinophilia

Treatment   (a) Avoidance of allergens where possible, e.g. freshly mown lawns, pollen-laden flower gardens, dusty bedrooms.
(b) Antihistamines. Newer long-acting antihistamines do not easily cross the blood–brain barrier and have less sedative effect, e.g. terfenadine, cetirizine
(c) Anti-inflammatory agents:

— drugs which inhibit mediator release from mast cells, e.g. sodium chromoglycate (Rynacrom nasal spray, Opticrom eye drops) or the newer, more potent Nedocromil sodium
— topical corticosteroid nasal sprays, e.g. beclomethasone diproprionate, fluticasone proprionate

(d) surgical excision of nasal polyps.

Respiratory infections   About 80% of illnesses in first 5 years are infective, of which two-thirds are respiratory.

1. *Upper respiratory tract infections*:

— coryza
— otitis

— tonsillitis
— laryngitis
— epiglottitis

2. *Lower respiratory tract infections*:

— bronchiolitis
— pneumonia

Coryza (common cold) Normal small children have at least 3–6 colds/year.

Symptoms Sneeze, mucoid nasal discharge, occasional fever. Nasal congestion may cause feeding difficulties or even apnoea. Postnasal drip may cause coughing.

Causative viruses Rhinovirus, coronavirus, RSV, influenza, parainfluenza and coxsackie.

Management No specific treatment. Antibiotics are not indicated unless complications develop, e.g. acute otitis media, secondary bacterial pneumonia. (Nose drops rarely help, and may increase nasal congestion and run down to the lower respiratory tract carrying infection.)

Tonsillitis and pharyngitis Common, particularly between 3–8 years.

Symptoms Sore throat, refusing feeds, fever. Occasionally: febrile convulsions, vomiting, halitosis.

Aetiology It is not possible to distinguish clinically between bacterial and viral causes. Purulent exudate may be present in both. Majority viral, e.g. adenovirus, influenza, parainfluenza, echo and coxsackie viruses. Often associated pharyngitis. Infectious mononucleosis (due to Epstein-Barr virus) may cause severe pharyngitis with tonsillar enlargement and exudate. Other features include lymphadenopathy (particularly posterior cervical and epitrochlear) and hepatosplenomegaly.

β-Haemolytic streptococci are the most common bacterial pathogens. Presence of submandibular tenderness and frontal headache and absence of other respiratory symptoms increases the likelihood of streptococcal infection.

Unilateral tonsillar enlargement accompanied by marked tenderness and trismus is suggestive of quinsy (peritonsillar abscess). Usually responds to benzylpenicillin but occasionally requires drainage and should be followed by tonsillectomy.

Other causes 1. *Herpes simplex tonsillopharyngitis* presents with fever and multiple, very painful ulcers on tongue, gums, buccal mucosa and throat. Severe cases may require parenteral fluids, acyclovir and local anaesthetic mouth washes. Acyclovir given early enhances the rate of healing of lesions and reduces virus shedding.

2. *Herpangina* causes less painful large, shallow, red-rimmed ulcers. Usually due to coxsackie A and B or echovirus.

Treatment   Streptococcal tonsillitis should be treated with a 10-day course of penicillin. (Use erythromycin or cotrimoxazole if sensitive to penicillin.)

Complications of bacterial tonsillitis
— abscess (peritonsillar/retropharyngeal)
— acute cervical lymphadenitis
— rheumatic fever
— acute glomerulonephritis

Indications
1. For *tonsillectomy*:
(a) Recurrent tonsillitis (>3–4 attacks/year), causing significant systemic illness, interference with growth and school loss.
(b) Recurrent cervical adenitis or peritonsillar abcess.
2. For *adenoidectomy*:
(a) Persistent nasal obstruction due to large adenoids.
(b) Evidence of Eustachian tube blockage causing recurrent otitis media and intermittent deafness.
3. For *adenotonsillectomy*:
(a) Sleep apnoea syndrome.
(b) Adenotonsillar hypertrophy causing UAWO-mouth breathers with nasal obstruction, snoring and short periods of sleep apnoea. (In severe cases pulmonary hypertension, right ventricular hypertrophy and right heart failure occur.)

Not indicated for:

— large asymptomatic tonsils
— allergic rhinitis
— tonsillitis which is part of a viral URTI

Contraindicated by short palate, cleft palate, bifid uvula (may aggravate nasal speech due to pharyngo-palatal incompetence).

Acute suppurative otitis media   Affects 1 in 4 children during the first 10 years; peak incidence 3–6 years. Commonest causes:

— *Haemophilus influenza*
— *Streptococcus pneumoniae*
— *Staphylococcus aureus*

Sources of infection
— from nasopharynx via Eustachian tube
— infected adenoid obstructing Eustachian tube
— mucopus from sinus
— from external ear through a perforation

(a) Analgesia, antipyretics, e.g. paracetamol.
(b) Amoxycillin or penicillin 7–10 days (though recent studies suggest a 2–3 day high dose course may be as effective). Alternative: cotrimoxazole/erythromycin if penicillin allergy.
(c) Occasionally aural toilet if persistent discharge of pus from ear canal, followed by antiseptic dressing.

    (d) Myringotomy if persistent collection of mucopus in middle ear.

    (e) Follow up at 6 weeks after acute episode in young children, including hearing assessment.

Complications

1. *Failure to resolve.* Consider

— wrong antibiotic
— inadequate course
— infected adenoid or sinusitis causing re-infection

2. *Secretory otitis media (glue ear).* Persistent middle ear effusion. May follow acute otitis media or obstruction of Eustachian tube due to enlarged adenoids or sinusitis, preventing air entering Eustachian tube. This causes a partial vacuum and a middle ear effusion. The tympanic membrane appears dull, retracted and is immobile. Bubbles or fluid levels may be visible. There is conductive hearing loss.

Treatment: myringotomy to remove fluid and insertion of grommets. (These usually stay in place for 6 months, but often fall out). Adenoidectomy if obstructing.

3. *Spread of infection* to adjacent structures:

— mastoiditis
— facial N palsy
— meningitis
— intracerebral abscess
— lateral sinus thrombosis

Causes of stridor

1. *Acute*

Common	Rare
Acute LTB	Foreign body
Acute epiglottitis	Retropharyngeal abscess
	Post-intubation
	Angioneurotic oedema
	Smoke, corrosives
	Diphtheria
	Tetany

2. *Recurrent*

Common	Rare
Laryngomalacia	Gross adenoid and tonsillar hypertrophy
Subglottic stenosis	Micrognathia, macroglossia
	Tracheomalacia
	Foreign body
	Vascular ring
	Cystic hygroma
	Vocal cord cyst or paralysis
	Laryngeal cyst, web, cleft or papilloma

Laryngotracheobronchitis
(LTB) (croup)

Incidence peaks at 6 months to 4 years. Majority of cases are viral in origin. Acute inflammatory changes include mucosal oedema and tenacious mucopurulent secretions, which in severe cases may form a coating membrane.
Causative viruses include:

— parainfluenza types 1, 2 and 3 in up to 50%
— RSV
— influenza A and B
— rhinovirus
— adenovirus
— echovirus
— coxsackie
— measles

Primary bacterial infection causing LTB is very rare; secondary bacterial infections occur occasionally, usually with *Staph. aureus* or *Haemophilus*, which is associated mainly with supraglottic infections and epiglottitis.

Symptoms

— coryzal for 1–2 days
— sudden onset of harsh barking cough, often at night
— hoarseness
— inspiratory stridor
— fever rarely >39°C

Differential diagnosis

From other causes of stridor, particularly:

— epiglottitis, which has a different onset with fever and lethargy, child looks iller, pale, toxic, sitting forward, drooling
— diphtheria: check if immunized
— foreign body
— acute anaphylaxis

Management

(a) Minimal disturbance. Examination of the pharynx can precipitate acute obstruction and should *not* be attempted.
(b) Humidification of the atmosphere is of unproven value but is widely practised.
(c) Oxygen. O_2 saturation can be monitored using an oximeter finger or ear clip without disturbance to the child and used as a guide to oxygen requirement. It may be necessary to overcome the airway obstruction by intubation or tracheostomy if there is increasing respiratory distress.

Both O_2 and humidity were traditionally provided in an O_2 tent with humidifier. These had disadvantages in isolating the child from parents, thereby increasing distress, and in obscuring the child from observation. In most cases an ultrasonic nebulizer with directable spray of mist together with O_2 by face mask or tubing held near to the child by the parent will be well tolerated.
(d) Nebulized adrenaline is useful in providing temporary relief of acute laryngeal obstruction but should be used only under close observation.

(e) Antibiotics are only indicated if there is evidence of secondary bacterial invasion.

(f) Corticosteroids have not been proven to be of benefit in acute LTB, but are sometimes used to reduce laryngeal oedema.

Epiglottitis   Incidence between 6 months and 6 years, with peak around 2 years. *Haemophilus influenza type B* is the usual pathogen (β-haemolytic streptococci cause a few cases).

Symptoms   Rapid onset of fever, toxicity, sore throat progressing within 3–6 h to respiratory obstruction with inspiratory stridor, drooling and increasing respiratory distress with cyanosis and restlessness. There is marked tachycardia and the child usually prefers to sit up with neck extended. The stridor may be softer and less obvious than in acute LTB.

Diagnosis   Should be made from history and general appearance, and the child taken immediately to hospital.

Management   (a) *Do not*

— attempt to examine the throat
— make the child lie flat on his back
— send the child unaccompanied for X-ray

Lateral X-ray of the neck is not routinely necessary. It may occasionally be helpful but should only be undertaken under close supervision with all intensive care facilities immediately to hand if needed.

(b) Examination of the epiglottis is performed in theatre by a doctor skilled in intubation and capable of performing a tracheostomy if necessary. The risk of acute obstruction and respiratory arrest is very high. The epiglottis is oedematous and cherry red. Maintenance of the airway by intubation is needed in many cases.

(c) *Haemophilus type B* is cultured from the blood as there is almost always accompanying septicaemia.

(d) i.v. antibiotics, e.g. chloramphenicol, ampicillin, cefotaxime.

(e) Supportive therapy includes i.v. fluids and antipyretics.

(f) Role of steroids is debated.

(g) In an acute emergency, the passage of a large bore needle into the trachea below the cricoid cartilage may be lifesaving.

Pertussis   Highly infectious disease seen worldwide. Declining incidence because of active immunization programmes over last 30 years and improved socioeconomic conditions. Incidence fluctuates considerably. There was a major epidemic between 1977 and 1979 with up to 66 000 cases/year. Further epidemics occurred in 1982 and 1986; there seems to be a 4-yearly cycle.

Commonest in pre-school children. Three causative organisms:

— *Bordetella pertussis* } no cross immunity
— *Bordetella parapertussis* } so second
— *Bordetella bronchiseptica* } attacks can occur

Incubation period 7–14 days.

Clinical course   — catarrhal stage — coryza ~1 week, cough develops in second week
— paroxysmal stage — spasmodic cough ± whoop and vomiting of tenacious mucus. Infants may not whoop but instead have choking or cyanotic apnoeic episodes. Usually lasts 4 weeks or more
— convalescent stage

Complications   — epistaxis, subconjunctival haemorrhage
— secondary bronchopneumonia/lobar or segmental collapse/ bronchiectasis, interstitial emphysema
— haemoptysis
— hypoxic convulsions
— encephalitis (incidence ~1 in 1000 *cf.* <1 in 100 000 post-vaccine, see p. 69)

Diagnosis   — pernasal swab plated on Bordet–Gengou medium
— cough plate
— *Bord. pertussis* antigen by IF on pharyngeal secretions
— supported by peripheral leucocytosis, usually about 40 000/ml, may be up to 200 000/ml

Prevention   See p. 68. Present vaccination uptake only 73% (Government target >90%). A new genetically engineered acellular vaccine is being developed which should be safer.

Treatment   (a) Erythromycin reduces the period of infectivity and may be useful given prophylactically to contacts before the disease has developed, but probably does not otherwise alter the course of the illness.
(b) Treat secondary bacterial complications.
(c) Cough suppressants are not of value.

Acute bronchiolitis   This is the most common serious lower respiratory tract infection of infancy. It is most frequent and severe in babies <6 months. Peak incidence in winter and early spring.

Clinical features   — harsh cough, coryzal symptoms, fever usually <38°C
— tachypnoea, hyperinflation
— wheezy, fine inspiratory crackles
— respiratory failure with hypercapnoea and hypoxaemia; apnoea
— CXR: hyperinflation with peribronchial thickening in ~50%. Areas of consolidation or segmental collapse seen in ~25%

Aetiology   — RSV (>70%)
— adenovirus
— rhinovirus

— parainfluenza 1, 2 and 3
— influenza A

Diagnosis Made on the clinical picture and in many cases can be confirmed within hours by direct detection of virus in nasopharyngeal secretions by immunofluorescence.

Management These infants may become exhausted with the increased work of breathing and should be admitted to hospital for close observation, including heart rate, apnoea and oxygen saturation monitors.

(a) Oxygen, e.g. via headbox attachment to babychair (Derbyshire chair) or nasal prongs.

(b) Nasogastric feeds or i.v. fluids may be necessary for several days.

(c) Intubation and ventilation may be needed either for apnoea or progressive respiratory distress.

(d) Ribavirin is an antiviral agent effective against RSV. It is a virostatic synthetic triazole nucleoside given by aerosol or by nebulization, using a Small Particle Aerosol Generator (SPAG) unit. Studies suggest more rapid resolution of symptoms in treated babies, with improvement in oxygenation in some cases. However, there is no evidence of shortened hospital stay or reduced mortality, which is in any case low (<1%). Ribavirin is expensive — £500 for a 5-day course — and is probably not justified in previously healthy babies. The American Academy of Pediatrics (1986) suggested that it should be considered for the following patients with RSV:

— 'high risk' babies — congenital heart disease, BPD and other chronic lung conditions, certain preterm infants, immune deficiency (specially SCID)
— severely ill infants — with PaO_2 <8.6 kPa or rising $PaCO_2$
— infants <6-weeks old or with underlying anomalies, neurological or metabolic disease

These guidelines are not universally accepted and are subject to revision as the results of further studies become available.

(e) Bronchodilator drugs. Salbutamol and theophylline have no effect on the airways obstruction of bronchiolitis. There is some evidence that nebulized ipratropium bromide may reduce the work of breathing. A high proportion of patients have persistent abnormal airways lability with 75% of babies having episodes of wheeze over the next 2 years, falling to 22% by 10 years. These episodes usually respond well to antiasthma therapy after the 1st year. Such children do not have an increased incidence of atopy and seem to form a different group from classical early childhood asthma.

(f) Antibiotics. If the illness is mild and diagnosis confirmed by IF, antibiotics are not indicated. They should be prescribed:

— in critically ill infants as it may be difficult to differentiate the condition from pneumonia, especially staphylococcal
— if there is any evidence of secondary bacterial infection

Prophylaxis Maternal IgG is protective against RSV, which is an enveloped paramyxovirus of which there are at least three antigenic subtypes. Trials in the 1960s with a killed vaccine showed no benefit conferred; in fact vaccinated children had more severe subsequent infections than controls. Work is in progress to produce a live attenuated vaccine but it is not yet available.

Pneumonia

Cause	Children affected	Typical features	Diagnosis	Treatment
Viral RSV Parainfluenza Influenza A1, A2, B Adeno, coxsackie, rhinovirus Chickenpox, measles	Common in infants and older children	Wide spectrum from coryza to severe pneumonia ± bronchospasm CXR: patchy consolidation infiltrating out from hilum ± effusion. Cx: febrile convulsions, GI symptoms, bronchiolitis obliterans	Respiratory viral antibody titres	None specific Supportive, including O_2, physiotherapy Antibiotics often given as virological Dx only possible in retrospect
Bacterial Pneumococcal	All ages but commonest 3–8 years particularly sickle cell disease, asplenia	Prodrome 2–3/7 ± conjunctivitis High fever, pleuritic pain, rapid shallow respirations CXR: lobar or segmental consolidation in older children, bronchopneumonia in infants Cx: pleurisy, herpes labialis, endocarditis, meningitis, cerebral abscess	CXR Blood culture Pleural fluid culture	Penicillin
Staph. aureus	Uncommon Children <2 years most severely affected	Severe constitutional disturbance, high fever, anaemia CXR: widespread consolidation	CXR Blood/pleural fluid culture	Flucloxacillin +2nd antibiotic, e.g. fusidic A

		± pleural fluid, pneumatoceles, Cx: empyema, pneumothorax, lung abscess, haematogenous spread		e.g. fusidic A
Haem. influenza type B	Mainly <3 years	Spasmodic cough Lobar/ bronchopneumonia ± haemorrhagic exudate Cx: empyema, bronchiectasis	CXR Blood/NP aspirate culture	Ampicillin (or co-trim/ cefataxime chloramphen if R-amp)
Mycoplasma pneumoniae	Common 5–15 years	Insidious onset headaches, fever, sore throat, cough ± haemoptysis and chest pain CXR: punctate mottling ± effusion May be non-resp manifestations: rash, haemolytic anaemia, splenomegaly, arthralgia, neurological Cx	CFT, cold agglut (in 50%)	Erythromycin or tetracyclin
Uncommon				
Chlamydia trachomatis	Rare, seen in infants	May be preceding conjunctivitis at 7–14 days Av. age presentation 6 weeks CXR: diffuse interstitial pneumonia	Conjunctival scrapings Cell culture	Erythromycin
Pneumocystis carinii	Immunosuppressed, e.g. ALL, AIDS Neonatal epidemics	Cough, low-grade fever, respiratory distress. CXR hyperexpanded, generalized granular infiltrate extending out from hilum Often fatal	Lung biopsy Tracheal aspirate CIEP for pneumocystis antigen	Cotrimox or pentamidine
Gram –ve organisms *Klebsiella Pseudomonas*	Rare: occasionally in neonates/ immunosuppressed	Severe fulminating illness Klebsiella causes lobar infiltrates with bulging fissure, abscesses	Blood culture Tracheal aspirate	aminoglyc/ cephalosporin or ticarcillin ±aminoglyc

Cystic fibrosis (CF)   Cystic fibrosis is a life-long multisystem disorder of the exocrine glands characterized chiefly by chronic respiratory obstruction and infection and by pancreatic insufficiency with consequent nutritional problems.

Inheritance   Autosomal recessive with gene carrier rate of 1 in 22 of Caucasian population.

Incidence   1 in 1800 in UK. The gene is most prevalent in north and central Europeans and is less common in other races.

Presentation   *Neonatal*

— meconium ileus
— prolonged jaundice

Infancy

— recurrent LRTI (± wheeze)
— failure to thrive
— loose stools, steatorrhoea
— heat prostration

Toddler

— recurrent LRTI (± wheeze)
— malabsorption
— rectal prolapse

School age

— meconium ileus equivalent
— portal hypertension
— chronic sinusitis, nasal polyps
— recurrent chest infections ± wheeze, pneumothorax
— short stature
— delayed puberty
— diabetes mellitus

Diagnosis   Can only be made if confirmed by a positive sweat test. Based on concentration of sodium and chloride in at least 100 mg of sweat collected after pilocarpine iontophoresis. Upper limit normal 60 mmol/l (higher in teenagers); values between 40 and 60 mmol/l are suspicious and should be repeated. Most children with CF have values between 80 and 125 mmol/l.

Conditions causing false positive sweat tests:

— Addison's disease
— ectodermal dysplasia
— nephrogenic diabetes insipidus
— glucose-6-phosphatase deficiency
— hypothyroidism
— mucopolysaccharidoses

It is difficult to obtain sufficient sweat in infants <6–8 weeks. Elevated serum immunoreactive trypsin (IRT) in neonates suggests the diagnosis and should then be confirmed by sweat test. (IRT gives false positive in 0.3%.) Pancreatic function should be documented in each case.

Complications   — Pneumothorax: 20%, mainly in teenagers
— gallstones: 10%, often asymptomatic, may cause cholecystitis in young adults

— cirrhosis, oesophageal varices and hypersplenism
— hypoxic pulmonary hypertension and cor pulmonale
— arthropathy: 10%, teenagers
— teenage rebellion, non-compliance, depression
— family stress, marital breakdown and parental psychiatric illness

Management   Aims:
(a) To enable the child to live as normal a life as possible.
(b) Optimal nutrition to maintain growth.
(c) Full immunization.
(d) Regular review and coordinated multidisciplinary management, which in most cases is best provided at a special CF clinic.
(e) Minimal hospitalization.
(f) Education of patient, family and school.
(g) Support of child and family in dealing with emotional consequences of the disease.

Treatment   1. *Respiratory*:

— monitoring every 2 weeks sputum culture
    every 6–12 weeks height, weight, PFT, review diet and physio technique
    every 6 months CXR
    every year abdominal US
    occasional lung scans
— full immunization including influenza
— physiotherapy. Usually done by parents twice/day — chest percussion, postural drainage and exercise followed by forced expiration (huffing) and coughing in the older child
— antibiotics. Some centres use anti-staphylococcal treatment from the outset but there is conflicting evidence regarding the efficacy of this policy. Choice is determined by the state of the patient and pathogens isolated, which commonly include *Haem. influenza*, *Staph. aureus*, *Klebsiella*, *Pseudomonas*. Aggressive i.v. regimens are often necessary. In some families, after careful training, i.v. antibiotics can be given at home.
— treatment of wheezing, which may be due to:
  • acute infection
  • bronchial hyperreactivity
  • allergic bronchopulmonary aspergillosis

and may respond variably to bronchodilators, steroids or antifungals, such as i.v. amphotericin B or miconazole for aspergillosis

— inhaled aerosol antibiotics or mucolytics are probably not effective.

2. *Nutrition*. Patients have above average energy requirements and need high protein diets. Restriction of dietary fat

is no longer advocated; instead the new pH-sensitive enteric-coated microsphere preparations of pancreatic enzymes (Creon, Duphar and Pancrease, Ortho-Cilag) are given in sufficient dosage to improve fat absorption and reduce faecal fat excretion to normal (5 g/day).

Dietary supplements may improve weight gain, e.g. CHO — Maxijul, Caloreen, Polycal; medium chain triglycerides — Liquigen. Multivitamin preparations, e.g. Ketovite and Vitamin E supplements are usually given.

3. *Psychosocial problems and family support*:

(a) Counselling and emotional support for child and parents involving nurses, paediatrician, GP, teachers and psychologist.

(b) The Cystic Fibrosis Research Trust has locally-based parent and adolescent groups; they provide literature and have holiday funds.

(c) Medical social workers can provide practical and financial help, including guidance about attendance allowance (payable to carers for children >2 years requiring frequent attention by day or night — leaflet NI 205 from DSS offices). Other allowances for diet, mobility and equipment, e.g. nebulizers may also be available.

(d) Education. Most CF children manage well in ordinary schools with the cooperation of the SMO, school nurse and teachers. Early careers guidance is important. The Disablement Advisory Service (DAS) and Disablement Resettlement Officer are valuable sources of advice about employment.

4. *Genetic counselling*. Referral should be made for genetic counselling after the diagnosis of the first affected child and should not be left until a further pregnancy occurs. Antenatal diagnosis is now possible in many families by analysis of fetal DNA obtained at chorionic villus biopsy in the 1st trimester (see p. 9). In a small proportion of families, gene probes are uninformative. In such cases a less specific test of amniotic fluid for microvillar enzymes can be carried out.

Recent advances Extensive genetic linkage analysis on affected families in many countries has resulted in the localization of the CF gene to the long arm of chromosome 7. A deletion in the coding region for phenylalanine at position 508 in the amino acid sequence of the protein coded for by the CF gene (delta F508) accounts for ~75–80% of the mutations in CF in the UK (though this frequency varies geographically, e.g. in Italy delta F508 accounts for only 37% of mutations; this has important implications for proposed screening programmes). Other rarer point mutations have also been identified.

Research has demonstrated a deficiency in chloride ion permeability of epithelia in CF. A model of the product of the CF gene has been generated, called the transmembrane conductance regulator protein (CFTR protein); this may be the chloride channel itself or a regulator of ion conductance in epithelial cells.

These advances have important implications for the feasibility of more accurate antenatal diagnosis, carrier detection and development of pharmacological agents, which may be able to restore membrane permeability and be used in treatment of CF patients.

Prognosis   Very variable and difficult to predict. Aggressive medical management has improved health and survival in recent years, although at the cost of considerable infringement on family life. 80–90% of children with CF now survive to adulthood.

A small number of CF children have had successful heart–lung transplants (1 year survival rate ~60%; higher incidence of pulmonary rejection and infection compared with adults). For most with progressive disease however, transplantation is not an option because of poor general condition or lack of suitable donors. When the disease reaches an advanced stage, recognition of this fact should be agreed with the family and most will prefer subsequent terminal care at home (see p. 310). Home oxygen will need to be supplied on prescription by the GP and the family will need continuing support through and following the death of the child.

12. Gastrointestinal disorders

Gastrointestinal symptoms are common in children and are often associated with disorders which do not primarily affect the gut. Presenting symptoms include:

— pain
— vomiting
— diarrhoea
— constipation
— gastrointestinal bleeding
— abdominal distension

Abdominal pain

Causes of acute pain

Common	*Uncommon*	*Rare*
Gastroenteritis	Intussusception	Testicular or
Mesenteric adenitis	Strangulated hernia	ovarian torsion
Urinary tract infection	Volvulus	Poisoning
Constipation	Appendicitis	Splenic rupture
Colic	Nephritis	Pancreatic
Henoch-Schönlein	Hydronephrosis	pseudocyst
purpura	Sickle cell crisis	Acute
Pneumonia	Cystic fibrosis	pancreatitis
Infestations		Cholecystitis
Diabetes mellitus		
Hepatitis		
Trauma		

Recurrent abdominal pain

Common problem affecting 10% of otherwise healthy children.

Causes

Common (95%)	*Rare (5%)*
Functional: constipation	Gastrointestinal
Abdominal: migraine	• infection, infestation
	• peptic ulceration
	• inflammatory bowel disease
	• malrotation
	• coeliac disease
	• pancreatitis
	Renal
	• pyelonephritis
	• hydronephrosis
	• calculi

Metabolic
- diabetes mellitus
- lead poisoning
- porphyria
- drugs

Mesenteric adenitis
Epilepsy
Food allergy
Referred pain, e.g. from hip, spine
Sexual abuse
Tumour

Presentation   Usually functional (95%) but many serious causes, therefore requires careful history and examination, attention to details of pain, associated symptoms, family and social history, e.g. family structure and dynamics, diet, pets, school, housing, travel.

Functional pain tends to be central, vague, lasting less than an hour and followed by quick recovery. Often retain good appetite despite pain.

Examination   (a) Check ENT, look for anaemia, lymphadenopathy, jaundice.
(b) Systemic examination, looking particularly for abdominal tenderness, hepatosplenomegaly, kidney enlargement. Check testes and hernial orifices, external genitalia, BP.
(c) Plot height and weight on centile chart.

Investigations   Should be kept to the minimum necessary to exclude organic causes, e.g.:

— FBC, ESR, U&E, LFTs, Ca, phosphate, glucose
— urinalysis and MSU
— stool culture
— plain abdominal X-ray
— abdominal US
— barium studies, endoscopy, etc. depending on history

Management   If investigations are normal and functional cause likely from history, explain to parents and reassure. Arrange to review after 2–4 weeks. Advise parents to acknowledge the child's symptoms but encourage normal daily activities.

Vomiting

Neonatal   See p. 36.

Causes in infants and children   — feeding problems
— infections, e.g. gastroenteritis, pneumonia, pertussis, otitis media, UTI, meningitis, septicaemia
— gastrointestinal
  - gastro-oesophageal reflux
  - obstruction: congenital malformation, pyloric stenosis, intussusception, strangulated inguinal hernia

- appendicitis
- cow's milk protein intolerance
- coeliac disease
— renal
  - UTI
  - uraemia
  - renal tubular acidosis
— cerebral
  - migraine
  - raised intracranial pressure
  - meningoencephalitis
— metabolic
  - diabetes mellitus
  - galactosaemia, aminoacidaemias
  - fructose intolerance
  - hypercalcaemia
  - congenital adrenal hyperplasia
— drugs

Diarrhoea

Causes	Acute	Chronic
	Gastroenteritis	Constipation with overflow
	Systemic infection	Post gastroenteritis, e.g. lactose intolerance
	Overfeeding in infancy	Cow's milk protein intolerance
	Medication	Infections, e.g. salmonella, giardia, amoebae, cryptosporidium
	Poisoning	Toddler diarrhoea

Causes

Acute
Gastroenteritis
Systemic infection
Overfeeding in infancy
Medication
Poisoning

Chronic
Constipation with overflow
Post gastroenteritis, e.g. lactose intolerance
Cow's milk protein intolerance
Infections, e.g. salmonella, giardia, amoebae, cryptosporidium
Toddler diarrhoea
Malabsorption
- small bowel enteropathy, including coeliac disease
- sugar malabsorption
- pancreatic insuffiency, e.g cystic fibrosis
- bile acid deficiency
- gut resections
Inflammatory bowel disorders, e.g. Crohn, ulcerative colitis
Other
- chloride losing diarrhoea
- endocrine disorders
- antibiotic therapy

Constipation

Causes
— functional: overzealous potty training, diet related
— anal fissure
— Hirschprung disease
— anal stenosis
— anal trauma, e.g. post surgery or sexual abuse

— medication
— dehydration
— malabsorption
— hypothyroidism
— hypercalcaemia
— spinal abnormalities, e.g. spina bifida

GI bleeding

Causes   1. *Haematemesis*:

— swallowed blood, e.g. maternal, nasopharyngeal
— oesophagitis, varices
— Mallory–Weiss tear
— peptic ulceration, gastric erosions, aspirin
— iron poisoning

2. *Rectal bleeding*:

— infections, e.g. camylobacter, shigella, salmonella
— anal fissures
— Henoch-Schönlein purpura
— chronic inflammatory bowel disease
— cow's milk protein intolerance
— toxic megacolon
— necrotizing enterocolitis
— Meckel's diverticulum
— intussusception, volvulus
— colonic polyps

3. *Either*:

— heamatological disorders, e.g. haemorrhagic disease of the newborn, thrombocytopenia, coagulopathies
— foreign body
— drugs

Food allergy   Allergy may occur to food proteins eaten in normal or large amounts which trigger IgE-mediated hypersensitivity reactions presenting with symptoms related to the GI tract or elsewhere. It may arise due to variation in mucosal passage and proteolytic handling of food proteins or in individual immune response after antigen ingestion.

M>F 2:1. Incidence decreases with age. Often family history of atopy or food allergy.

Cow's milk allergy (CMA) is the commonest food allergy, affecting 3.5–7.5% of children. 75% of these children have hypersensitivity to other foods as well.

Presentation   Onset of symptoms can be within minutes (type I hypersensitivity) or delayed for hours or days (type III or IV hypersensitivity).

Clinically, food allergy tends to affect the GI tract, skin or lungs.

1. *GI symptoms*:

— abdominal pain, colic
— vomiting
— diarrhoea
— rectal bleeding or colitis (especially in children <2 years)

2. *Cutaneous*:

— urticaria
— circumoral or perianal rashes
— eczema

3. *Respiratory*:

— allergic rhinitis
— asthma
— angioedema

4. *Other*:

— behavioural disturbance, see p. 117
— CNS symptoms: headache, migraine
— arthritis
— failure to thrive

Food proteins most commonly provoking hypersensitivity reactions:

— cow's milk   — citrus fruit
— soya   — fish
— cereals   — nuts
— eggs   — colourings

Colourings and preservatives probably cause food intolerance mediated by pharmacological mechanisms, which is different from immunologically-mediated food allergy.

Diagnosis There are as yet no good diagnostic tests for food allergy. Diagnosis is based on:

— unequivocal clinical reaction to food challenge with elimination of symptoms on dietary exclusion
— in infants with malabsorption associated with cow's milk allergy, serial jejunal biopsies documenting enteropathy on normal diet with changes on exclusion and after challenge, strongly support the diagnosis
— skin tests: false positives common, false negatives rare
— dietary and symptom record
— circulating IgE antibodies to specific food antigens, demonstrated by radioallergasorbent test (RAST)

Treatment Primarily by avoidance of implicated foods.
   Exclusive breast feeding with avoidance of antigens in maternal diet is best treatment for infants. Formula-fed infants with cow's milk allergy should be changed to a hypoallergenic low osmotic formula with low molecular

weight peptides, e.g. Prejomin, Alfaré (soya milks are not suitable if there is mucosal injury as ~20% of infants will also be intolerant of soya protein).

Exclusion diets with sequential challenges may identify offending foods but must be supervised by a dietician. Risks: malnutrition, social disruption, anaphylaxis, Munchhausen-by-proxy syndrome.

Oral Sodium Chromoglycate or Ketotifen may have a role in children with definite clinical and immunological features of IgE-mediated food allergy.

Gastrointestinal reflux

Presentation Most babies under 3 months regurgitate frequently with no apparent ill effects. This is thought to be due to lowered oesophageal sphincter pressure. More severe reflux may cause oesophagitis, haematemeis, anaemia or failure to thrive. Occasionally presents with persistent cough, chest infections, recurrent wheeze, or apnoeic episodes.

Investigation In severe cases reflux may be quantitated by lower oesophageal pH monitoring; manometry and contrast studies are used to check motility and for anatomical abnormalities.

Treatment 1. *Simple measures*:

— nurse semi-prone with head raised
— thickening agents, e.g. Carobel, Nestargel, added to feeds

2. *Medication*:

— infant Gaviscon (antacid and mucosal protectant)
— cisapride (affects oesophageal motility and gastric emptying)

3. *Surgery*. Reserved for intractable cases, e.g. those with underlying neuromuscular disorders.

Gastroenteritis Children <2 years are chiefly affected, with acute onset of watery diarrhoea ± vomiting, fever and dehydration. Can progress very rapidly in babies.

Causes Commonest pathogens are viral, e.g. rotavirus, adenovirus, small round virus. Bacterial causes include: *E. coli*, salmonella, shigella, campylobacter, yersinia, *Giardia lamblia*, *Entamoeba histolytica*.

Treatment (a) Initially 24 h oral rehydration solutions (ORS), e.g. Dioralyte, Rehidrat, containing glucose and electrolytes. Ileal absorption of glucose draws sodium and water into the enterocytes. (Breast feeding should continue if tolerated).
(b) Reintroduce feeds after 24 h of ORS.
(c) Admission to hospital is needed with moderate to severe dehydration or with persistence of symptoms after a trial of ORS as above.

(d) Secondary lactose intolerance may require non-lactose containing milk substitution.

(e) Antibiotics are indicated in some infections:

Giardia	metronidazole
Campylobacter	erythromycin
Entamoeba	metronidazole
Shigella	cotrimoxazole, nalidixic acid

Complications — dehydration
— secondary lactose intolerance
— convulsions
— extra-intestinal infection, e.g. salmonellosis
— renal: pre-renal failure, renal vein thrombosis, medullary necrosis
— hypokalaemia
— cerebral oedema

Dehydration Three types:

— isotonic: water and sodium depleted in equivalent amounts
— hypotonic: sodium loss exceeds water loss
— hypertonic: water loss exceeds sodium loss

Causes — excess losses:
  • GI: diarrhoea, vomiting, fistulae
  • renal: diabetes mellitus or insipidus, tubular disorders
  • insensible: heat stroke
— deficient intake: coma, fluid restriction

Features of different types of dehydration

	Isotonic	Hypotonic	Hypertonic
Plasma sodium (mmol/l)	130–150	<130	>150
Skin texture	Reduced elasticity	Reduced elasticity	Doughy, thick
Blood pressure	Low	Very low	Normal until late stage
Peripheral perfusion	Poor	Poor	Preserved until late stage
Sunken eyes	Present	Present	Not obvious
Pulse	Rapid	Rapid	Rapid
Anterior fontanelle	Depressed	Depressed	Depressed
Convulsions	No	Rarely	Prominent feature
Fluid replacement (see below)	1/3 in 4 h, 2/3 in next 16 h	1/3 in 4 h, 2/3 in next 16 h	Slowly and steadily over 2–3 days
Type of fluid	If circulatory failure at presentation, expand plasma volume with 20 ml/kg plasma, plasma substitute or 0.9% saline over 1–2 h then		
	4% dextrose, 0.18% saline	0.45% saline until Na deficit replenished	0.45% saline with 2.5% glucose, not 5% dextrose

Hypertonic dehydration   Common cause of death or disability until infant-feeding practices changed in the UK in the 1970s. Affects mainly infants with gastroenteritis given excessively concentrated feeds; can also occur in diabetic ketosis and heat stroke.

Important to be aware that presentation is different from other types of dehydration: clinical signs may be less obvious until a later stage when serious neurological symptoms develop.

(a) Excess water loss in frequent hypotonic stools or severe febrile and/or respiratory illness leaves the plasma more concentrated and hypernatraemic.

(b) Continuing concentrated feeds require more water for excretion; this interferes with water conservation (which is the normal renal compensatory mechanisms as plasma sodium rises).

(c) Since water moves more rapidly than solute between body fluid compartments, it is drawn from the ICF to the hypertonic ECF and intracellular dehydration results. This may cause brain shrinkage and tearing of cerebral vessels leading to haemorrhage.

(d) The brain then adapts to hyperosmolality by generating osmoles from peptide breakdown to increase intracellular osmolality, so water is drawn back into the neural cells. This can happen rapidly, especially if there is acute reduction in plasma osmolality (e.g. as a result of injudicious use of hypo-osmolar fluids, e.g. dextrose 5%, in rehydration) causing cerebral oedema.

(e) Intracellular dehydration and renal dysfunction result in metabolic acidosis.

(f) Resulting complications may include convulsion, coma, intracerebral haemorrhage, subdural effusions, pre-renal failure and renal vein thrombosis.

Estimation of dehydration   — mild (5%)   Dry mucous membranes
(hypotonic/isotonic)   — moderate (10%)   Ill child, sunken eyes and fontanelles
                                               Poor peripheral perfusion
                          — severe (10–15%)   Shock: tachycardia, hypotension, oliguria/anuria, hyperventilation, drowsiness

Management   Mild cases can be managed at home with ORS as long as parents can cope. Persistent vomiting or refusal of fluids requires admission and change to i.v. route; all moderate or severely dehydrated children require i.v. fluids and careful monitoring in hospital.

Replacement volumes per day are calculated from:

Deficit (rough guide: deficit (ml) =
% dehydration × wt (kg) × 10)

+

Maintenance (rough guide*: allow

100 ml/kg for first 10 kg b. wt
+
50 ml/kg for next 10 kg b. wt
+
25 ml/kg thereafter

*Reduce rate in hypertonic dehydration to max. 100 ml/kg/day)
+
Replace continuing losses with fluid of similar composition, reassessing 6–8 hourly

— monitor vital signs including BP. Weigh daily and compare with previous known weights
— careful recording of all intake and output including urine output and GI losses
— investigations:
  • serum U&E, creatinine, glucose, calcium, osmolality
  • urine SG or osmolality
  • + if >5% dehydrated:
    Astrup
    urine electrolytes, microscopy
    tests for infection as indicated by clinical presentation
  • ±ECG

Metabolic acidosis will usually correct spontaneously as circulation is restored. If very severe, persistent or progressive, sodium bicarbonate may be indicated.

Potassium supplementation will often be required once urine flow is established (maintenance 2–3 mmol/kg/day; concentration not >40 mmol/1 of i.v. fluid).

Malabsorption

Causes   1. *Small bowel mucosal abnormality*:

— *morphological*: non-specific   coeliac disease
cow's milk protein
   intolerance
giardiasis
post-gastroenteritis
protein energy
   malnutrition
tropical sprue
immunodeficiency
   states

specific   intestinal
   lymphangiectasis
congenital
   microvillus
   atrophy
abetalipoproteinaemia

— *functional*:   lactose deficiency   primary or secondary
to morphologic
changes
sucrose–isomaltase deficiency
glucose–galactose malabsorption
chloride–losing diarrhoea

2. *Intraluminal abnormalities*:

— pancreatic insufficiency   cystic fibrosis
Shwachman–
Diamond syndrome
(+ neutropenia and
bone abnormalities)

— altered enterohepatic circulation   prematurity
cholestasis
cirrhosis
blind loop syndrome
ileal resection
Crohn's disease of
ileum

— anatomical   short bowel
malrotation
altered motility

Presentation
— failure to thrive
— abdominal distension
— diarrhoea/steatorrhoea
— anaemia

Investigation
— FBC and film, ESR, U&E, LFTs, iron, B12 and folate, Igs, serum proteins, RAST, antigliadin antibodies
— xylose and fat absorption studies, or differential sugar absorption tests, e.g. cellobiose–mannitol test
— stool microscopy and culture; stool reducing sugars, chloride
— X-ray wrist for bone age
— consider sweat test, jejunal biopsy, contrast studies, US, etc.

Coeliac disease
Malabsorption disorder caused by sensitivity to the protein α-gliadin in gluten in wheat and rye, which results in damage to the small bowel mucosa characterized by villous atrophy.

Incidence 1 in 2000 with slight family clustering. Commoner in girls. Associated with HLA-DR3, DR7 and DQW2.

Presentation
— usually age 9 months to 3 years, although mild cases may not be recognized until adult life
— insidious onset of failure to thrive associated with anorexia, loose, frequent stool, steatorrhoea, anaemia
— if undiagnosed, progresses to abdominal distension, stunted growth, muscle wasting — especially buttocks

— older children may have fewer symptoms and signs but usually have some growth impairment
— rarely
  • dermatitis herpetiformis, rickets
  • increased incidence of bowel malignancy in adult life (though strict adherence to gluten-free diet may have a protective effect)

Diagnosis   Currently based on the revised criteria of the European Society of Pediatric Gastroenterology and Nutrition (ESPGAN criteria, 1990).
(a) Characteristic small intestinal mucosal appearance of hyperplastic villous atrophy on jejunal biopsy of patient eating gluten.
(b) Clearcut clinical remission on strict gluten-free diet (within weeks).
(c) Diagnosis supported by finding of circulating IgA anti-gliadin, IgA anti-reticulin and IgA anti-endomysium antibodies, and by their disappearance on gluten-free diet.
(d) Serial jejunal biopsies before and after gluten challenge is no longer deemed mandatory to make the diagnosis, but must be performed if there is doubt about the initial diagnosis, e.g. difficulty excluding other causes of enteropathy, particularly in children <2 years.
    Challenge is preferably left until after age 6 years, because of risk of dental damage if done earlier.

Management   (a) Dietary advice to ensure nutritionally adequate gluten-free diet. Gluten-free products are available on prescription, e.g. biscuits, spaghetti, flour, bread mix. The prescription should be marked ACBS.
(b) Put parents in touch with local branch of the Coeliac Society for ongoing support. The Society produces leaflets listing well-known supermarket foods that are gluten free.
(c) Anticipate psychological difficulties long-term particularly with teenagers.

Cystic fibrosis   See p. 177.

Lactose intolerance   Lactose is normally broken down in the small intestine by lactase. Lactase deficiency results in excessive lactose in the colon which draws water into the bowel, giving an explosive, loose, acidic stool (pH <5.5, clinitest positive). Lactase deficiency may be primary or secondary.

Primary lactase deficiency (rare) is present from birth and symptoms begin as soon as breast feeding starts. These babies present with diarrhoea, vomiting, failure to thrive and irritant perianal erythema due to acidic stool.

Secondary lactose intolerance (common) usually results

from gastroenteritis or other small bowel enteropathies. It is usually transient and lactose can be re-introduced after 2–4-weeks treatment with a lactose-free milk, see p. 50.

Diagnosis — pH stools
— clinitest stool — if positive, do sugar chromatography to differentiate from sucrase–isomaltase deficiency or glucose–galactase malabsorption
— lactose challenge

Toddler diarrhoea   Children aged 1–3 years sometimes develop frequent loose stools with no pathological cause. On examination they are healthy with good weight gain. Often associated with dietary changes or concurrent minor illness of respiratory tract.

Natural history is of intermittent attacks that may persist for years. Possible correlation with adult irritable bowel syndrome.

Investigations — stool MC&S to exclude giardiasis or other chronic infestation. Check stool pH and reducing substances, FBC, and urine culture
— centile measurements over a period of months to confirm normal growth velocity

Management (a) Reassure parent about normal growth and health, and that disorder is benign and self limiting.
(b) Refer if abnormal growth or other signs of disease.

Ulcerative colitis   Characterized by diffuse inflammation and ulceration of mucosa of rectum and colon.

Incidence: rare in childhood (5 in 100 000)

Presentation   Presents either in 1st year of life or around age 8–10 years with:

— intermittent attacks of bloody diarrhoea and abdominal pain
— general malaise with fever
— poor growth
— extra-intestinal features, e.g. finger clubbing, mouth ulcers, anaemia, arthritis, pyoderma gangrenosum, erythema nodosum
— toxic dilatation of the colon

Investigations — malabsorption screen; exclude infection
— double contrast barium enema
— colonoscopy and biopsies

Management (a) Correct anaemia, fluid and electrolyte disturbances.
(b) High-energy diet with supplementary vitamins.
(c) Drug treatment: steroids (oral/enemas), sulphasalazine or in severe cases, immunosuppressives, e.g. cyclosporin.
(d) Surgery is indicated for failure to respond to medical treatment, or for toxic dilatation, severe haemorrhage or

perforation. Increaed risk of malignancy associated with early onset and prolonged disease.

(e) Psychological support is important in this chronic relapsing disease.

Crohn's disease   Inflammation of the whole thickness of the bowel wall affecting the terminal ileum and proximal colon most commonly but can affect any part of the small bowel. Rectum is usually spared but may have perianal fissures, fistulae and abscess formation.

Incidence: increased in recent decades, now 5–6 per 100 000. Aetiology obscure.

Presentation   — anorexia, lethargy
— failure to thrive, sexual immaturity
— mouth ulcers, orofacial granulomatosis
— abdominal pain
— intermittent fever
— diarrhoea
— perianal lesions
— extra intestinal features: erythema nodosum, arthritis, clubbing, anaemia

Investigations   — malabsorption screen; exclude infection
— barium meal and follow through. Classical X-ray changes are narrowing of the lumen ('string sign'), patchy involvement ('skip lesions') and 'rose thorn' ulcers
— endoscopy and biopsy

Management   (a) Elemental diet effective in inducing remission and avoiding growth failure. High-energy, low-fibre diet with or without overnight nasogastric supplements improves subsequent growth velocity.

(b) Drugs: sulphasalazine or mesalazine, immunosuppressives, e.g. azothiaprine, steroids.

(c) Surgical resection for complications, e.g. obstruction, perforation.

Constipation   Term commonly used when there is infrequent passage of stools, but is more properly a description of hard dry stools causing distress to the child. Breast-fed babies may pass soft or liquid stools infrequently; this is not constipation and mothers should be reassured.

Causes   See p. 185.

Management   (a) Detailed history, including diet.

(b) Examination including ano-rectal, spine, neurological examination, height and weight.

(c) Investigations may include

— plain abdominal X-ray
— serum electrolytes, including calcium, TFTs, blood

lead contrast studies, manometry, biopsy, etc. if neuromyenteric abnormality suspected

(d) Empty rectum and colon, then soften stool with, e.g. lactulose, and encourage regular emptying using stimulants, e.g. senna, bisacodyl. Frequent relapses, so encourage parents to persist. Often need laxative treatment for several months to regain normal bowel habit.

(e) Refer if
   — early onset (delayed passage of meconium or constipation from first week)
   — failure to thrive, vomiting, abdominal distension
   — gush of faeces after rectal examination
   — ribbon stools
   — failure to respond to well-ordered laxative treatment

Hirschsprung's disease Congenital absence of intestinal autonomic ganglion cells of Auerbach and Meissner plexus with concomitant hypertrophy of extrinsic autonomic nerves. The resulting lack of gut peristalsis leads to chronic constipation and dilatation of the proximal bowel.

Incidence 1 in 5000 (increased in Down's syndrome); M:F 5:1.

Presentation — delay in passage of first meconium after 24 h
   — chronic and/or recurrent intestinal obstruction
   — ribbon-like stools
   — failure to thrive
   — abdominal distension
   — empty rectum on PR

Investigation — barium enema shows aganglionic narrow segment with dilated proximal bowel
   — ano-rectal manometry shows failure of sphincter relaxation in response to rectal distension
   — rectal biopsy reveals absence of the submucosal ganglion cells, hypertrophy of nerve fibres and increased acetylcholinesterase activity in the lamina propria

Treatment Relief of obstruction by colostomy, then excision of affected segment and re-anastomosis or pull-through operation.

Appendicitis Rare in children <2 years old.

Presentation — pyrexia
   — anorexia
   — coated tongue and foetor
   — central abdominal pain localizing in right iliac fossa with tenderness and guarding
   — may have constipation or diarrhoea
   — retrocaecal appendicitis may not cause any localizing signs but rectal examination reveals tenderness anteriorly

— may present with urinary signs if pelvic appendix is inflammed

Differential diagnosis   1. Mesenteric addenitis:

— usually associated with URTI, lymphadenopathy elsewhere, especially neck and axillae, may have had previous episodes
— usually higher fever
— abdominal pain is vague, generalized, intermittent

2. *UTI*:

— usually urinary symptoms of dysuria and frequency
— need urgent urine microscopy and culture

3. *Intussusception*:

— more acute onset with obstructive symptoms
— younger age group

4. *Lower lobe pneumonia*:

— chest signs
— vomiting often starts before abdominal pain
— no guarding on abdominal examination

5. *Infectious hepatitis*.
6. *Diabetes mellitus*.

Investigations   — FBC, differential, ESR
— U&E, creatinine, glucose, LFTs, serum amylase
— plain abdominal X-ray
— MSU

Management   (a) Appendicectomy.
(b) Intravenous fluids.
(c) Antibiotic cover if suspicion of perforation or peritonitis, e.g. metronidazole and third-generation cephalosporin.

Intussusception   Due to one segment of bowel telescoping into the adjacent, usually distal, segment. Ileocolic intussusception is the most common but ileoileal and colocolic forms also occur rarely.

90% of cases in children <3 years; commonest between 3 months and 2 years. In older children more often associated with lead point (e.g. polyp, Meckel diverticulum, lymphosarcoma or cyst at the apex of the intussuscepted gut), but in most cases no obvious cause. May be associated with hyperplastic intestinal lymphoid tissues causing local disturbance of peristalsis. May follow viral illness.

Presentation   Sudden onset of colicky abdominal pain and screaming followed by vomiting, pallor and opening of the bowels; stools appear normal early but later develop classical 'redcurrent jelly' stool containing blood and mucus. Abdominal palpation may reveal 'sausage-shaped' mass lying in the line of the colon. Late presentation may be with signs of small bowel obstruction with bilious vomiting, pyrexia and dehydration.

Management   (a) Pass NGT and correct fluid and electrolyte disturbances intravenously. Transfusion may be required.

(b) Plain abdominal X-ray.

(c) Urgent barium enema. Used not only for diagnostic purposes but also therapeutically, as the bolus of barium often reduces the intussusception by hydrostatic pressure. Most successful in fit children with a short history.

(d) Operative reduction, after adequate resuscitation, if:

— signs of peritoneal irritation or bowel perforation
— rectal bleeding plus symptoms for longer than 48 h
— child has been shocked

Prognosis   Mortality ~1%. Recurrence rate ~1–3% (higher if lead point present).

Pyloric stenosis   Incidence M:F 5:1. More common in first-born males. Incidence 3 in 1000 in the UK.

Caused by hypertrophy of the pylorus resulting in delayed gastric emptying.

Presentation   Onset between 2nd and 6th week of life. Recurrent non-bilious vomiting, increasing in frequency and amount, and eventually, usually around 6–8 weeks, becoming projectile. Hungry baby with initially good weight gain but then starts to lose weight, and may become dehydrated and alkalotic. Constipation is usual.

On examination visible peristalsis may be seen, with a palpable pyloric tumour — just lateral to right rectus muscle. Only intermittently palpable, best felt during feed or just after vomit.

Management   (a) Admit to hospital. Clinical diagnosis may be confirmed by US or barium meal but these are not always necessary.

(b) Correct dehydration and hypochloraemia, hypokalaemic alkalosis if present.

(c) Surgery — Ramstedt's operation (pyloromyotomy). Post-op rapid return to oral feeding.

Testicular torsion

Presentation   Sudden onset of testicular pain. Young children may present with abdominal pain only. Testicular examination reveals the swollen tender scrotum and must not be omitted in any boy presenting with acute abdominal pain. Torsion may be major (twisting of whole testis and epididymis) or minor (twisting of hydatid of Morgagni only, more common in younger boys).

Management   Urgent exploration, reduction and orchidopexy. The other testis is usually fixed in the scrotum at the same time as the recurrence rate is high. Late diagnosis may necessitate removal of the testis due to irreversible necrosis.

In torsion minor, the hydatid (a vestigial remnant on the upper pole of the testis) is excised.

Liver disorders   Commonest presentations of hepatic disease in childhood are jaundice and hepatomegaly.

Causes of jaundice   (Neonatal jaundice, see p. 37)
  1. *Infective*:

— viral: hepatitis A, B, C, CMV, infectious mononucleosis
— bacterial: septicaemia, leptospirosis
— protozoa: malaria, toxoplasmosis
— helminths: ascariasis, schistosomiasis

  2. *Haemolytic*:

— sickle cell anaemia
— thalassaemia
— congenital spherocytosis
— G6PD deficiency
— acquired haemolytic anaemia

  3. *Toxic*:

— paracetamol poisoning
— halothane
— iron

  4. *Obstructive*:

— biliary
— cirrhosis of the liver
— gallstones
— acute pancreatitis

  5. *Metabolic*:

— Wilson disease
— galactosaemia
— cystic fibrosis
— α-1-antitrypsin deficiency
— storage disorders
— Dubin–Johnson, Rotor syndrome

  6. *Chronic inflammatory*:

— chronic acute hepatitis
— inflammatory bowel disease

Causes of hepatomegaly   1. *Infection*: congenital infections, infectious mononucleosis, hepatitis, malaria, septicaemia, parasitic infection.

2. *Haematologic*: thalassaemia, spherocytosis, iron deficiency, thrombocytopenia, sickle cell anaemia, leukaemia.
3. *Chronic active hepatitis.*
4. *Congestive heart failure.*
5. *Malignancy, abscess, cyst.*
6. *Metabolic*: mucopolysaccharidoses, Reye's syndrome, galactosaemia, alpha-l-antitrypsin deficiency.
7. *Cystic fibrosis.*
8. *Portal hypertension.*

Chronic hepatitis   Defined as hepatitis for >3 months.

1. *Persistent*: good prognosis, although children may show poor growth until recovery.

2. *Active*: onset acute, with jaundice, fever, anorexia, hepatosplenomegaly in up to 80%, or insidious, with fever, arthralgia and autoimmune extrahepatic manifestations, e.g. erythema nodosum. Liver biopsy is necessary to confirm the diagnosis. 70% of children with chronic active hepatitis achieve remission in response to corticosteroids, with azathioprine added in difficult cases.

Complications include acute hepatocellular failure and cirrhosis.

Hepatic cirrhosis

Presentation
— general malaise
— poor growth
— hepatomegaly, jaundice, bruising
— clubbing, liver palms, spider naevi (rare in children)
— ascites
— splenomegaly and hypersplenism
— varices

Causes
— post-hepatitis: viral, chronic active hepatitis, toxic
— venous congestion: CCF, constrictive pericarditis, Budd–Chiari syndrome
— metabolic: Wilson's disease, storage disorders, α-l-antitrypsin deficiency
— biliary cirrhosis: biliary atresia, cystic fibrosis, ulcerative colitis, familial intrahepatic cholestasis
— Indian childhood cirrhosis

Reye's syndrome

Acute encephalopathy with fatty degeneration of the liver, kidneys and pancreas. High mortality. Pathogenesis uncertain; usually follows a viral illness, and an association with aspirin exposure led to withdrawal of its use in young children in 1986. Since that time there has been a steady decline in incidence.

Presentation   Commonest under 2 years of age. After a short prodromal illness, vomiting, delirium, fits and coma supervene. Other features include:

— hepatomegaly
— hypoglycaemia
— hyperammonaemia
— cerebral oedema

Differential diagnosis is from infection, inborn errors of metabolism, poisoning, pancreatitis and fulminating hepatitis.

Management   (a) General supportive measures:

— fluid and electrolyte balance, dextrose infusion
— treatment of coagulopathy with vitamin K, FFP
— treatment of hyperammonaemia with lactulose, neomycin
— control temperature

(b) Raised intracranial pressure:

— hyperventilation with sedation and muscle paralysis
— mannitol, hypothermia, barbiturate coma

(c) Treat complications, e.g. renal failure, GI haemorrhage, pancreatitis.

Splenomegaly

Causes   — haematological: haemolytic anaemias, iron deficiency anaemia, leukaemia
— infection: viral, bacterial, protozoal (kala-azar, schistosomiasis), parasites, infective endocarditis
— malignancy: lymphoma, histiocytosis
— other: portal hypertension, lipid storage disorders, Still's disease

13. Cardiology

Changes in circulation at birth	Normally the lungs fill with air in the first few minutes after birth. Lung expansion is accompanied by:

(a) fall in pulmonary vascular resistance (PVR) rapidly in first few minutes, then gradually over next days and weeks of life

(b) Increased blood flow to lungs.

(c) Gas exchange across alveolar capillary bed.

(d) Increased venous return from lungs to left atrium, (LA).

(e) Reduced return to right atrium (RA), due to interruption of umbilical flow as umbilical vessels functionally close within a few minutes of birth.

(f) LA pressure rises to above RA pressure and the foramen ovale closes functionally soon after birth (anatomical closure takes up to a year or more).

(g) In term babies the ductus arteriosus also rapidly constricts after birth (influenced by oxygen and PGE amongst other factors) but remains partially open with potential for shunt for about 18 h, closing functionally by the end of the first day. Anatomical closure follows over a period of weeks.

Congenital heart disease

Incidence: 8 in 1000 live births. Proportion of individual major lesions:

Ventriculoseptal defect (VSD)	25%
Patent ductus arteriosus (PDA)	12%
Tetralogy of Fallot	10%
Atrial septal defect (ASD)	7%
Pulmonary stenosis	7%
Transposition of great arteries (TGA)	7%
Aortic stenosis	5%
Coarctation	5%
Others	22%

Causes of congenital heart malformations

In most cases no specific cause is found. In a minority, genetic or environmental aetiological factors can be identified:

1. *Genetic*:

— chromosomal aberrations with multiple phenotypic effects. e.g. Down's syndrome (associated particularly with AV canal defects present in 30–40%), Turner's syndrome (coarctation of aorta in approximately 30%).

— monogenic — very rare.

• ASD
• supravalvar aortic stenosis
$\left.\begin{array}{c}\\\\\\\\\end{array}\right\}$ autosomal dominant with variable penetrance in some families

2. *Environmental* (< 1%):

— rubella in 1st trimester can cause PDA, pulmonary or aortic stenosis or VSD
— Drugs, e.g. thalidomide, cytotoxics, anticonvulsants, cocaine in first 28 weeks — septal defects
— fetal alcohol syndrome — ASD or VSD, PDA
— Maternal illness — PKU, diabetes

Modes of presentation
— murmur
— dyspnoea
— cyanosis
— failure to feed/thrive
— cardiac failure

Features of cardiac failure
— tachycardia (HR >180 at rest)
— respiratory distress
— excessive weight gain
— sweating
— hepatomegaly
— gallop rhythm

Causes of cardiac failure in infants

Cardiac	Non-cardiac
Coarctation	Sepsis
Hypoplastic left heart	Anaemia
Severe aortic stenosis	Acidosis
Persistent truncus arteriosus	Fluid overload
Double outlet right ventricle without pulmonary stenosis	Hypothyroidism
Complete AV septal defect	Polycythaemia
Cor triatriatum	Hypoglycaemia —
Complex combined lesions	(especially infants of diabetic mothers)
Myocarditis (e.g. coxsackie, echovirus)	
Arrhythmias	
Endocardial fibroelastosis (± associated lesion, e.g. coarction, aortic stenosis in two thirds).	

Causes of central cyanosis in first weeks of life
— transposition of great vessels
— pulmonary atresia or severe pulmonary stenosis with intact ventricular septum
— pulmonary atresia or severe pulmonary stenosis with VSD
— total anomalous pulmonary venous drainage with obstructed venous return

— tricuspid atresia
— Ebstein anomaly

Physical examination

(a) Height and weight.
(b) Any characteristic facial features or dysmorphism.
(c) Pulse — rate, volume, character, presence of radiofemoral delay.
(d) BP

— use correct cuff (width approx. two-thirds length of upper arm)
— in infants easier to use US Doppler or flush methods
— check all four limbs in infants or if any suspicion of coarctation
— check against graph of normal value for age
— if BP (correctly taken and checked) > mean for age by more than 2 SD, investigate cause of hypertension (see p. 215)

Average blood pressure in children at rest	Systolic (mm Hg)	Diastolic (mm Hg)
Newborn	60	35
Neonate (term)	75	45
1–12 months	95	60
2 years	95	60
6 years	97	62
8 years	105	65
15 years	120	75

(e) Inspect the thorax for asymmetry, scars, etc.
(f) Check the position of the apex beat:

— children <4 years — 4th ICS in midclavicular line
— children >4 years — 5th ICS in midclavicular line

(g) Auscultation:

Heart sounds: I Mitral and tricuspid closure usually single sound. Best heard lower left sternal edge or apex.

II Normally two components generated by asynchronous closure of aortic then pulmonary valve. Splitting usually only audible in inspiration (as a greater volume of blood returns to the R heart in inspiration, so RV ejection time is longer and pulmonary valve closure lags further behind aortic closure than in expiration).

Causes of abnormally wide splitting of II: ASD, pulmonary stenosis, RBBB.

III Ventricular filling sound. Normal in up to 50% of children.

IV Atrial contraction. Abnormal.

Ejection clicks: added sounds in early systole when the semi-lunar valves open. In children most frequently heard with aortic or pulmonary valve stenosis with dilatation of the ascending aorta or pulmonary artery.

Description of murmurs

1. *Timing* in cardiac cycle:

Systolic

— pan systolic (PSM) — equal intensity throughout systole. Usually best heard at apex or LSE. May be due to VSD, mitral regurgitation or, less often, tricuspid regurgitation

— ejection systolic (ESM) — maximal in mid-systole. Usually best heard in aortic or pulmonary areas associated with obstruction to flow across stenosed semi-lunar valves (or increased flow across normal semi-lunar valves)

Continuous

Murmurs which continue from systole into diastole. Usually produced by flow communication between a systemic artery and another channel at lower pressure throughout the cardiac cycle, allowing continuous shunt, e.g. PDA, cerebral AV fistula, Blalock-Taussig shunt.

Diastolic

Less common than other types in children and usually indicative of organic heart disease.

— early diastolic (EDM) — loudest immediately after 2nd sound. Reflects either aortic or pulmonary regurgitation (AoR/PR) (listen over upper praecordium with patient leaning forward; loudest end-expiration with AoR, end-inspiration with PR)

— Mid-diastolic (MDM). Occurs during ventricular filling with increased flow across the M/T valve (e.g. due to large L–R shunt) or, less commonly in paediatrics, with normal flow across stenosed M/T valve

2. *Intensity*. The conventional grading system is:

I   just audible
II   soft but easily heard } no thrill
III   moderately loud
IV   loud murmur + soft thrill
V   loud murmur + easily felt thrill
VI   audible with stethoscope off chest wall

3. *Location* of point of maximal intensity and radiation of murmur.

Functional (innocent) murmurs

Very common at all ages; heard in up to 70% of normal neonates and 50% of infants and children.

Features suggesting a murmur is innocent:

— no significant cardiac symptoms
— heart sounds normal
— heart size normal
— low amplitude, no thrill
— no diastolic component
— no ejection click
— normal CXR and ECG

Functional murmurs

Murmur	Timing	Site	Features	Differential diagnosis
Stills	ESM	Lower praecordium	Probably originates in LV outfow tract. Often buzzing or vibratory. Accentuated by squatting	VSD
Pulmonary flow murmur	ESM	Pulmonary area	No thrill No ejection click Common in normal neonates	ASD Pulmonary stenosis
Aortic arch murmur	ESM	Neck, base	No thrill No ejection click	Aortic stenosis
Venous hum	Continuous	Neck, sternoclavicular junctions	Due to turbulent flow in jugular venous system. Best heard with patient sitting. Diminished when child lies flat. Changes intensity with position of head and neck or compression of ipsilateral jugular V (unlike PDA which varies little with posture or respiration)	

The diagnosis of functional murmur is always one of probability. Before labelling a murmur as functional, the doctor should try to exclude an organic basis for it. In many cases this will include doing some basic investigations such as CXR, ECG and sometimes echocardiography. Once it has been decided that a murmur is innocent on the basis of all available facts, the doctor must be prepared to commit himself and reassure the parents as strongly as necessary that there is no evidence of any organic defect.

Congenital heart lesions

Ventriculoseptal defect (VSD) Commonest congenital heart defect.

Signs — PSM, maximal LSE (3–5th ICS)
— thrill (often)
— LV+, RV+ (often)

— loud P2 (occasionally)
— apical MDM (occasionally)
— signs of cardiac failure (occasionally)
— CXR: cardiomegaly, plethora
— ECG: LV or biventricular hypertrophy

History In many children with VSD a murmur is not heard until the 6-week check, because by this time the PVR has fallen sufficiently that enough blood flows through the defect (L→R) to generate a murmur. Patients with small or medium size VSDs are asymptomatic; the majority of such defects close spontaneously during the first 6 years. Up to 50% close by 18 months. (Maladie de Roger is a small asymptomatic VSD with no CXR or ECG changes.)

Those with larger defects (greater than the size of the aortic annulus) develop congestive cardiac failure by 2–3 months of age. Subsequently:

— ~5% of large defects close spontaneously
— pulmonary vascular disease may develop, with medial hypertrophy and later intimal proliferation causing progressive elevation of PVR. Once PVR > systemic vascular resistance (SVR) the shunt changes to R→L, there is decreased pulmonary blood flow and cyanosis develops (the Eisenmenger complex)
— infundibular pulmonary stenosis may develop

Treatment of large VSDs (a) Cardiac failure is treated mainly with diuretics; other drugs, e.g. captopril may be effective. NG feeds and caloric supplements may be needed for failure to thrive.
(b) Antibiotics for respiratory infections.
(c) Prophylaxis against endocarditis (see p. 213).
(d) Surgical closure is indicated for:

— large defects causing failure not responding to medical treatment
— VSD with increasing PVR and significant L→R shunt
— VSD with RV outflow tract obstruction
— VSD with aortic regurgitation (and cusp prolapse)
— VSD with LV→RA shunt (Gerbode defect) and tricuspid regurgitation

Operative mortality of primary repair in infancy is 5–10%. After age 2 years, mortality is < 2%.

Atrial septal defect (ASD)

Types — ostium secundum (70%)
— ostium primum (15–20%) (defect in lower part of septum, may be associated with abnormality in AV valve; worse prognosis)
— complete AV septal defect (10–15%)

Signs — soft ESM maximal P area, radiating to back
— wide fixed split II
— tricuspid MDM (often)
— RV+ (often)
— apical PSM (occasionally)
— CXR: cardiomegaly, plethora
— ECG: incomplete RBBB + RAD (secundum defect) + RVH
  or
  incomplete RBBB + LAD (primum defect) + BVH

History Often asymptomatic, not presenting until 2nd/3rd decade. May present with SVT in infancy or gradual onset dyspnoea on exertion.

Treatment (a) Medical control of cardiac failure.
(b) Antibiotics for respiratory infections.
(c) Prophylaxis against endocarditis.
(d) Closure by direct suture, patching using cardiopulmonary bypass or umbrella devices inserted during catheterization (e.g. clamshell). Results are excellent though mortality is higher for more complex defects. Usually performed before school entry; occasionally necessary in infancy.

Patent ductus arteriosus (PDA) Develops from the left 6th aortic arch. Normally closes functionally within 10–15 h of birth and anatomically obliterated over next 2–3 weeks. Delayed closure frequently seen in premature babies.

Signs — continuous murmur in P area radiating to L clavicle and back (though in infancy only the systolic component may be audible)
— thrill (often)
— collapsing pulses (often)
— LV+ (often)
— apical MDM (occasionally)
— loud P2 (occasionally)
— signs of cardiac failure (occasionally)
— CXR: cardiomegaly, plethora, prominent pulmonary A
— ECG: normal if small shunt; LV hypertrophy if large

Treatment (a) Ducts in preterm infants between 28 and 32 weeks may close with indomethacin, a prostaglandin synthetase antagonist.
(b) If PDA causes cardiomegaly, recurrent respiratory infection or failure to thrive, surgery is performed in infancy.
(c) The majority, which are asymptomatic, are closed in 2nd/3rd year of life. Methods not requiring surgery are being developed, e.g. Rashkind umbrella device for trans-catheter insertion.

Pulmonary stenosis Usually at valvar level; occasionally subvalvar, supravalvar or branch artery stenosis is found. May be mild, moderate or severe (critical).

Signs — ESM maximal P area, radiating to back
— thrill (often)
— RV+ (often)
— ejection click (absent in severe stenosis) (often)
— wide split S2 (often)
— CXR: prominent pulmonary conus (post-stenotic dilatation)
— ECG: RVH, P pulmonale

Treatment Valvotomy (performed when catheterization shows gradient across valve >40–50 mmHg). Alternatively balloon angioplasty valvotomy is possible even for quite severe cases.

Aortic stenosis May be valvar (70%), subvalvar (25%) or supravalvar (5% — frequently combined with peripheral pulmonary stenosis and typical elfin-like facies (William syndrome); may be associated with idiopathic hypercalcaemia).

Signs — rough ESM maximal in aortic area, radiating to neck
— thrill (often)
— ejection click (often)
— CXR: usually normal
— ECG: LVH

History Most are asymptomatic until adulthood when dyspnoea, syncope and angina may develop, but all forms of aortic stenosis carry the risk of sudden death, probably due to ventricular fibrillation which occurs in 7% of patients. In severe cases (systolic pressure gradient of >70 mmHg across obstruction) competitive exercise should be banned. There is a high risk of bacterial endocarditis.

Treatment Valvotomy or valve replacement (indication resting gradient >50 mmHg)
Mortality rate in infants ~20%, later in childhood <5%. After valvotomy may have aortic regurgitation and need aortic valve replacement.

Coarctation of the aorta Narrowing of the aorta classified by relation to the ductus arteriosus: pre-, juxta- or post-ductal. Male predominance 5:1.

Signs — higher BP in arms than legs (difference > 20 mmHg)
— femoral pulses absent, diminished or delayed
— ESM maximal LSE, apex and between scapulae
— hypertension
— ejection click
— systolic/continuous murmur between scapulae, over clavicles
— CXR: cardiomegaly in severe cases and may be visible indentation at site of coarctation; rib-notching (in children >9 years)
— ECG: RV+ in infants; LV+ in older children

History   Patients presenting in infancy usually have pre-ductal narrowing of the aortic arch ('tubular hypoplasia') and often have additional anomalies. They develop severe congestive failure which may respond to aggressive medical treatment but usually requires surgery. Mortality varies with associated lesion, severity of aortic hypoplasia and age at presentation with rates over 60% in first 6 weeks, falling to 25% between 3 and 6 months.

Coarctation presenting in older children is more likely to be juxta-ductal or post-ductal, localized and isolated. May present on routine examination with discovery of murmur or hypertension.

Indications for surgical resection are resting gradient >40–50 mmHg or hypertension.

Fallot's tetralogy

Features   — pulmonary stenosis
— VSD
— RV hypertrophy
— aortic override

Signs   — cyanosis
— ESM at LSE, maximal 3–4 ICS (due to infundibular pulmonary stenosis, not VSD)
— single 2nd sound (often): (aortic valve closure — loud because aorta more anterior. P valve closure delayed and rarely detectable
— clubbing
— thrill
— RV+
— CXR: small or normal size heart with uptilted apex (boot-shaped heart or *'coeur en sabot'*), oligaemia, concave pulmonary artery segment, right aortic arch in 25%
— ECG: RV+

History   Onset of cyanosis related to severity of pulmonary outflow tract obstruction. Some present in neonatal period but more often noted later in 1st year. Often have hypercyanotic spells and squat during exertion (increases SVR and so reduces R→L shunt). Risk of cerebral thrombosis or brain abscess.

Treatment   Emergency palliative procedures are often necessary in infancy, before radical correction with relief of pulmonary stenosis and closure of VSD under cardiopulmonary bypass, which is performed around 4 years. (Some surgeons now prefer primary total correction in infants >5 kg.)
Palliative procedures include:
— Blalock-Taussig shunt (subclavian A to pulmonary A anastomosis)
— Waterston shunt (R PA to ascending aorta)
— Potts procedure (L PA to ascending aorta)
— Balloon dilatation of infundibular pulmonary stenosis

Transposition of great arteries

In this condition the aorta arises from the RV and the pulmonary artery from the LV (arterial discordance). Survival depends on communication between the independent pulmonary and systemic circuits. Fortunately the foramen ovale and sometimes the ductus arteriosus or a coexistent septal defect enable the infant to survive for a few days during which time palliative procedures can be performed.

Signs

— cyanosis — usually marked from birth
— may be no other signs
— with associated VSD (~25%) may be systolic murmur
— CXR: may be normal; may be large heart, 'egg-on-side', narrow pedicle, plethora (variable)
— ECG: may be normal, RV+

Treatment

(a) *Palliative.* Prostaglandin E to keep ductus open. Urgent catheterization, with Rashkind procedure (balloon atrial septostomy).

(b) *Corrective.* Usually performed between 9 and 12 months. Most widely employed procedure is Mustard operation (excision of existing atrial septum and insertion of atrial baffle to redirect venous return). Alternatively some centres now performing arterial switch operations, usually within the 1st month of life.

Infective endocarditis

This infection of the endocardium or endothelium of great vessels usually complicates congenital or rheumatic heart disease but occasionally affects normal hearts. It is rare in children <3 years old. The anomalies involving highest risk of endocarditis are:

— VSD
— PDA
— coarctation of the aorta
— aortic stenosis
— tetralogy of Fallot
— patients with aorto-pulmonary shunts, intracardiac prostheses (valves, patches, stents, umbrellas)

The commonest infecting organisms are: *Streptococcus viridans* (after dental extraction) and staphylococci (after cardiac surgery).

Clinical features

— fever, rigors
— anaemia
— splenomegaly
— signs of embolization, e.g. splinter haemorrhages, haematuria
— weight loss

Investigations

— repeated blood cultures
— ESR and CRP (elevated)
— leucocytosis

— check for haematuria
— echocardiography

Treatment   Antibiotics for 4–8 weeks. Surgery is occasionally required for myocardial abscess, refractory prosthetic valve infection or heart failure.

Prevention   The following patients must be prescribed antimicrobial cover for dental extractions, scaling and surgery:

— known congenital heart lesion
— rheumatic heart disease
— surgical systemic to pulmonary shunt
— prosthetic heart valve ⎫ *'special risk'*
— previous endocarditis ⎭

Patients needing a GA + history of penicillin allergy *or* have received course of penicillin more than once in previous month, are also deemed at 'special risk' and require parenteral prophylaxis; consult Regional Paediatric Cardiac Unit.

Acute rheumatic fever   Sharp decline in incidence over last 20–30 years in western world, though still common in some developing countries. Systemic inflammatory connective tissue disorder affecting particularly the heart, with tendency to recur. Occurs in school age children (5–15 years).

Aetiology   Related to infection with *Haemolytic streptococcus, Lancefield Gp A*, but only ~0.3% of such infections lead to rheumatic fever. Factors responsible for rheumatic sequelae in individual cases are poorly understood. There is a familial predisposition. Susceptible individuals may produce antibodies to Gp A streptococcal cell-wall polysaccharide which cross-react with glycoproteins of human heart tissue, and also in some cases with synovial and/or brain tissue.

Clinical features   Usually sore throat 2–3 weeks preceding onset of malaise, pyrexia and flitting large joint pains.

Diagnosis   Based on modified Duckett–Jones criteria (American Heart Association 1965)

Major	*Minor*
Carditis	Fever
Polyarthritis	Arthralgia
Chorea	Previous history of rheumatic fever
Subcutaneous nodules	Elevated acute phase reactants
Erythema Marginatum	Prolonged PR interval

Diagnosis requires two major or one major and two minor criteria

\+

evidence of preceding streptococcal infection

— recent scarlet fever

— raised ASOT or other streptococcal antibodies
— positive throat swab culture for Gp A streptococcus

Rheumatic carditis   Occurs in less than half of cases of acute rheumatic fever and this proportion seems to be falling. It is a pancarditis with histopathological findings of:

— endocarditis, with thrombotic vegetations on valves, particularly mitral
— myocarditis, with Aschoff bodies
— pericarditis

Evidence of cardiac involvement in rheumatic fever may include:

— tachycardia or bradycardia
— cardiac enlargement
— pericardial friction rub
— heart murmur
— heart failure
— ECG—prolonged PR and QT interval; ST and T wave changes with pericarditis
— echocardiographic findings — ventricular enlargement, vegetations, pericardial fluid, etc.

Treatment   (a) Bed rest during acute stage.
(b) Penicillin initially parenterally then orally at high doses for 10 days. Subsequently continued in prophylactic doses *indefinitely* to prevent relapse.
(c) Salicylates in high anti-inflammatory doses relieve joint pains.
(d) Steroids are sometimes given for severe carditis but their efficacy is debated.
(e) Treatment of valve disease may include balloon valvotomy, valve replacement and antimicrobial prophylaxis against endocarditis.

Arrhythmias   1. *Disturbances of conduction* (mostly at level of AV node):

— shortened AV conduction, associated with abnormal conducting pathway across AV junction, e.g. Wolff–Parkinson–White syndrome:
  • short PR interval
  • wide QRS complex
  • delta wave (slurring of upstroke of R wave)
— prolonged AV conduction: heart block
  • 1st degree found in normal children, ASD, Ebstein anomaly, acute infections, acute rheumatic fever, digoxin treatment
  • 2nd and 3rd degree associated with congenital heart disease, myocarditis, postoperative, maternal lupus

2. *Pacemaker disturbances:*

— atrial
- sinus arrhythmia; normal variant; HR increases with inspiration and slows with expiration
- premature atrial extrasystole. From ectopic focus; no treatment required
- paroxysmal supraventricular tachycardia (SVT) — commonest arrhythmia in children (1 in 25 000). Atrio-ventricular re-entry tachycardia (with accessory connexion between atrium and ventricle) is usual mechanism.

  May present with poor feeding, sweating and tach-ypnoea with HR 200–350 bpm. Prognosis good. Some remit spontaneously. Effective treatments include cold water plunge, DC shock, digoxin, flecainide, adenosine.

  Infants with underlying abnormalities causing SVTs such as Ebstein's anomaly or Wolff–Parkinson–White syndrome may have recurrent episodes
- atrial flutter or fibrillation are very rare except in association with cardiomyopathy, endocardial fibro-elastosis or Ebstein's anomaly

— ventricular
- Ventricular premature extrasystoles. These are usually unifocal and benign. Multifocal premature ventricular contractions are often related to myocardial disease
- ventricular tachycardia is rare but serious in children. In ~50% of cases a cause is found, e.g. congenital heart disease, drugs (digoxin), myocarditis, heart tumours

Hypertension

1. *Renal*

Causes
— congenital: dysplastic or polycystic kidneys
— acquired: glomerulonephritis, chronic pyelonephritis, reflux nephropathy, haemolytic–uraemic syndrome, Henoch-Schönlein purpura, Wilm's tumour

2. *Vascular*

— coarctation of aorta
— renal A stenosis or embolization
— renal V thrombosis

3. *Essential*

4. *Endocrine*

— phaeochromocytoma, neuroblastoma
— Cushing's syndrome
— Conn's syndrome
— diabetes mellitus
— adrenogenital syndrome
— hyperthyroidism

5. *Neurological*

— neurofibromatosis
— raised intracranial pressure
— encephalitis

6. *Miscellaneous*

— lead poisoning
— obesity
— porphyria
— drugs (e.g. corticosteroids)

Assessment　1. *Clinical evaluation*, including especially fundoscopy, full CVS exam including 4-limb BP, serial measurement of BP.

2. *Investigations:*

— FBC, ESR
— serum urea and electrolytes, creatinine
— urinalysis
— creatinine clearance
— CXR
— renal US
— ECG, echo
— IVU
— plasma hormone levels (renin, aldosterone, catecholamines, thyroxine, cortisol)
— urine hormone levels (catecholamines and their metabolites, e.g. vanillyl mandelic acid, VMA or homovanillic acid, HVA)
— renal angiography

Chest pain

Causes　1. *Musculoskeletal*

— 'stitch' (?strain on peritoneal ligaments attached to diaphragm)
— trauma, including rib fractures
— costo-chondritis (Tietze syndrome)
— osteitis

2. *Pulmonary*

— pneumonia
— asthma
— pneumothorax
— pleurodynia (Bornholm disease)
— infarction (sickle cell disease)

3. *Cardiac* (rare)

— pericarditis

— valve disease: aortic stenosis, Marfan syndrome (dissecting aortic aneurysm), mitral valve prolapse
— anomalous origin left coronary A

4. Gastrointestinal

— oesophagitis
— subdiaphragmatic abscess
— peptic ulcer

Role of the GP in care of child with cardiac disease

(a) Involvement in coordinated medical care of the child. In collaboration with the paediatric cardiologist and local paediatrician the GP has an important role in the care of the child in the community between hospital visits and admissions.

— monitoring growth and advising about feeding difficulties. Guidance about expected intake and growth rates may prevent parental anxiety and guilt that poor growth is due to their inadequate care
— awareness of possible medical complications and recognition of early signs, e.g. of heart failure or endocarditis
— vigilant antibacterial prophylaxis against endocarditis
— administration of routine immunizations
— prescription and monitoring of necessary drugs and awareness of possible side-effects
— close liaison with cardiologist and reiteration of their explanations, advice and plans for future management

(b) Helping the child and family to deal with likely psychosocial complications of cardiac disease

— after birth of child with congenital heart disease. Parents will usually feel very shocked and will have difficulty comprehending and remembering information. They will often need a lot of time and repeated explanations to absorb the implications of the diagnosis. Feelings of guilt and self-blame are common and it must be stressed that few causes of CHD are known. In cases where there is a recognizable syndrome or family history associated with cardiac disease, specific genetic counselling is needed
— parental anxiety. Parents are understandably invariably very anxious about such children, sometimes fearing that the child may collapse and die at any minute. This results in excessive concern and over-protectiveness, and they may find it difficult to follow the doctor's advice that the child should not be restricted but should be allowed to find his own level of activity. Working with the clinic doctor and health

visitor in the pre-school years, the GP should encourage the parents in allowing the child freedom to develop, explore and become self-reliant.

— education. Enforced school absence and limited parental expectations may result in educational difficulties. The range of intelligence of children with CHD is wider than normal, but the mean intelligence is within the normal range.

Schools must be given clear instructions about any restrictions in activity which are advised, including postoperatively, and when a return to normal activities can safely be encouraged.

— hospitalization and surgery. Such times are very stressful for the child and the whole family. Familiarity with the hospital team and anticipatory preparation for investigative and operative procedures, together with emotional and practical support from nursing staff and social workers, can help to reduce anxiety

— terminal care. When a child dies after a long illness or postoperatively, parents and siblings need opportunities to discuss their feelings and questions and continuing support through the grieving process

14. Nephrology

Urinary tract infection (UTI)

Incidence Commonest in 1st year. Incidence higher in boys in 1st month of life; more common in girls from age 6 months. Frequency of symptomatic infection up to 3% through childhood and adolescence. Asymptomatic (covert) bacteriuria also common, affecting up to 5% of girls but <1% of boys.

Aetiology Causative organisms include *Escherichia coli* (70–80%), *Klebsiella*, *Staph.albus*, *Proteus*, viruses, e.g. adenovirus type II.

Pathogenesis In the neonate, most UTIs are haematogenous; in older infants and children, organisms are usually derived from colonic flora by the ascending route. Mechanisms to prevent ascending infection depend on:

— ability to complete emptying of the urinary system
— bactericidal effect of bladder wall, possibly mediated by secretory IgA

Interference with these mechanisms accounts for the high prevalence of UTIs seen in children with:

— vesico-ureteric reflux
— neurogenic bladder
— renal calculi

However, many UTIs occur in children with apparently normal urinary tracts. Nephropathogenic bacteria such as *E. coli* ascend the urinary tract using fimbriae, which adhere to urothelial cells. Bacterial endotoxins affect ureteral peristalsis leading to intrarenal reflux, nephron damage and subsequent scarring. Renal scarring is initiated by the first UTI and may be prevented or reduced by prompt antibiotic treatment.

Vesico-ureteric reflux is found in 30–50% of children with UTI. There is a significant risk of progressive renal damage in children under 5 years with reflux nephropathy, whereas the development of new scarring after this age is relatively uncommon. Accurate diagnosis and prompt treatment for UTIs are therefore essential in children, as the potential sequelae are much more serious than in adults.

Presentation It is important always to be alert to the possibility of UTI in children who may present with:
1. Non-specific symptoms, e.g.:

— fever, febrile convulsions
— screaming attacks, irritability

— vomiting
— feeding problems
— recurrent abdominal pain

2. Symptoms related to urinary tract, e.g.:

— frequency, dysuria, haematuria
— loin pain

3. Some children with UTIs are asymptomatic.

Confirmation of diagnosis depends on examination of urine which must be carefully collected to avoid contamination. Suitable methods include:

1. *Clean catch*: The perineum is cleaned with water or a non-irritant antiseptic (with particular attention to the preputial folds in boys, which harbour large numbers of bacteria especially proteus) then a specimen is caught into a clean bowl. Bacteria multiply rapidly at room temperature so it is essential that specimens are plated within an hour of collection. If storage is unavoidable, specimens can be refrigerated at 0–4°C for up to 24 h. Dipslide cultures, innoculated during voiding, can be done at home and do not need to be kept cold. Unfortunately there is a high rate of technical failures and false positives with dipslides.

2. *Suprapubic bladder aspiration (SPA)*. When satisfactory catch specimens cannot be obtained (e.g. when there have been repeated growths of mixed organisms, in acutely ill children where rapid diagnosis is needed, or if there is obstruction of bladder outflow) direct suprapubic bladder puncture is performed after a feed when the bladder is filled and palpable.

3. *Catheter specimens (CSU)*. Catheterization carries a risk of introducing infection or contaminants and of trauma to the urethra.

4. *'Bag' specimens*. Collecting urine into a plastic bag applied to the perineum is often unsatisfactory because of contamination. Careful skin cleaning and removal of the bag immediately after voiding improve accuracy to some extent and a negative result is helpful (provided no antibiotics or antiseptics have been used). Positive results should always be confirmed by clean catch or suprapubic specimens.

Examination of urine:

1. *Bacteriuria*: Usually significant when $>10^5$ bacteria/ml (but for SPA $>10^3$/ml regarded as probably significant).

2. *Pyuria*: Occurs in about 50% of UTIs. Degree varies during time course of infection. Absence of pyuria does not disprove UTI; conversely its presence does not prove UTI. Other causes of pyuria include:

— fever due to other causes
— trauma
— drugs, e.g. cyclophosphamide, analgesics, diuretics
— calculi, nephrocalcinosis

— renal tuberculosis
— renal tubular acidosis

3. *Haematuria*: >10 RBC/mm^3 is suspicious. Not un-common in UTI.

4. *Proteinuria*: >300 mg/24 h. Non-specific finding which is of little diagnostic help in UTI. May be:

— associated with fever of any cause
— orthostatic (i.e. present in upright active child but absent when recumbent). 2–5% of normal adolescents are affected. Early manifestation of renal disease in some children
— persistent isolated proteinuria

Management   1. *Treatment of acute infection*:
• Assess for systemic toxicity, dehydration, electrolyte im-balance and treat as necessary with i.v. fluids, antipyretics, etc.
• Once diagnosis established (on basis of urine microscopy and culture), acutely unwell children should be treated with i.v. antimicrobials for up to 10 days (e.g. ampicillin, cephalosporins, aminoglycosides); most children improve rapidly and can be converted to a suitable oral antibiotic after 48 h.
• Many children with UTI are not systemically unwell. They do not require hospital admission but confirmation of the diagnosis and initiation of treatment should be performed as a matter of urgency, a course of antibiotics prescribed (e.g. amoxycillin/trimethoprim for 7 days) and arrange-ments made for investigation in all first infections as discussed below.
• Single-dose or short-course treatment has been found to be effective in adolescent girls and adults, but is not as successful as conventional regimens in children, where it is associated with increased incidence of early recurrence. It is therefore not advocated for young children, or those with systemic symptoms or abnormal urinary tracts.

2. *Evaluation of renal function*:
(a) U & E, serum creatinine.
(b) glomerular filtration rate (GFR) measured by

— inulin clearance
— radionuclide plasma disappearance curves e.g. ^{51}Cr-EDTA
— creatinine clearance test
— derived from plasma creatinine

3. *Investigation for predisposing and complicating factors*:
(a) *Preliminary* investigations

— plain X-ray of abdomen: look for renal calcification, spinal abnormalities

— renal US: check kidney size, configuration and location. US can detect reflux of Grade II or worse, changes in renal echogenicity and renal or perirenal abscesses. Provides no information about kidney function

(b) *Further* investigations may include:

— micturating cysto-urethrogram (MCUG). Bladder is catheterized and filled with contrast medium under fluoroscopic control. Provides information about:
  • bladder outline and capacity
  • post-voiding residual capacity
  • vesico-ureteric reflux (VUR). It is the definitive method to detect presence and extent of VUR, and provides information about urethra, bladder neck or calyceal anatomy

  Unpopular with patients and parents, and involves risk of introduction of infection or occasionally urethral strictures. Should only be performed after child has been free from UTI for at least 2 weeks and under antibiotic cover.

— excretory urography. Requires a cooperative child, i.v. injection of contrast medium and exposure to ionizing radiation. Provides information about:
  • renal outlines
  • parenchymal thickness, cortical scars
  • reflux; calyceal clubbing, dilatation of pericalyceal system and ureter
— Renal isotope scans. Intravenous injection of ^{99m}Tc bound to either diethylene triamine penta-acetic acid (DTPA) or dimercaptosuccinic acid (DMSA).

  DPTA is handled like inulin by the kidney; provides a measure of differential function between both kidneys and between different areas of the same kidney. Can also be used to detect reflux after voiding (but up to 20% of reflux occurs during filling and would be missed by this method).
  DMSA is taken up by functioning renal tubular epithelial cells and shows areas of renal parenchymal damage. Sensitive for detecting scarring. Gives better results in neonates than excretory urography.

— Videocystometrogram. Video recording of bladder and urethra during filling is accompanied by measurement of intravesical and detrusor pressures using bladder and rectal catheters. Provides information about intravesical pressure, presence of unstable contractions, residual volumes, reflux, bladder

outline and urine flow rate. Particularly useful in children with neuropathic bladder.
— Radionuclide voiding cystography. Alternative to MCU. The bladder is catheterized and filled with ^{99m}Tc-pertechnetate and saline. Isotope detected in upper tracts indicates reflux. Sensitive; involves less radiation than MCU. Fails to provide anatomical details about bladder and urethra so is not suitable as initial investigation, but may be useful in follow-up of reflux in children old enough to cooperate (>3–4 years).
— cystoscopy. Provides information about the trigone and ureteral orifices; important in assessing prognosis in severe VUR, and helpful in cases of severe chronic cystitis.

The best scheme for investigation varies according to age of patient, clinical circumstances and facilities available locally. The following guidelines are suggested for investigation after first UTI:

Infants		1–7 years	7 years +
AXR + US + MCU +DMSA	all cases	AXR + US + DMSA + MCU if: — above investigation abnormal — first infection was acute pyelonephritis — recurrence of infection — family history of chronic atrophic pyelonephritis	AXR + US

If expertise or facilities for US or DMSA are not available, excretory urography may be substituted but may give unsatisfactory visualization in infants.

Serial US is useful in follow-up, with repeat DMSA scans helpful in following the progress of renal scarring.

4. *Prophylaxis against recurrence.* After treatment of a proven UTI, low-dose chemoprophylaxis should be continued in all cases until investigation of the urinary tract is complete.

— if MCU is planned, the risk of infection entailed by catheterization should be covered by prescription of trimethoprim at full dosage for 48 h from time of procedure
— long-term low-dose prophylactic antibiotics appreciably reduce re-infection rates. Drugs which are effective and usually well tolerated include trimethoprim and nitrofurantion (doses 1–2 mg/kg/day) usually given as a single

dose at night, so drug remains in bladder urine for several hours overnight. Prophylaxis is advisable for:
- children <5 years with VUR
- children with obstructive lesions of urinary tract, urolithiasis, renal scarring, neurogenic bladder (often difficult to eradicate bacteriuria; only treat when symptomatic)
  Surgical correction of urological anomalies often necessary before infection can be cleared.
- recurrent symptomatic UTI not associated with any detectable anatomical anomaly.

5. *Monitoring for recurrence.* Urine should be cultured after completion of treatment of first UTI to ensure infection eradicated, then at regular intervals for at least 2 years. Repeated infections are common in children; more than 50% of recurrences occur within 6 months, but the risk of recurrence continues for up to 5 years.

In addition, regular monitoring of blood pressure and growth is important in children with recurrent UTIs, together with serial US and renal isotope studies to monitor renal growth and function, as above.

Vesico-ureteric reflux (VUR)

VUR is found in about one-third of children investigated following a UTI. In some cases it may be familial. It is generally regarded as an abnormal finding though it has been found in up to 30% of healthy children under 5 years and its significance probably depends on its severity and the coexistence of infection. The combination of reflux and infection can produce segmental renal scarring (reflux nephropathy) which is the most important cause of renal hypertension and chronic renal failure in childhood.

Classification

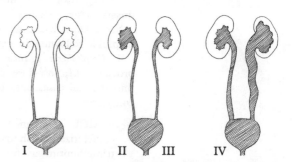

Fig. 3 Grades of reflux. Grade I — reflux into lower end of ureter without dilatation; grade II — reflux entering up to kidney on micturition only; grade III — reflux entering up to kidney both during bladder filling and during voiding; grade IV — reflux with dilatation of ureter or renal pelvis

Natural history   Tends to improve with time; complete spontaneous remission in up to 60%. Resolution is less likely with more severe grades of reflux. Renal scarring is most frequent with infections in the first 2 years of life, particularly with severe reflux, but it may develop later and may be associated even with milder degrees of reflux.

Management   (a) After treatment of first UTI, low-dose chemoprophylaxis should be continued with regular urine monitoring for as long as reflux persists.
(b) Monitor renal growth and morphology with serial US scans. DTPA or radionuclide voiding cystography are a useful alternative to repeating MCUG when monitoring progress of VUR
(c) Management of severe (Grade IV) reflux remains contentious; such cases should be referred for expert urological opinion. Options are:
— consevative medical management including chemoprophylaxis
— surgical re-implantation of ureters
— endoscopic submucosal Teflon injection

Haematuria

Definition   >10 erythrocytes/mm^3 urine. Reagent strips (e.g. Hematest, Labstix) give positive results in the presence of haemoglobin, usually in the erythrocytes but occasionally as free haemoglobin or myoglobin, so urine microscopy is essential to confirm erythrocyturia and to look for red cell casts which indicate a renal cause for the bleeding.

Causes   1. Common

— benign recurrent haematuria
— contamination: menstrual
— haematologic: sickle cell disease
— hypoxia, asphyxia, hypovolaemia: acute tubular necrosis, cortical necrosis
— infections: pyelonephritis, cystitis, urethritis
— meatal stenosis
— phimosis
— post-infectious glomerulonephritis
— trauma
• accidental: fractured pelvis, renal contusion, post-catheterization/circumcision
• non-accidental

2. Uncommon

— allergy
— diabetic nephropathy
— drug-induced: analgesic nephropathy, cyclophosphamide
— exercise

— glomerulonephritis: membranous, membrano-proliferative with vasculitis–HSP, HUS, SLE, etc.
— haematologic: thrombocytopenia, haemophilia, DIC
— hydronephrosis
— hypercalciuria
— infections: malaria, schistosomiasis, TB etc
— neoplasms: Wilm's tumour
— polycystic kidneys
— recurrent haematuria syndromes: Alport's syndrome, IgA nephropathy
— renal calculi
— renal vein thrombosis
— urethral foreign body

Acute nephritis   A variety of glomerular lesions ranging in extent and severity are seen in this disease. In some forms renal involvement is the primary event; in others the nephropathy is just one feature of a generalized systemic disorder.

Primary glomerulonephritis may present with:

— acute nephritis
— nephrotic syndrome
— asymptomatic proteinuria
— recurrent haematuria

There are seven types of glomerulonephritis (GN).

1. Minimal change   On light microscopy glomeruli look normal or show minimal changes of mesangial hypertrophy and occasional patchy glomerulosclerosis. Electron microscopy (EM) shows (reversible) fusion of glomerular epithelial cell foot processes. Usually presents with nephrotic syndrome (q.v.). Occasionally causes only asymptomatic proteinuria or benign recurrent haematuria.

2. Membranous   Diffuse thickening of glomerular capillary walls. EM shows subepithelial deposits of IgG and C3 with the basement membrane extending between them as spiky finger-like processes.

Causative agent not established. Associated antigens include Hep B_sAg, syphilis, SLE, drugs.

Often has very prolonged course and may become quiescent but 50% of adults progress to renal failure over 10 years. Very uncommon in children and their prognosis is better, with only ~15% developing renal failure.

3. Diffuse endocapillary proliferative   Most common cause of acute nephritis in children, though incidence is declining. Most cases are the immunological consequences of infection of respiratory tract or skin with nephritogenic strains of Gp A haemolytic streptococcus (though occasionally precipitated by viral infection).

Incidence: peaks at 3–7 years. M:F 2:1.

Histopathology
— polymorphonuclear infiltrate and oedema of glomeruli
— increased cellularity of endothelium and mesangium
— infrequently, epithelial crescent formation

Antibodies produced in response to infection probably cross-react with endogenous basement membrane to form immune complexes visible on EM as deposits within the capillary walls.

Clinical features
May be history of pharyngitis or impetigo 7–14 days previously, followed by abrupt onset of:

— malaise
— haematuria (smoky-brown urine colour)
— oedema, usually periorbital initially
— oliguria
— acute hypertension which may cause headaches, seizures, encephalopathy or acute LVF with pulmonary oedema

Usually two stages:
(a) Oliguria with hypervolaemia, hypertension, uraemia (1–2 weeks)
(b) Diuresis and natriuresis

Investigations
— haematuria with casts, leucocyturia, proteinuria (usually <1 g/24 h)
— mild anaemia (usually due to haemodilution)
— raised ESR
— raised serum urea and creatinine
— Evidence of preceding streptococcal infection
  • on throat/skin swab
  • raised ASOT > 200 Todd unit/ml
  • positive anti-streptococcal deoxyribonuclease B (anti-DNase B)
  • reduced plasma C3 concentrations (bad prognosis if low for >1 month)

Management
(a) *Antibiotics.* Penicillin for at least 2 weeks (unless allergic).
(b) *Acute renal insufficicency*:

— fluid restriction during oliguric phase (see p. 234)
— provision of adequate calories (~400/m^2/day)
— restrict protein (0.5–1 g/kg/day) if increasing urea >25 mmol/l
— monitor for and treat hyperkalaemia

(c) *Acute hypertension*:

— bed rest
— drugs, e.g. hydrallazine, reserpine; diazoxide in acute hypertensive emergency, e.g. seizures, encephalopathy
— sodium restriction

(d) *Recovery*. During the diuretic phase, diet can return to normal. Once hypertension, oliguria and gross haematuria have abated activity can be increased gradually as tolerated, with a return to school about a week after normal activity is resumed at home.

Prognosis   Outcome for most children is very good. Histological changes usually start to resolve after 2–3 weeks and have disappeared by about 2 months. 5–10% develop rapidly progressive glomerulonephritis and chronic renal failure.

4. Diffuse mesangial proliferative   Commonest form of GN worldwide. Histological increase in mesangial cells and matrix with deposition of mesangial IgA and IgG. (Also known as mesangial IgA nephropathy or Berger disease). Usually presents with recurrent macroscopic haematuria. Benign in majority but ~15% of children develop renal insufficiency or sustained hypertension (particularly those who have persistent proteinuria between episodes of haematuria).

5. Diffuse mesangiocapillary (membranoproliferative)   Although relatively uncommon overall, this disorder causes about 25% of cases of progressive GN in childhood. Characterized by:

— persistent hypocomplementaemia
— histology shows thickened hypercellular capillary loops with splintering of the basement membrane (tramline effect). EM shows dense deposits in subendothelium (type I) or basement membrane (type II)
— presence of C3-nephritic factor (a 7s globulin autoantibody which interferes with feedback control of the enzymes of the alternate complement activation pathway)

Onset usually after age 6 years. May be familial. May complicate *Staph. albus* infection of ventriculo-atrial shunts.
    Variable course; most cases progress to renal failure over 5–10 years.

Treatment   Steroids, cyclophosphamide, dipyridamole and anticoagulants are under study but no treatment yet proven to be effective. (Shunt nephritits usually resolves after removal of the shunt and treatment with antibiotics.)

6. Diffuse crescentic (rapidly progressive GN (RPGN))   May be superimposed on any underlying pattern of GN, or is often a feature of systemic disorder e.g. SLE, Henoch-Schönlein purpura, infective endocarditis.

Histology   Crescentic aggregations of proliferating epithelial cells which become fibrosed and scarred.

Treatment   In severe cases immunosuppressants have been tried, particularly cyclophosphamide, and also plasmapheresis. Transplant may be successful but sometimes the disease recurs in the graft.

Prognosis   Depends on extent of crescent formation. If >80% glomeruli affected, rapid deterioration is seen. If few crescents, may heal with only local scars.

7. **Focal and segmental glomerulosclerosis**   Non-specific pattern of scarring involving only parts of some glomeruli. Seen in generalized systemic disorders, Henoch-Schönlein purpura and idiopathic nephrotic syndrome. Variable prognosis.

Henoch-Schönlein nephritis   See also p. 228.

The majority of children with HSP have some renal involvement. About half have microscopic haematuria which resolves spontaneously; more serious kidney disease occurs in a smaller proportion. 20–30% have gross haematuria. Heavy proteinuria may indicate diffuse RPGN, often with a nephrotic phase. A small number develop severe hypertension and ARF requiring dialysis. No treatment is of proven value, but in the severely ill patient with life-threatening GN, combined therapy with cytotoxics, anticoagulants and corticosteroids has been tried.

Follow-up should continue for at least 3 months and until all urinary abnormalities have disappeared.

Nephrotic syndrome (NS)   Manifestation of a variety of disease processes which involve increased permeability of the glomerular basement membrane with resultant proteinuria.

Clinical features   — proteinuria
— hypoalbuminaemia
— generalized oedema
— hyperlipidaemia

Major complications   — hypovolaemia: may lead to circulatory collapse and ARF
— thrombotic tendency:
  • increased clotting factors, V, VII, VIII, X, fibrinogen
  • thrombocytosis and increased platelet aggregability
  • decreased plasma concentration of antithrombin III
  • hypovolaemia
— increased susceptibility to infection:
  • low plasma IgG
  • decreased serum factor B
  • improved opsonization
  • protein malnutrition
  • immunosuppressant drugs

Causes   1. *Congenital*

— Finnish type
— diffuse mesangial sclerosis
— syphilis

2. *Idiopathic* (primary NS)

— minimal change GN (70–80%)
— focal segmental glomerulosclerosis (10%)
— diffuse proliferative GN (10%)
— membranous (2%)

3. *Secondary*

— HSP
— infection: shunt nephritis, bacterial endocarditis malaria, leprosy, schistosomiasis
— collagen disorders e.g. SLE
— diabetes mellitus
— sickle cell disease
— toxins, e.g. drugs-penicillamine, captopril; heavy metals
— allergy, e.g. bee stings, pollens
— mechanical, e.g. RVT, constrictive pericarditis
— lymphoproliferative neoplasia, e.g. Hodgkin's

Minimal change NS (steroid responsive) In children the majority of cases of NS have only minimal changes on LM; >90% of these respond to steroid therapy. Incidence: 2 in 100 000 (UK). M:F 2:1. Peak 2–5 years.

Presentation History of preceding URTI in one-third. Usually insidious onset with periorbital oedema, then ankles, scrotum, ascites, pleural effusions. In severe cases, intravascular volume depletion leads to poor renal perfusion and hypovolaemic circulatory failure, characterized by abdominal pain and vomiting with reduced CVP and cold peripheries. Note that paradoxical hypertension is sometimes seen in response to severe hypovolaemia.

Investigation — urine protein > 1 g/m^2/24 h
— serum albumin <25 g/l
— highly selective proteinuria (i.e. clearance (C) of low m. wt proteins, e.g. transferrin or albumin, is greater than that of high m. wt protein, e.g. IgG.

$$\frac{C_{IgG}}{C_{transferrin}} \quad <0.1 = \text{highly selective proteinuria}$$

— haematuria in <10%
— increased serum cholesterol, triglycerides
— C3 normal in minimal change nephrotic syndrome whereas persistently low in nephrotics with underlying mesangiocapillary or post-streptococcal GN
— in patients with circulating volume contraction, very low urine sodium concentration (<10 mmol/l) and increased PCV

Management Hospital admission is necessary for assessment and treatment of presenting episode.

1. *Corticosteroids.* Oral prednisolone (dosage 60 mg/m^2/24 h) until proteinuria disappears for 3 consecutive days. Dosage reduced to 40 mg/m^2/24 h, then reduced to alternate day regimen and tapered down gradually over 2–3 months.

Most steroid-responsive patients enter remission within 2 weeks; if there is no response at 4 weeks, renal biopsy is indicated.

2. *Antimicrobials*:

— suspect infection in every sick nephrotic child; they are specially prone to pneumococcal peritonitis, cellulitis, UTI and Gram negative septicaemia (particularly after steroid treatment). Prophylactic penicillin during the acute phase is sometimes advocated but is of unproven value

— immunization with pneumococcal vaccine may be protective

— specific globulin should be given to nephrotics exposed to viral infections such as varicella or measles

3. *Diet and fluids*:

— urgent plasma infusion is required for those with evidence of volume contraction

— if there is progressive oedema, a no-added-salt diet is given (reducing sodium intake to 40–80 mmol/day). Some advise fluid restriction to ~1 l/day but it is preferable to normalize the sodium concentration and so reduce thirst

— adequate protein and calorie intake is important and will be supplied if the child will eat a normal balanced diet

4. *Diuretics*:

— used in acute stage concommitantly with intravenous albumin in children with severe oedema

— useful in chronic oedema in steroid-dependent children.

5. *Family education and support.* It is important to help the child and family to understand the nature of the disease and to prepare them for the possibility of relapses. They need to learn how to monitor for proteinuria at home. Practical and emotional support will be needed for families where the child's illness runs a chronic course.

6. *Management of relapses.*

(a) Treated with steroids, aiming to tail off completely each time but if there are frequent relapses (3 or more in 12 months), the child is considered steroid-dependent and is maintained on alternate day prednisolone for at least 6 months. Side-effects of steroids must be watched for. These include:

— growth retardation (less with alternate day regimens)
— hypertension and oedema

— Cushingoid obesity with moon face, buffalo hump and striae
— osteoporosis
— increased protein catabolism (associated with increased appetite)
— altered psychological state, usually euphoria
— diabetes mellitus
— GI complications, including peptic ulcer, pancreatitis
— intracranial hypertension
— sudden adrenal insufficiency (Addisonian crisis)

Contraindications to steroids:

— persistent hypocomplementaemia ⎫ biopsy
— haematuria, systemic hypertension, uraemia ⎬ advised
— exposure to varicella or measles (temporary)
— bacterial infection
— other disease, e.g. peptic ulcer

(b) Immunosuppressive agents such as cyclophosphamide are a valuable adjunct to treatment in the frequent relapser suffering unacceptable steroid effects, though cyclophosphamide also has side-effects (including reversible baldness, increased vulnerability to infection and sterility).

Prognosis   It should be remembered that there is a tendency for spontaneous complete remission in a considerable proportion even without treatment. Long-term prognosis is good for the majority of children with steroid-responsive disease.

Haemolytic-uraemic syndrome (HUS)   Characterized by acute haemolysis and acute renal failure. Leading cause of acute renal failure in children.
      Incidence and natural history vary with geographical area. Clusters occur. Verocytotoxin-producing *Escherichia coli* (VTEC, serotype 0157:H7) is the most common infectious trigger. May be due to hypersensitivity to infection, often enteral, triggering an abnormal platelet-vascular interaction, causing intravascular coagulation with microangiopathy seen in the kidney, where there are fibrin thrombi in capillaries and arterioles. Recent evidence suggests defective release of prostacyclin, the natural inhibitor of platelet aggregation.

Clinical features   — prodrome-diarrhoea, often bloody + abdominal pain ±vomiting, fever. May last from 1 day to >2 weeks
      — acute renal disease: haematuria, proteinuria, acute microangiopathic haemolytic anaemia with burr cells and fragmented cells + thrombocytopenia in 85%
            ±Complications of ARF: hypertension, severe acidosis, hyperkalaemia, heart failure, coma, severe anaemia
      — pallor, bruising, purpura
      — jaundice

— splenomegaly
— neurolgical: tremor, hemiparesis, fits

Management   (a) Management of acute renal failure as below.

(b) Transfusion may be required if Hb falls below ~7 g/dl. Use small volumes to avoid aggravating hypertension; with severe anaemia transfusion should be given by partial exchange transfusion or accompanied by dialysis to remove excess fluid.

(c) i.v. heparin has been used because of the underlying thrombotic microangiopathy but its value is not proven.

(d) other experimental approaches under evaluation include:

— fibrinolytic agents, e.g. streptokinase
— plasmapheresis
— prostacyclin infusion

Prognosis   Mortality rate has fallen from 50 to 5% as recognition and management have improved. Recovery of renal function usually starts within 21 days, may take up to a year. Residual CRF in 10–30%.

Acute renal failure (ARF)

Characterized by sudden disruption of kidney function resulting in oliguria (defined as urine output <300 ml/m^2/day) and or rising serum urea and creatinine.

Causes in childhood   1. *Pre-renal*:

— hypovolaemia
  • acute gastroenteritis
  • post-surgery, particularly cardiopulmonary bypass
  • burns
  • nephrotic syndrome
  • salt wasting disorders
— hypotension
  • Septicaemia
  • Hypothermia

2. *Renal*:

— Haemolytic-uraemic syndrome
— acute glomerulonephritis
— renal vein thrombosis
— nephrotoxins
— congenital glomerular or tubular disorder

3. *Post-renal*:

— congenital obstructive uropathy, e.g. posterior urethral valves
— acquired — calculi, pelvic mass

Management   (a) Assess circulation and resuscitate as necessary, e.g. plasma expanders, ventilation (needed in about 25% of patients with ARF).

(b) Establish cause of ARF from history, examination and investigations, including serum and urine biochemistry, FBC, film, urinalysis, infection screen, renal imaging).

(c) Hyperkalaemia

— Calcium gluconate i.v.
— calcium resonium oral/rectal
— correct metabolic acidosis
— glucose/insulin infusion
— dialysis if severe hyperkalaemia not responding quickly to above measures

(d) Fluid overload (hypertension, pulmonary oedema, raised JVP, raised CVP). During oliguria restrict fluid intake to replacement of insensible water losses plus measured urine output. Challenge with i.v. frusemide; if response poor, dialysis probably required.

(e) Hypocalcaemia, hypomagnesaemia: may cause convulsions or tetany. Hyperphosphataemia treated with aluminium hydroxide gel.

(f) Treat sepsis with i.v. antibiotics

(g) Nutrition: maintain adequate calories with restricted protein. TPN often necessary.

(h) Dialysis. Decision to dialyse based on assessment of clinical course and laboratory data. Indications include:
— diuretic-resistant hypervolaemia with hypertension and pulmonary oedema
— uraemia (>54 mmol/l)
— dialysable nephrotoxin
— hyperkalaemia
— hyperphosphataemia and hypocalaemia ⎱ relative indications — can usually be
— severe metabolic acidosis ⎰ controlled by above measures

Chronic renal failure (CRF)

Definition   Glomerular filtration rate <25% normal for at least 3 months

Prevalence   20–50 cases per million children (Europe).

Causes in childhood   In order of frequency:

— congenital malformations — obstructive uropathy, reflux nephropathy, hypoplasia-dysplasia
— glomerulonephritis
— hereditary nephropathies
— vascular disorders — haemolytic–uraemic syndrome, renal vein thrombosis
— other — renal tumours, unknown

Symptoms   Often vague: lassitude, anorexia, nausea, headache. May present with anaemia, hypertension, growth failure, haematuria or proteinuria.

Management   1. *General management* includes regular monitoring and assessment of potential problems:

— biochemical disturbances
— nutrition and growth
— hypertension
— renal osteodystrophy
— infection
— anaemia
— social and emotional development
— family relationships
— progress in school

2. *Dialysis*. Usually undertaken when plasma creatinine >500 µmol/l. Peritoneal dialysis (PD) more often used in acute situations: children in end-stage CRF have usually been managed by haemodialysis (HD). Continuous ambulatory peritoneal dialysis (CAPD) is an alternative form of long-term therapy becoming more widely used in children.

(a) HD requires vascular access using either external arteriovenous shunt or internal arteriovenous fistula. Usually done 3 times per week. Though complex, can be performed at home by suitably motivated parents but requires a high degree of commitment and discipline from family.

(b) PD may be performed by continuous cycling machine via indwelling peritoneal catheter overnight as child sleeping or by CAPD, which involves four exchanges of peritoneal fluid daily.

As effective as HD, especially in children, in whom the peritoneal surface area per unit body weight is larger than in adults.

Advantages of CAPD include psychosocial, decreased transfusion requirement and more normal blood pressure. The main disadvantage is the risk of peritonitis. Used in up to 25% of children with end-stage CRF in recent years.

Though there is evidence of reduction in levels of emotional disturbance in children dialysed at home, this is at the expense of parental stress and disruption of family relationships. A well-integrated support service is essential and children do better if management is supervised at specialized centres (those managing >3 children with CRF per annum) with resources of a paediatric nephrologist, psychiatrist, dietician, hospital school. Because of the relative rarity of the problem and difficulty of frequent travelling, <40% of children are managed in such centres.

3. *Renal transplantation*. Preferred treatment and feasible for most children, with good chance of success. 3-year graft survival: 65% cadaveric grafts; 87% live-related donor.

However, there are many potential problems:

— supply of donor kidneys

— hazards of immunosuppression e.g. increased susceptibility to infection, and to neoplasia, steroid effects, e.g.
growth failure, cataracts. A combination of immunosuppressants is used, including: prednisolone, AZTP,
cyclosporin, monoclonal antibodies (e.g. OKT3), e.g.
antithymocyte globulin (ATG)
— graft rejection: symptoms may include fever, graft
tenderness, hypertension, oliguria and deterioration of
renal function. Managed with bolus corticosteroids,
ATG
— emotional. Dialysis and transplantation programmes involve considerable psychological stress for the child and
family resulting in difficulties with social and emotional
adaptation. Problem areas include obesity, stature and
other cosmetic effects of treatment resulting in low self
esteem and poor compliance. Prolonged and frequent
hospitalization and restricted activities impair social
development and family relationships. Anxiety regarding
the status of the graft, with the overshadowing threat that
it may fail at any time, contributes to the high rate of
psychiatric morbidity in children with end-stage CRF
and their parents

A renal replacement programme must integrate all these
aspects of management with the aims of:

— optimizing the child's physical and emotional health and
development
— helping the family to deal with the strains imposed by
chronic illness while preserving as far as possible a
normal family life

15. Paediatric gynaecology

Many gynaecological problems in childhood reflect the endocrine changes evolving from the perinatal period through to adolescence and sexual maturity. Increasing sexual awareness and activity in adolescence in contemporary society, with associated increase in venereal disease and teenage pregnancies, make it imperative that sex education, sympathetic counselling and accessible contraception are readily available to this age group, though the provision of such services may raise difficult issues of morality and confidentiality.

Gynaecological examination

Examination of the genitalia should always be part of the neonatal check in order to detect developmental abnormalities and also to become familiar with the normal anatomical appearance in the newborn. When necessary in older children, gynaecological examination should be preceded by history taking and done as part of a complete physical examination in the presence of a parent or other trusted adult. Some teenagers may prefer their mother not to be present; their wishes for privacy must be respected.

With small children it is often least traumatic to perform the examination with the child on mother's knee, with hips flexed and knees drawn up and spread. For older girls the Sims position is usually most comfortable; adequate drapes and a good examination light are important. Any swabs, slides or instruments which may be needed should be readily to hand; a tape measure is occasionally helpful.

Normal variations in the newborn

(a) Transplacental passage of maternal oestrogens may cause several effects in the neonate:

— breast swelling
— vulval congestion
— prominent hymen, hymeneal tags
— white vaginal discharge
— vaginal bleeding

These changes disappear quickly and require no treatment.

(b) Premature babies often have a relatively prominent clitoris and labia minora.

(c) Labial adhesions are rare and are only important because the resulting appearance of a flat vulva with no tissue visible below the clitoris is occasionally mistaken for congenital absence of the vagina, which causes much parental anxiety. The adhesions usually separate after the application of oestrogen cream topically for 2 weeks, revealing normal underlying anatomy. They sometimes recur.

Normal variations in older children

See p. 134.

Causes of vulval irritation/vaginal discharge

1. Vulvovaginitis

Commonest gynaecological disorder of children. Arises because the vagina of the child lacks the protective acid secretion of the reproductive period and because pathogenic organisms gain access to the vagina with relative ease owing to:

— proximity of vagina and anus
— lack of labial fat pads protecting vaginal orifice
— wrong wiping direction
— bottom-shuffling and crawling round floors, sandpits, etc.
— dirty fingers

Infecting organisms are often mixed flora of low virulence but may be spread from focus elsewhere, e.g. *Haemolytic streptococcus*. Organisms most commonly cultured in children and adolescents are *Gardnerella vaginalis*, *Candida albicans* and *trichomonas*. Threadworm infestation may also cause vulvovaginitis.

A vaginal foreign body should be considered if discharge is blood-stained or offensive.

Treatment

(a) If a specific organism is present, antibiotics may be indicated.
(b) Exclude underlying cause, e.g. diabetes mellitus, broad-spectrum antibiotics, sexual abuse or ectopic ureter.
(c) Attention to vulval hygiene, with daily baths, clean cotton pants and avoidance of irritant antiseptics, bubble baths and bath oils.
(d) In refractory cases dienoestrol cream topically may help to clear infection by improving acidity.

2. Local skin disorders

(a) Lichen sclerosis et atrophicus. Usually affects post-menopausal women but may present in childhood with a white wrinkled dystrophic appearance of the vulva and associated irritation. Mainly affects vulva and perineum but may appear on any part of body, so it is important to examine child thoroughly. Cause not known but age distribution suggests low oestrogen levels as predisposing factor. Up to 30% of patients have an accompanying autoimmune disorder. A similar appearance may result from chronic friction, which in some cases may raise the suspicion of child sexual abuse.

Treatment:

— vulval hygiene
— topical steroids for troublesome cases
— treat secondary infection
— often regresses spontaneously at puberty

(b) Eczema.
(c) Vulval psoriasis.
(d) Seborrhoeic dermatitis.
(e) Erythema multiforme.

Vaginal bleeding in the prepubertal child

This important symptom should never be ignored. Possible causes include:

— trauma
  • accidental: straddle injuries
  • sexual abuse
  • vaginal foreign body
  • local vulval lesions: scratching of lichen sclerosis or threadworms; prolapsed urethra
— infection, e.g. streptococcus, shigella, enterobiasis (pinworm), schistosomiasis
— precocious puberty (see p. 90)
— tumour
— structural: urethral/vaginal prolapse

Disorders of menstruation

Excessive menstrual bleeding (Menorrhagia)

Irregular and heavy periods are common in the first 2 years post-menarche and are due to anovulatory cycles, resulting in continuous endometrial proliferation with eventual heavy shedding. The cycle usually becomes regular with time and treatment is rarely needed. If there is no improvement after 6 months the patient should be referred for assessment. Hormone therapy is occasionally necessary and rare causes should be excluded (hypothyroidism, bleeding disorder, endometriosis, IUCD).

Painful periods (dysmenorrhoea)

Colicky cramps usually on day 1 of bleeding affect up to two-thirds of teenage girls and are a major cause of school absenteeism. Due to endometrial production of $PGF2_\alpha$ and E2 causing smooth muscle stimulation.

Treatment
• Analgesics and antispasmodics, e.g. Buscopan.
• Prostaglandin inhibitors, e.g. mefenamic acid (Ponstan).
• Oral contraceptives (OC) to inhibit ovulation.

Amenorrhoea

Primary   Never menstruated.

Normal age range for menarche in UK is 10–16 years. Average weight at menarche is 47 kg. Clues as to likely cause of amenorrhoea provided by development of secondary sexual characteristics.

(a) Sexual development otherwise normal; consider:

— absent vagina: check chromosomes
  • XY (testicular feminization)
  • XX (abdominal US and IVP, check uterus and kidneys)
— imperforate hymen: retained menstrual blood accumulates in vagina (haematocolpos). May present as emergency with abdominal pain, mass, acute retention. Treat by incision of membrane to release fluid

(b) Poor/absent sexual development:

— constitutional
— hypothalamic/pituitary lesion, e.g. tumour, Laurence-Moon-Biedl syndrome
— gonadal dysgenesis, e.g. 45XO (Turner syndrome)

(c) Heterosexual pubertal changes. Signs of virilization may be due to:

— intersex
— congenital adrenal hyperplasia
— tumour (adrenal or ovarian)

Secondary   Cessation of periods >6 months in non-pregnant patient between ages of 16 and 40 years.

Causes:

(a) Hypothalamic/pituitary

— emotional stress   ⎫
— acute weight loss, anorexia nervosa ⎬ 45%
— post treatment with combined OC
— tumour

(b) Ovarian

— premature ovarian failure
— polycystic ovary syndrome (Stein–Leventhal)
— androgen-producing tumour

(c) Adrenal

— congenital adrenal hyperplasia
— Cushing syndrome

(d) Hypothyroidism.
(e) Uterine

— pelvic infection, e.g. TB
— intrauterine adhesions (Aschermann syndrome)

Sexual activity and contraception in the adolescent

Accurate data about sexual activity in young people is difficult to gather, but UK studies suggest that the percentage of teenage girls who are sexually active increases from about 10% at 13 years to 50% at 19 years, with an increasing trend towards sexual initiation at a younger age. Live birth rates in teenage mothers of 15 years or less remain about 8 in 1000 and abortion rates in the same group are rising (10 in 1000 in 1985). Pregnancy rates in 16–19-year olds are even higher.

These statistics emphasize the need for contraceptive advice for teenagers in whom contraceptive usage rates are alarmingly low due to lack of knowledge about, and availability of, contraception.

Contraceptive clinics can encourage adolescent attendence by an informal setting and well-trained non-judgemental staff able to counsel young people of either sex about any type of sexual problem with assured privacy and confidentiality.

Legal aspects

When prescribing contraceptives to adolescents under 16 years, the doctor should be guided by the advice of Lord Fraser in the Gillick case, which has been endorsed by the General Medical Council. The doctor must be satisfied that the girl understands the advice, that she is very likely to begin or continue to have sexual intercourse with or without contraceptive treatment, and that her physical and/or mental health is likely to suffer unless she receives contraceptive advice or treatment. The doctor should discuss with the patient the desirability of informing her parents, but refusal to do so does not preclude the prescribing of contraception and confidentiality is paramount.

Special groups

Teenagers in foster care are particularly likely to be in need of counselling; they are 50% more likely to have sexual intercourse before the age of 18 years, are twice as likely to have been pregnant, and are less likely to use contraceptives.

Another group whose needs for sex education have not been adequately met are those with chronic disabilities. A recent study of young adults with myelomeningocele found that only 1 in 5 had received information regarding their sexual or reproductive function though a quarter had experienced sexual activity. There was evidence of increased sexual awareness and improved social life in this group compared with earlier studies.

Mentally handicapped

Contraception may be requested in this group because of signs of increasing sexual awareness or occasionally because of the risk of sexual abuse. It is important that young people with minor mental handicap be educated about sex and encouraged to enjoy physical relationships; but they are at increased risk of having retarded offspring and should be advised about suitable contraceptive methods like any other sexually active teenager.

OCs are suitable providing the pills can be administered regularly. Many of these patients are taking anticonvulsants and may therefore need a higher oestrogen dose (e.g. 50 µg). IUCDs are useful if there are not menstrual disorders. If both of these methods are contraindicated, depot progestogens are useful. Barrier methods are not suitable.

Sterilization is sometimes requested but preferable alternative methods can usually be found. If no other solution seems possible, legal advice should be sought; if the teenager is >16-years old, court approval is required.

Contraceptive methods in adolescence	Choice of method must be made on an individual basis.
Barrier methods, e.g. condom + spermicide	Very suitable in this age group as they provide some protection against STDs, and the risk of AIDS has prompted many teenagers to change their sexual behaviour. Widely available but proper use requires motivation and adequate knowledge.
Diaphragm + spermicide	Only suitable for highly motivated teenager after detailed instruction; many find them awkward to fit and high failure rate in teenagers.
Oral contraceptives (OC)	Generally reliable method, though remembering to take the pill regularly is not always compatible with adolescent lifestyles. Caution recommended in very young girls because of concern regarding possible neoplastic effects (cervix, breast) associated with long-term use of the combined OC.
Intrauterine devices (IUD)	Associated with increased risk of pelvic infection and not a method of choice in adolescents.
Post-coital contraception	Generally used only as emergency measure; carries a theoretical risk of teratogenicity. Useful for teenager presenting within 72 h after unprotected intercourse.
Possible consequences of adolescent motherhood	(a) Increased risk of preterm and low birth weight infants.
	(b) Interruption of maternal education and frustration of ambitions.
	(c) Single parenting; only 50% of under 16 year olds maintain a relationship with the father of their child after delivery.
	(d) Increased risk of poor mothering skills and child abuse.

16. Neurology

Normal CSF

	WBC ($\times 10^6$/l)	Glucose (mmol/1)		Protein (g/l)	Pressure (mmH$_2$0)
Pre-term	<20	1.3–3.4	>50% of	<1.5	40–150
Term	<10	1.9–6.6	blood	<1.0	
>1 year	<5	2.8–4.8	glucose	0.2–0.4	70–180

Volume		
	Infants	40–60 ml
	Young children	60–100 ml
	Older children	80–120 ml
	Adults	120–160 ml

CSF findings in CNS infections

	Leucocytes/ml	Protein (g/l)	Glucose (mmol/1)	Smear	Comments
Acute bacterial meningitis	100–2000+ PMN predominate	↑	↓	Organisms may be seen	Countercurrent immunoelectrophoresis (CIE) or Latex agglutination for bacterial antigen in CSF may help if cultures negative (e.g. if pre-treated with antibiotics)
Viral meningitis	100–1000 PMN early then lymphocytes predominate	Normal or slightly ↑	Normal (low in mumps in 20% of cases)	Negative	Virus culture from CSF e.g. enterovirus Paired sera for antibodies
Tuberculosis	10–500 PMN early then lymphocytes	↑ (0.6–5)	↑		Ziehl–Nielsen and immunofluorescence

Meningitis Infectious meningitis may be due to bacteria, viruses, myco-plasmas, fungi, spirochaetes or protozoa.

Pathogenesis Organisms may reach the meninges either by haematogenous spread or from a contiguous focus of infection such as otitis media or sinusitis. Bacterial invasion causes inflammation of the meninges which become covered by a thick fibrinopurulent exudate, usually thickest at the base of the brain where it may:

— obstruct CSF circulation causing hydrocephalus
— interfere with diffusion of drugs through the CSF
— damage the cranial nerves
— lead to thrombosis of cerebral vessels

Other complications   — subdural effusion may develop (particularly in haemophilus meningitis)
— pus may become encapsulated (particularly in pneumococcal meningitis)
— ventriculitis (particularly in infants with myelomeningoceles)

Epidemiology   Bacterial meningitis is more common:

— in winter and spring
— between 2 months and 2 years
— in boys

Organisms responsible vary with the age of the child.

	Common	Less common
Neonate	Group B strep.	*List. monocytogenes*
	E. coli	*Pseudomonas, proteus*
Infants and children	*Haem. influenza*	*Staph. aureus/epidermidis*
	N. meningitidis	Gram negative enteric bacilli
	Strep. pneumoniae	*M. tuberculosis*

After the neonatal period *Haem. Influenza* is the commonest cause of bacterial meningitis in children in the USA and Australia, whereas meningococcus is the commonest in the UK (risk ~1 in 1000 for children <10 years.)

Clinical manifestations

Neonates	*Infants*	*Children*
Signs may be non-specific or minimal	Fever	Fever
Irritability	Irritability	Irritability
Restlessness	Lethargy	Headache
Poor feeding	Vomiting	Vomiting
vomiting	Convulsions	Neck stiffness
Apnoea, bradycardia	Bulging fontanelle	Back pain
Temperature instability	High pitched cry	photophobia
Hypotonia	Nuchal rigidity	Febrile convulsions
Bulging fontanelle	Rash	Rash
High pitched cry	Coma	Coma
Fever		
Convulsions		
Jaundice		
Diarrhoea		

A number of small epidemics (such as that in Stroud, Gloucestershire) have resulted in considerable public concern in recent years. The overall mortality is about 9%. Although mortality from haemophilus is rather lower (5%), sequelae are common. *Strep. pneumoniae* meningitis occurs at all ages but is most common in adult life and has the highest mortality (>20%).

Meningococcal infection
Meningococci are Gram negative diplococci which are divided into nine serotypes, the commonest of which are B, C, A, Y and W135. Group B strains account for ~60% of notified infections.

There are irregular periodic surges in meningococcal infection in the UK, e.g. 1940–45, the mid-1970s and 1986–88.

The incidence is highest in infants followed by 1–5-year olds, but a recent epidemic of Group B 15 PI.16 and the new B4 strain was associated with an increased incidence in teenagers.

The carriage rate in the population is about 10% but varies with age. Meningococci are transmitted by droplet spread or direct contact from carriers or those in early stages of illness. The incubation period is variable because infection may follow colonization but is 2–3 days for infection by a newly acquired organism.

Haemophilus influenza
This is a small Gram negative coccobacillus classified into capsular serotypes A–F and non-capsulated strains. In children, 95% of infections are caused by serotype B. Asymptomatic colonization of the upper respiratory tract is common, usually with non-capsulated organisms, but ~5% of individuals are colonized by encapsulated strains. Transmission is by droplet inhalation. This organism shows increasing antibiotic resistance, with 3% of invasive isolates resistant to chloramphenicol and at least 15% resistant to ampicillin in the UK, with even higher levels elsewhere (e.g. the USA, Spain).

Pneumococcal infections
Strep. pneumoniae is a Gram positive diplococcus (pneumococcus). The pathogenic strains are encapsulated, with some 80 serotypes related to the capsular polysaccharide composition. Pneumococci are found in the nasopharynx of about 30% of the healthy population. Spread may be by inhalation or direct contact with fingers, handkerchieves, etc. soiled with respiratory tract secretions. Incubation period 1–3 days.

Management of meningitis
1. Children in whom meningococcal infection is suspected should be given an intravenous dose of benzyl-penicillin by their GP before transfer to hospital.

2. Lumbar puncture (LP) should be performed whenever meningitis is suspected, but three reasons may justify withholding or delaying LP:

— signs of raised intracranial pressure
— cardiorespiratory instability
— infection in the area the needle would have to traverse to obtain CSF

If there is evidence of raised intracranial pressure in a suspected case of meningitis, antibacterial therapy should be started immediately whilst arrangements are made for urgent cranial CT scan. Microbiological diagnosis may be possible from blood or urine cultures. Gram-stained smears from petechial skin lesions may provide immediate clues in meningococcal meningitis.

3. Initial antimicrobial therapy is selected using a regimen broad enough to cover the most likely pathogens for the age group involved, e.g.:

neonates:	benzyl-penicillin or ampicillin + an aminoglycoside	or	ampicillin + cefotaxime
1–3 months:	ampicillin + chloramphenicol	or	ampicillin + cefotaxime
3 months–6 years:	benzylpenicillin or ampicillin + chloramphenicol	or	cefotaxime

Once the results of cultures and sensitivities are available the treatment regimen can be modified accordingly.

4. Supportive care. Intensive monitoring of:

— vital signs
— fluid balance and urine output
— neurological function
— daily head circumference and transillumination

5. Monitor for and treat possible complications, e.g.

— hypotension
— inappropriate ADH secretion
— seizures
— hypoglycaemia
— raised intracranial pressure
— apnoea
— arrhythmias
— subdural effusion

6. Adjunctive therapy. As understanding of the pathophysiology of sepsis develops, other possible therapeutic agents are being evaluated including:
(a) Corticosteroids. There is considerable evidence that dexamethasone probably reduces the risk of deafness after *Haem. Influenza* meningitis when administered at the

time of the first dose of antibiotics and continued for the first 4 days of treatment, but its efficacy in other types of meningitis is not yet clear and results of additional studies are awaited.

(b) FFP.

(c) Immunoglobulins.

(d) Prostacyclin.

(e) Monoclonal antibodies *vs*, e.g. tumour necrosis factor, (TNF) (a cytokine believed to participate in the host's inflammatory response).

7. Control of infection in the family and the community:

(a) Meningococcal:

— chemoprophylaxis. As soon as the diagnosis is established, rifampicin should be given to all family members and household contacts (attack rate up to 800 times greater than the general population); all day care and school contacts; and the index case should also be treated with rifampicin prior to discharge

— notification. The diagnosis must be notified to the local community medicine specialist (Consultant in Communicable Disease Control or Public Health Medicine), initially by telephone. A GP referring a suspected case to hospital should liaise with hospital staff later the same day to find out if the diagnosis has been confirmed and notified.

The Community Medicine Specialist will advise GPs on administration of chemoprophylaxis and coordinate the implementation of the antibiotic policy in schools, day care centres and other local general practices where necessary

— vaccination. Vaccination should be considered if there is a local outbreak of infection. Vaccines against groups A, C, Y and W135 are available but only that against Group A is effective under the age of 2 years. Close contacts over the age of 2 years of patients with Group A or C infections should be vaccinated. However, many recent cases have been caused by B serotypes for which no effective vaccine is available, although one is being evaluated. Advice on the use of meningococcal vaccines is available from the Communicable Disease Surveillance Centre (081–200 6868) or the Public Health Laboratory Service Meningococcal Reference Laboratory (061–445 2416)

(b) *Haemophilus influenza*:

— chemoprophylaxis. For 30 days after contact with *Haem. influenza* meningitis the risk for household contacts is 585 times greater than in the general population, with special risk to those under 2 years. The recommendation of the British Paediatric Association and The American Academy of

Pediatrics is that where there is another pre-school child in the house of a case of invasive type infection, rifampicin prophylaxis is recommended for all household contacts and for the index case (since standard treatment does not erradicate nasopharyngeal carriage).

— Immunization–see Chapter 4.

(c) Pneumococcus:

— chemoprophylaxis. Not recommended for pneumococcal infection routinely
— vaccination. Antipneumococcal vaccine (pneumovax) is routinely recommended for prevention of pneumococcal infections in special children at high risk:
— sickle cell anaemia
— asplenia
— nephrotic syndrome

The vaccine alone will not confer complete protection against pneumococcal disease, particularly in children with sickle cell disease where extra protection with oral penicillin is advised. The efficacy of Pneumovax in preventing meningitis has not been established.

Complications of meningitis

	Incidence	Comments
Seizures	30% in acute phase 2–8% develop permanent seizure disorder	If persist >4 days or difficult to control, more likely to be associated with permanent neurological sequelae
Sensorineural hearing loss	12% (mild impairment in 25%)	May occur early or be undetectable until months later. *All* children recovering from meningitis should have audiological assessment
Subdural	Up to 30% particularly in infants with *Haem. influenza*	Confirm by CT scan. Most resolve spontaneously. Drainage is required if there is: — clinical suspicion that effusion is infected (subdural empyema) — rapidly enlarging head circumference without hydrocephalus — focal neurological signs — evidence of raised ICP
Brain abscess	Very rare	Confirm by CT scan. EEG may show localized slow wave activity. Treatment: antibiotics and surgical drainage
Ventriculitis	Commonest in neonates	High risk of mortality or handicap. Treatment: intraventricular antibiotics via Rickham reservoir and surgical drainage
Impaired vision	2–4%	
Hemi-/quadriparesis	Up to 10% acutely but <2% after 1 year	Significant but unpredictable resolution with time
Mental retardation	2–3%	
Behavioural problems	About 10%	

Epilepsy   Epilepsy is a condition in which there is a tendency to recurrent seizures. Incidence is 0.5–1% of the population.

Causes of childhood seizures   Idiopathic: 70–80%.

Secondary:
(a) Perinatal

   — hypoxic–ischaemic
   — cerebral malformations
   — birth trauma
   — intrauterine infections
   — haemorrhage

(b) Infections

   — meningitis
   — encephalitis
   — abscess

(c) Neuro-cutaneous Syndromes

   — tuberose sclerosis
   — neurofibromatosis, etc.

(d) Metabolic abnormalities

   — hypoglycaemia
   — degenerative disorders
   — porphyria

(e) Poisoning

   — drug withdrawal
   — lead

(f) Systemic disorders

   — encephalopathy
   — vasculitis

(g) Trauma.
(h) Tumours.

Management   1. *Starting anticonvulsant therapy.* Having one seizure does not constitute epilepsy. It is essential to take a careful history of the episodes, including any apparent precipitating factors, and to talk to an eyewitness if possible, to establish whether the episodes are truly epileptic or not. Investigations such as EEG, skull X-ray and CT scan may be helpful in some cases in revealing, e.g. neoplasia, calcification, porencephalic cysts or localized cerebral atrophy. Biochemical and metabolic disorders should also be excluded.

It is usual not to treat after a single seizure in most cases (although the presence of a known progressive cerebral disorder or a very abnormal EEG might indicate early treatment to be advisable in an individual patient). If there is a clear

Classification of seizures

(Adapted from International Classification of Epilepsy.)

Type	Clinical features	Aetiology	Most effective treatment
I Partial seizures (those beginning focally)			
(a) Simple partial seizures	No loss of consciousness + elementary symptoms — motor — sensory, inc. special sensory — autonomic — psychic	Focal anatomical lesion, e.g. cyst, tumour, abscess, AV malformation, scar	Carbamezepine Phenytoin
(b) Complex partial seizures (temporal lobe epilepsy)	Impaired conciousness + complex symptoms	Temporal lobe sclerosis, cyst, tumour	Carbamezepine Phenytoin
(c) Secondarily generalized partial seizures	Initially focal then grand mal		Valproate Phenytoin Carbamezepine
II Generalized seizures (those without focal onset)			
(a) Petit mal	Absences EEG bilateral symmetrical 3 cps spike and wave	Idiopathic	Valproate Ethosuximide
(b) Grand mal	Tonic–clonic seizures	Idiopathic	Valproate Carbamezepine Phenobarbitone Phenytoin
(c) Myoclonic	Often on waking or going off to sleep. May be very frequent	Degenerative disorders Idiopathic	Valproate Clonazepam Carbamezepine
(d) Infantile spasms (West syndrome)	Salaam or jack-knife spasms EEG: hypsarrhythmia	Perinatal factors Tuberose sclerosis (up to 30%) Metals Idiopathic	ACTH Nitrazepam/clonazepam Valproate
(e) Akinetic	Drop attacks	Perinatal factors Idiopathic	Valproate Clonazepam/Nitrazepam
III Unilateral seizures	Unilateral grand mal	Focal anatomical lesion Tumour, AV malformation, cyst	Carbamezepine Phenytoin
IV Unclassified			

pattern of recurring seizures which are of potential risk to the child and causing concern to child, parents and/or teachers, anticonvulsants are indicated.

Once the diagnosis is established, it must be explained to the family and to the patient where he or she is able to understand. Considerable mythology still surrounds epilepsy, and parental fears about underlying causes, social aspects, effects of treatment and likely outcome for the future must be fully discussed.

Side-effects of anticonvulsants

	Side-effects	Serious toxicity
Carbamezepine	Rashes Ataxia Leucopenia, usually reversible	Aplastic anaemia Agranulocytosis
Clonazepam	Somnolence, hypotonia Overactivity, ataxia Salivary and bronchial hypersecretion	Respiratory depression (intravenous)
Ethosuximide	Vomiting, rashes	Blood dyscrasias, rare
Phenobarbitone	Sedation. Reduced cognitive ability in 30%+ Hyperactivity Rash Rickets	
Phenytoin	Gum hypertrophy 93% Hirsutism 75% Ataxia, nystagmus Rickets Rash	Megaloblastic anaemia Lymphoma Choreoathetosis SLE Stevens–Johnson
Sodium valproate	Nausea, epigastric pain Tremor, drowsiness Transient hair loss Increased appetite, obesity	Pancreatitis Liver failure

Other modes of treatment for epilepsy:

(a) Ketogenic diet. This dietary treatment restricts protein and carbohydrate, supplying >80% of daily calories as fat. It is unpalatable and difficult to enforce, although somewhat easier since the introduction of medium-chain triglycerides which are tasteless and water-miscible. Beneficial in some children with intractable seizures, especially of the minor motor type.

(b) Surgery. In a small number of selected children with refractory epilepsy, surgery may give good results, e.g. where optimal medical treatment has been inadequate to control seizures and permit acceptable quality of life and where there is a discharging epileptogenic lesion localized by serial EEG or more specialized methods to a surgically accessible area of the brain. Surgery is particularly effective for some children with mesial temporal sclerosis related to past history of recurrent febrile convulsions or with temporal lobe hamartomas.

2. *Advice about living with epilepsy*:

(a) Parents should be taught the principles of maintaining the airway and appropriate posture to prevent aspiration. In selected cases they are taught to administer rectal diazepam. Clear written guidelines should be given about when medical advice should be sought.

(b) Education, learning and behaviour. Most children with epilepsy can be educated in normal schools. Clinical medical officers and teachers should be kept informed about progress and drug treatment. Both the disorder itself and the treatment may affect school performance. Learning problems in such children require careful assessment and often special remedial help.

In a few cases the frequency or severity of seizures, or the presence of accompanying problems such as mental retardation (in one-third of children with epilepsy) or cerebral palsy, result in the need for placement in a special school.

Parents and teachers should be counselled against being over-protective towards the child with epilepsy and against identifying the child as different. Wherever possible he or she should be treated the same as other children and encouraged to take part in a full range of activities. Restrictions should be kept to a minimum:

— swimming is allowed if supervised by someone who is aware the child has epilepsy
— cycling and riding also should be performed under supervision, avoiding busy roads and wearing a protective helmet
— it is safest to discourage at an early stage an interest in sports such as mountain climbing, parachuting or ski jumping

(c) Advice and counselling from psychologists, child guidance clinics and support groups are helpful for some children and their families, particularly during adolescence when potential constraints on career opportunities, driving and leisure activities may result in difficulties in etablishing independence and cause frustration and rebelliousness. It is important that the teenager retains ready access to a trusted physician, social worker or psychologist during this period so that transfer of care from paediatric to adult services around this age must be carefully coordinated.

Headache   Headache is a common symptom in childhood; up to 20% of schoolchildren complain recurrently of headache. Chronic headaches are most commonly associated with psychological factors or migraine, but other causes must be considered.

Causes   1. *Acute*

— simple febrile illness
— earache, toothache, acute sinusitis
— poisoning
— subarachnoid haemorrhage or acute subdural haemorrhage
— concussion

2. *Recurrent*

— psychogenic
— migraine
— related to epilepsy
— raised intracranial pressure

- space occupying lesion, e.g. tumour, cyst, abscess
- benign intracranial hypertension
- hypertensive encephalopathy
- lead poisoning
— depression
— eye strain
— drugs inc. antihistamines, carbamezepine, indomethacin, antibiotics, anti-tuberculous therapy, vincristine
— cervical spondylosis
— malocclusion

Assessment   1. Careful history:

— including nature, site, duration, timing and frequency of headache and the degree to which it interferes with daily activities
— any associated symptoms, e.g. vomiting, visual disturbance, clumsiness, weight loss
— family history including of headaches, migraine
— social and school history: any recent changes, problems, truancy, illness amongst friends
— drug history, dietary history

2. Examination. Full general examination including BP, urinalysis, check ears, teeth + neurological examination, including fundoscopy, plus OFC and examination of sutures and fontanelles in infants.

3. Significant features in history which may be associated with underlying pathology include:

— headaches which wake child at night or are most severe on waking in the morning
— acute severe headaches with no history of headaches
— headache accompanied by vomiting, stiff neck, etc.
— headache exacerbated by coughing or bending
— daily headaches getting worse in a crescendo pattern

Migraine   One of the commonest causes of chronic recurrent headache in children and adolescents.
Incidence: 5% of school children, increasing to 10% in adults.

Pathogenesis   Not well understood but related to stimulation of pain fibres in walls of cerebral vessels which are abnormally labile and liable to constrict or dilate under influence of various factors, including diet, hormones and psychological stress.

Clinical features   — unilateral headache, throbbing, often frontal or temporal (but bifrontal or generalized migraine headaches also occur)
— preceded by aura: type depends on which arteries are affected and the degree of vasoconstriction:
• ophthalmic A commonest. Visual aura may consist of

scintillating scotomata and zigzag lines ('fortification phenomenon'), field defects, micropsia
- mesenteric A — nausea, vomiting, sense of fullness
- cranial As — oculomotor N palsy, transient ataxia, hemiparesis, aphasia

— duration variable — usually last a few hours and ended by sleep but may last several days
— positive family history in 80% of cases

Complicated migraine Term applied to rare cases which involve longer-lasting neurological dysfunction. Includes:

— ophthalmoplegic migraine
— hemiplegic/alternating hemiplegic migraine
— basilar A migraine

Migraine variants (a) Abdominal migraine, periodic syndrome. May include recurrent abdominal pain, cyclical vomiting and/or headache or vasomotor disturbances.

(b) Rarely migraine attacks may be associated with loss of consciousness and convulsions probably due to syncope. Epileptic seizures may involve abdominal pain or headache. The distinction between migraine and epilepsy may thus be difficult. The two conditions may coexist.

Management (a) Detailed history and examination to exclude other causes of symptoms and to identify provoking factors particularly dietary or stress.

(b) Allay child's and parents' anxiety about other feared pathology.

(c) Consider possible dietary triggers. There is good evidence that foods may be the factors provoking vasomotor instability in a proportion of cases of childhood migraine. The commonest provoking foods in one study of 76 cases were:

cow's milk	39%	wheat	31%
chocolate	37%	cheese	31%
benzoic acid	37%	citrus	30%
eggs	36%	coffee	24%
tartrazine	33%		

If the history suggests sensitivity to particular foods a trial of dietary exclusion is merited, avoiding likely provoking food items in series for 2 weeks at a time, with the child or parent keeping a diary of frequency and severity of symptoms during each exclusion period. If symptoms occur reproducibly with a certain food, it is withdrawn. If symptoms are very severe and food sensitivity is suspected, a trial of an oligo-antigenic diet under the supervision of the dietician should be arranged.

(d) Drug treatment can be reduced or avoided altogether in many children by the above plus symptomatic measures, e.g. rest in a dark quiet room, simple analgesics, antiemetics.

Ergotamine tartrate may shorten attacks by causing vaso-constriction and preventing the vasodilation which underlies the headache phase *but* its use should be restricted in children because it can itself cause headaches, it is a potentially toxic drug, with risks of habituation or accidental overdosage and it is contraindicated in complicated migraine as it may increase symptoms due to excessive vasoconstriction.

Prophylaxis: Pizotifen (5-HT antagonist) or propanolol may be helpful in prevention of severe or frequent attacks which cannot be reduced by the above measures to less than one every 2–4 weeks.

Other drugs used in adults such as methysergide have a high risk of side-effects (such as vascular stenoses and retro-peritoneal fibrosis) and should not be used in children.

Head injury In the western world, accidents are the most important single cause of death in children aged between 1 and 14 years. Most fatal accidents, particularly road traffic accidents, involve craniocerebral trauma.

The nature of head injury in children differs from that in adults because of the structural and maturational changes which occur during childhood.

(a) The greater plasticity of the infant's skull enables it to absorb physical impact better than that of the adult.

(b) In infants, rising intracranial pressure (ICP) produces tension in the fontanelle, separation of sutures and increasing head circumference. With increasing age and especially after fontanelle closure there is distortion of the brain as ICP rises, with development of signs of compression of the brain stem at the tentorial hiatus and foramen magnum (coning).

(c) One-third of children with mild head injury have associated linear fractures. As a rule their presence does not alter the clinical course and they heal over 3–4 months.

(d) 'Growing fractures' of the skull occur only in children. These are characterized by a dural tear beneath a fracture, usually diastatic and predominantly parietal. Herniation of the leptomeninges may cause erosion of the overlying bone so that the fracture enlarges to form a cranial defect. Seizures may result from pressure on the underlying cortex. Cranioplasty is required in most cases.

(e) Basal skull fractures. Relatively uncommon in children. Signs may include:

— bleeding from nasopharynx
— CSF leak from nose or ears
— haemorrhage around the eyes + exophthalmos and subconjunctival haemorrhages
— post-auricular bruising (Battle's sign)

(f) Extradural haemorrhages (EDH) in infants and young children are more common than was previously recognized. Usually result from tears of the dural veins, even after mild injury with no fracture, and therefore symptoms develop more slowly than in adults where middle meningeal artery haemorrhage into the extradural space causes rapid deterioration. In infants the middle meningeal artery is less indented into the inner skull table so it is less susceptible to trauma.

(g) Subdural haemorrhage (SDH). Acute SDH may occur at any age and usually coexists with other serious cerebral damage.

Chronic SDH is an important cause of serious disability and should be suspected in infants presenting with irritability, failure to gain weight and an enlarged head with a biparietal bulge and tense fontanelle. Later signs will include evidence of raised ICP such as vomiting and seizures. May be associated with a relatively minor degree of trauma, such as shaking which may cause shearing stresses to tear cortical veins bridging the subdural space as they drain into the dural sinuses. Such tears may occur during precipitate delivery or result from later trauma. They are frequently associated with retinal haemorrhages and the possibility of NAI must be considered (see p. 129).

SDH must be differentiated from a post-meningitic subdural effusion containing clear or xanthochromic fluid.

If associated with intracranial hypertension or signs of brainstem shift, repeated subdural taps are usually sufficient treatment. Shunting is rarely necessary.

Management (a) *Initial assessment* must obviously include history of injury from family or other witnesses. Ask about condition of child before injury (including any history of fits, recent infection, blood disorders, drug treatment, etc.). Determine whether any circumstances suggest NAI.

(b) *Full examination* of whole child, including vital signs and neurological examination, plus check for other injuries.

Examination of the head should include inspection of scalp for swellings, depressed fractures, fontanelles, sutures, measure OFC. Inspect nose and ears for escape of blood or CSF (which can be differentiated from nasal secretions by using Clinistix to detect glucose in CSF). Tilt head back to examine nasal septum for haematoma. Check facial contours. Examine ears for haemotympanum or Battle's sign.

(c) *Mild head injury*. If examination is normal the child may return home, provided observation by a reliable adult can be guarenteed. The child should be awakened 2–3 times during the night and reviewed the next day to check all is well. A card should be given to the parents outlining danger signs and symptoms indicating the need for further medical attention.

(d) *Children should be admitted to hospital after head injury if:*

— injury associated with loss of consciousness or confusion
— there is a skull fracture or penetrating injury
— there are focal neurological signs
— there is persistent vomiting
— there is concern about aetiology of head injury or ability of parent to observe child adequately because of social or other problems
— there are coexisting medical problems, e.g. coagulation disorders

(e) *X-rays* are only requested after full examination. Routine views are posteroanterior, lateral and, if history of occipital injury, a Townes view. If depressed fracture is suspected, request a tangential view, indicating clearly the area of concern.

Indications for skull X-ray include:

— neurological signs or symptoms
— tense fontanelle
— history of unconsciousness
— penetrating injury, e.g. fall onto sharp object
— falls from height >60 cm or onto hard surface
— palpable depression in scalp
— laceration >5 cm or down to bone
— cephalohaematoma
— injury with haemorrhage around the eyes/CSF rhinorrhoea/otorrhoea/haemotympanum
— <1 year of age
— suspected NAI

(f) *Moderate and severe head injury.* The first priority is to stabilize airway, oxygenation and circulation and prevent further secondary cerebral damage. The risks of secondary complications are then assessed and a decision made regarding transfer to a neurosurgical centre (e.g. the likely risk of an intracranial haematoma requiring urgent evacuation in a child with coma and a skull fracture is 1 in 12, so all such children should be discussed with a neurosurgeon with a view to urgent transfer for CT scan and treatment; many would advocate that all children with skull fractures should have cranial CT scans, as should any child whose condition is deteriorating after a head injury). Serial assessments of vital signs and conscious level are recorded, including e.g. the Paediatric Glasgow Coma Scale (eye opening, best motor and verbal response).

Further management may include:

— assisted ventilation with blood gas monitoring
— treatment of hypovolaemia
— control of seizures with, e.g. phenytoin, clonazepam (be prepared to provide respiratory support if not already ventilated)
— consultation with neurosurgeon
— emergency CT scan
— antibiotics; prophylactic only for basal fracture, compound vault fracture, suspected meningitis
— intracranial pressure monitoring and control of cerebral oedema, e.g. mannitol
— if transfer is necessary, it is essential to resuscitate fully and stabilize the patient first and to ensure that a suitably experienced doctor accompanies the patient

Intracranial tumours   Brain tumours account for almost 20% of all paediatric neoplasms, being second only to leukaemia in overall incidence of childhood malignancy. There are about 24 new cases per million children each year. In children, 60% of brain tumours are infratentorial with the commonest types being low-grade astrocytomas and embryonic neoplasms, whereas in adults most CNS tumours are supratentorial (malignant astrocytomas or metastatic carcinomas).

Clinical manifestations   The commonest presenting symptoms are:

— headache
— vomiting
— unsteadiness
— impaired conciousness

Other presenting features may include strabismus, diplopia, large head, nystagmus, cranial N deficits, failure to thrive, weight loss, personality changes, deterioration in school performance and endocrine abnormalities.

Long-term sequelae of treatment   (a) Intellectual and emotional changes. Much variation between individuals after similar treatment programmes. Significant mental impairment ensues in ~20–30% of children with emotional disturbance in 25–90%. Some of the factors influencing the degree of psychological disturbance during treatment include:

— age at time of treatment
— site and extent of tumour
— extent of surgery
— presence, degree and duration of hydrocephalus
— volume and time-dose factors in radiotherapy
— combined irradiation and chemotherapy
— dose, duration and route of administration of cytotoxic agents

Primary CNS tumours

Site	Manifestations	Treatment	5-year survival rate
Infratentorial Cerebellar astrocytoma	2–8 years Raised ICP Cerebellar signs	Surgical excision Radiation if incomplete resection Corticosteroids to reduce tumour oedema	90%
Medulloblastoma	2–5 years M:F 2:1 Midline-cerebellar vermis and floor 4th ventricle, raised ICP, hydrocephalus, cerebellar signs, spinal cord compression Rapid growing, seeds along cerebrospinal axis and may metastasize to extraneural tissues	Surgical excision and radiotherapy to posterior fossa + low dose radiation to whole neuraxis over 7–8 weeks + chemotherapy 12–18 months, e.g. CCNU + vincristine	30–50%
Ependymoma of 4th ventricle	From floor 4th ventricle Hydrocephalus and raised ICP, may calcify, spinal seeding 12%	Surgical excision + radiotherapy + ?adjuvant chemotherapy e.g. CCNU + vincristine (under evaluation)	Depends on degree of differentiation 30–50%
Brain stem glioma	Presents 5–8 years. Usually arise in pons. Multiple bilateral cranial N palsies, pyramidal signs, ataxia	Excision impossible Palliative radiotherapy Experimental chemotherapy — no benefit shown as yet Corticosteroids to reduce oedema	Poor prognosis 15–20%
Supratentorial Craniopharyngioma	Growth failure, impairment of vision, raised ICP. Endocrine abnormality — rare initially. D. insipidus 10% preop.	Pre- and postop. steroids Total excision + adjuvant radiotherapy or chemotherapy Treat D. insipidus post-op. and monitor vision	70–90%
Optic glioma	Associated in 25% with neurofibromatosis Usually <5 years. Visual loss, proptosis, slow growing	Surgical excision ± radiotherapy	50–90%
Cerebral hemisphere tumours Astrocytoma/ oligodendroglioma Glioblastoma multiforme	Convulsions, hemiparesis, hemisensory deficit, raised ICP late. Rapidly progressive focal signs and raised ICP	Surgery or radiotherapy depending on location and extent Chemotherapy, e.g. CCNU, vincristine + prednisolone Anticonvulsants, steroids	10–50% 0–5%
Choroid plexus papilloma	Presents in first 3 years with hydrocephalus	Surgical excision, treatment of persistent hydrocephalus may be needed	60–80%

— associated physical handicaps, e.g. impairment of vision or hearing
— opportunities for rehabilitation

(b) Secondary infection.
(c) Hepatotoxicity, e.g. MTX, 6MP.
(d) Pituitary dysfunction-isolated growth hormone deficiency or panhypopituitarism after cranial irradiation.
(e) Necrotizing leucoencephalopathy affects a small percentage of patients given MTX with or after brain irradiation, presenting with confusion, ataxia, spasticity and fits.
(f) Second primary tumours.

Progress in management Advances in neurodiagnostic techniques such as CT and NMRI have greatly improved the accuracy of diagnosis and localization of intracranial masses. Modern surgical and precise megavoltage irradiation techniques have improved the prognosis for many children. The large number of continuing national and international multicentre trials of adjuvant combination chemotherapy and immunotherapy may lead to even better results in the future. Such progress depends on close collaboration of multidisciplinary teams taking coordinated overall care of children not only during treatment but throughout their subsequent follow-up and rehabilitation including education and employment.

Acute encephalopathy

Presentation
— clouding of conciousness
— coma
— fits
— raised ICP
— ataxia
— acute hemiplegia
— decerebration

Causes 1. *Infection*, e.g.

— meningitis, encephalitis
— fungal infections, e.g. cryptococcus
— rickettsia, e.g. typhus, Rocky Mountain spotted fever
— protozoa, e.g. malaria
— post-viral encephalopathy
— slow-viral encephalopathy

+ non-infectious encephalopathies probably precipitated by viral infections, e.g.

— Reye's syndrome
— haemolytic–uraemic syndrome
— exacerbations of IEM under stress of infection, e.g. Leigh's encephalopathy, MSUD

2. *Hypoxic–ischaemic encephalopathy*, e.g.

— birth asphyxia

— cardiorespiratory arrest
— near miss cot death
— near drowning
— shock

3. *Status epilepticus.*
4. *Cerebrovascular disorders*:

— intracranial haemorrhage, thrombosis, embolism
— hypertensive encephalopathy

5. *Toxic encephalopathy*:
(a) Endogenous, e.g.

— hypoglycaemia, diabetic ketoacidosis
— hepatic or renal failure, adrenal insufficiency
— Reye's syndrome
— hypercalcaemia
— scalds
— IEM

(b) Exogenous, e.g.

— drugs:
  • accidental ingestion — iron, salicylates
  • side-effects — chemotherapeutic agents, e.g. MTX, vincristine, particularly when combined with cranial irradiation
  • abuse — solvents, alcohol, narcotics
— heavy metals, e.g. lead, mercury
— plants, mushrooms
— bites and stings

6. *Cerebral trauma.*
7. *Tumours.*

The floppy infant   This term refers to babies with persistent hypotonia inappropriate to their stage of development.

Causes   1. *General.* Many infants who are acutely unwell (e.g. with acute infection or electrolyte imbalance, etc.) will be apathetic and floppy.
2. *CNS*

— birth asphyxia
— cerebral palsy
— chromosomal anomalies, particularly Down's syndrome, Prader–Willi (15q deletion in up to 50%)
— metabolic:
  • aminoacidurias
  • storage disorders
  • Lowe's oculocerebrorenal syndrome
  • Zellweger's cerebrohepatorenal syndrome

3. *Neuromuscular*

— these diseases produce floppiness associated with weakness, manifesting as reduced spontaneous movements, weak cry, poor suck and poor respiratory effort.

(a) Spinal cord

— trauma, e.g. birth injury
— infantile spinal muscular atrophy (Werdnig–Hoffmann)

(b) Neuropathy

— congenital sensory neuropathy
— Guillain–Barré syndrome

(c) Neuromuscular junction:

— myasthenia gravis
— infantile botulism

(d) Myopathy (congenital):

— structural:
  • central core
  • nemaline
  • centronuclear
  • fibre type disproportion
  • mitochondrial myopathies
— metabolic:
  • storage disorders, e.g. glycogen storage disease type II, V
  • abnormalities of lipid metabolism
  • periodic paralysis
  • congenital muscular dystrophy
  • congenital myotonic dystrophy (Steinert)

Guillain-Barré syndrome (acute post-infective polyneuritis)

Pathogenesis   Acute or sub-acute diffuse disorder of nerve roots and peripheral nerves which may follow about 2 weeks after a viral infection or rarely after immunization. Up to one-third have no history of preceding illness. May follow post-infectious sensitization of lymphocytes to a protein component of myelin.

Presentation   Sudden onset symmetrical weakness, hypotonia and hyporeflexia usually most severe in lower limbs:

±   meningism in one-third of children
±   respiratory muscle paralysis; ventilation required in up to 25%
±   cranial nerve involvement, particularly facial palsy

—   sensory involvement usually minimal; may be muscle tenderness and parasthesiae

Investigations CSF shows high protein level with normal cell count. Peripheral nerve conduction velocity is slow.

Differential diagnosis
— poliomyelitis
— polymyositis
— transverse myelopathy
— spinal cord tumour

Treatment Supportive. Corticosteroids make little difference in the acute stage but may improve outcome in those following a chronic course.

Prognosis Complete recovery in 95%; usually begins after 1 week, may continue for up to 2 years.

Myasthenia

Characterized by muscular weakness due to defect in neuromuscular transmission.

Pathogenesis Autoimmune reaction producing circulating IgG antibodies against acetylcholine (AC) receptor sites in motor end-plates.

Presentations
1. *Transient neonatal myasthenia.* Passive transfer of maternal AC receptor antibodies causes transient myasthenia in about 15% of infants born to myasthenic mothers. May present with feeding or respiratory difficulties including apnoea. Improves over 4–6 weeks.

2. *Infantile myasthenia.* Very rare with equal sex incidence. Often familial (autosomal recessive). Usually mild, mainly ocular involvement.

3. *Juvenile myasthenia gravis.* Rare. Usually starts after age 10 years. Commoner in girls (6:1)

Symptoms: ptosis, diplopia, difficulty swallowing, dysarthria, generalized weakness worsening through the day. May be sudden exacerbations at times of stress (myasthenic crises).

Diagnosis confirmed by increase in muscle strength in response to anticholinesterse drugs, e.g. edrophonium chloride (Tensilon) or neostigmine.

Treatment: Pyridostigmine 4 hourly. For severe cases — thymectomy, steroids, plasmapheresis. Avoid drugs which exacerbate neuromuscular block, e.g., aminoglycosides, phenytoin.

4. *Symptomatic myasthenia.* Rare association with acute leukaemia in children.

Muscular dystrophies

Duchenne

A group of familial disorders involving progressive muscle degeneration.

Presentation Affects 1 in 4000 boys (and can very rarely affect girls). Inheritance is X-linked recessive with about one-third due to new mutations.

— slow motor development
— may have mild mental retardation and speech delay (mean IQ 80)

— waddling gait, falls
— progressive weakness more marked proximally
— muscle pseudohypertrophy (due to fatty infiltration)
— Gower's sign (getting up from floor by rolling prone, pushing up on all fours and then to standing by pushing with hands against shins, knees then thighs), late sign rarely developed before 4–5 years

Early diagnosis is essential so that effective genetic counselling can be given to prevent avoidable spread of disease through the family. All boys who are not walking by 18 months or who have unexplained motor and speech delay should have a serum creatinine kinase assay (raised in Duchenne patients to >10 times normal even in infancy before weakness is evident).

Prenatal diagnosis DNA analysis is performed on chorionic villus samples at 9–12 weeks gestation. The combined use of RFLP linkage and dystrophin cDNA deletion analysis offers a highly accurate method for prenatal diagnosis and carrier detection.

Management Families need considerable help in coming to terms with this diagnosis and planning their lives around it. Assessment and support from a unit specializing in muscular dystrophy is usually advisable. Families may also obtain information and help from the Muscular Dystrophy Group of Great Britain.

During the ambulatory phase advice is needed about exercise, prevention of contractures and scoliosis, avoidance of undue immobilization and obesity. In selected cases orthopaedic procedures may prolong ambulation for a few years. A wheelchair becomes necessary by about 12 years in most cases. Practical help should include anticipation of the need for lifting facilities, wheelchair ramps and suitable transport.

Most boys can start education in an ordinary school but as their handicap progresses each must be assessed individually. Some will prefer to battle on with the help of their school friends and teachers: others will be depressed by their inability to keep up with their peers and will be happier in a physically handicapped school with other boys with similar problems.

Death may occur any time from late teens to early 20s as a result of either respiratory disease or cardiomyopathy.

Becker Also X-linked recessive; less severe, later presentation but usually progresses until wheelchair required in adult life.

Limb girdle dystrophy — pelvic girdle type
— facio-scapulo humeral type

Dementia Presents with developmental regression and intellectual impairment, manifestations depending on child's age:

Infant:

— loss or slowing down in aquisition of skills
— loss of interest in surroundings
— less sociable
— may develop hypotonia, decerebrate rigidity or seizures

Toddler:

— unsteadiness, slurring of speech
— irritability, temper outbursts
— slow deterioration of language
— hypotonia or spastic tetraplegia

School age:

— deterioration in school performance
— poor coordination
— apathy or aggression
— seizures

Causes of regression   (a) Progressive degenerative disorders:

— poliodystrophies (neuronal destruction), e.g. Alper's disease, Leigh's disease, CNS storage disorders
— leucodystrophies and leucoencephalopathies (demyelination), e.g. metachromatic leucodystrophy, Krabbe's disease, adrenoleukodystrophy

(b) Disintegrative pyschoses.
(c) Unrecognized status epilepticus.
(d) Toxic encephalopathy.
(e) Drug treatment.
(f) Depression.
(g) Severe adverse social conditions.

17. Metabolic and endocrine disorders

Diabetes mellitus

Definition Disorder of energy metabolism characterized by altered homeostasis of carbohydrate, fat and protein, and due to a relative deficiency of insulin or of its action.

Epidemiology The annual incidence rate has nearly doubled over the last 15 years, with 13.5 cases in 100 000 age-related population reported in 1988. A quarter were under 5 years old. There is considerable geographic variation, probably due to a combination of genetic and environmental (particularly dietary) factors. Finland has the highest incidence and Japan the lowest.

Classification Diabetes mellitus is a heterogenous group of disorders within which there are distinct genetic and pathophysiologic patterns. Primary diabetes in children is predominantly insulin-dependent (type I, 'juvenile onset', JOD). Non-insulin-dependent diabetes (type II, 'maturity onset', MOD) also rarely occurs in young people.

Aetiology Development of diabetes in a susceptible person depends on environmental factors, such as viral infections, triggering an abnormal autoimmune response which causes progressive pancreatic islet β-cell damage, resulting in insulin deficiency.

Genetic susceptibility to IDDM is associated with a group of major histocompatibility antigens located in lymphocytes (HLA antigens), which are coded for on the 6th chromosome. These HLA antigens may serve as markers of gene loci (A, B, C, D), which in some way confer susceptibility to islet cell damage. HLA-D and HLA-DR antigens are associated with increased risk. 90–98% of childhood-onset diabetics express DR3, DR4 antigens (although many apparently healthy people also possess these markers, with <1% of them developing diabetes).

Cell-mediated immune mechanisms involving T-cells appear to be of greater importance in initiating β-cell destruction than antibody-mediated damage. Various constituents of β-cells have been identified as auto-antigens in IDDM, including membrane-associated glycolipids and proteins (e.g. a protein called 64K after its molecular weight and recently identified as glutamic acid decarboxylase, GAD). Characterizing these antibodies is an important step in development of new immunotherapeutic approaches to prevent the disease.

Presentation   There is considerable variation in speed of onset of the clinical disorder. Metabolic disturbance may precede the clinical disorder by months or even years in some cases.

Usual presentation is a short clinical history of a few days or weeks of malaise, polyuria, bedwetting, polydipsia, weight loss and poor appetite. As the disease progresses the development of ketoacidosis is associated with increasing abdominal pain, vomiting, dehydration and hyperventiliation with Kussmaul respiration. Circulatory collapse, oliguria and coma may ensue.

Differential diagnosis includes:

— UTI
— compulsive drinking
— diabetes insipidus
— acute abdomen
— pneumonia
— salicylate poisoning

Diabetic ketoacidosis (DKA)   This is a life-threatening condition with a mortality rate of 1%, usually due to cerebral oedema. It is important to diagnose diabetes early; if it is suspected the child should be sent immediately to hospital to be seen the same day.

Initial management   (a) Rapid history, clinical examination and blood glucose by test strip to confirm diagnosis.

(b) Clinical assessment of state of hydration — if severely ill with evidence of circulatory collapse, i.v. plasma or 0.9% saline (20 ml/kg) should be given over 30–60 min.

(c) Investigations (blood glucose, U&E, plasma osmolality, arterial blood gases, FBC and infection screen) as infusion is set up.

(d) Pass NGT.

(e) Once circulating volumes are restored, fluid requirements are assessed to calculate remaining deficit due to dehydration + maintenance requirements + replacement of continuing losses, e.g. GI, and cautious rehydration is completed slowly using 0.9% saline initially with regular clinical and biochemical reassessments.

(f) Total body potassium is depleted. Plasma potassium will fall as acidosis is corrected. KCl should be added to infusion fluid (initial concentration 26 mmol/l). Insulin treatment should be started before KCl is added; if there is evidence of peripheral circulatory failure, potassium supplementation is deferred until urine has been passed. ECG and serum potassium are monitored.

(g) After i.v. fluids have been started, insulin is given. A continuous i.v. infusion at 0.05–0.1u/kg/h is the safest and least uncomfortable route. Alternatively small intramuscular doses may be given hourly. The subcutaneous route should *not* be used as absorption will be irregular in a dehydrated child.

(h) Once blood glucose is <14 mmol/1 fluids are changed to 0.45% saline 5% dextrose.

(i) Use of sodium bicarbonate is controversial. Arguments against its use in DKA include:

— HCO_3^- combines with H^+, dissociating to H_2O and CO_2. Cessation of hyperventilation leads to retention of CO_2, which diffuses freely across the blood–brain barrier in comparison to HCO_3^-, which crosses it slowly. Blood pH rises and a relative cerebral acidosis remains, creating a pH gradient and exacerbating cerebral depression.

— rising pH leads to decreased dissociation of O_2 from haemoglobin, with impaired oxygen release to the tissues so predisposing to lactic acidosis.

However, severe acidosis with pH <7.1 is associated with:

— decreased respiratory minute volume
— decreased myocardial contractility
— danger of arrhythmias

Therefore, sodium bicarbonate should only be given in severe acidosis (pH <7.1) and then used sparingly over at least 30 min.

$$\text{mmol bicarbonate} = \frac{\text{wt (kg)} \times \text{base deficit (mmol/l)}}{10}$$

(j) Oxygen if PaO_2 <11 kPa in air.

(k) Biochemical monitoring:

— Lab. blood glucose hourly for 4 h, then hourly reagent strips plus 4 hourly lab checks. Glucose should be brought down slowly, falling not >5 mmol/h
— check K^+ at 1, 2 and 4 h, 4 hourly for 12 h, then 6–8 hourly with electrolytes and osmolality
— blood gases hourly until pH >7.25
— check urine for glucose and ketones

(l) Antibiotics if suspected sepsis.

Subsequent management   (a) Oral fluids are re-introduced as tolerated any time after 12–24 h and the i.v. line discontinued when the child is drinking well and urine is ketone-free. Oral potassium supplements are given for about 4 days until diet is adequate.

(b) Subcutaneous insulin is started 30 min before the i.v. infusion is stopped (approx. 1 u/kg/24 h 6–8 hourly, modified according to blood glucose). After 48–60 h, a twice daily regime may be adopted, e.g. combination of short (soluble) and intermediate acting (isophane) insulin 1.0–1.5 u/kg/24 h with approx. two-thirds before breakfast (ratio sol: isophane <1:1) and one-third before evening meal (ratio sol: isophane <1:3). Highly purified human or porcine insulins should be used. Dose required often decreases rapidly after control is achieved and must be regularly revised in the first few weeks.

(c) Education of child and family about diabetes usually starts during the initial stay following presentation with ketoacidosis. Some new diabetics presenting with early symptoms and without ketoacidosis can be managed without hospital admission if there is a diabetes nurse specialist, liaison nurse or specialist health visitor who can make daily home visits for supervision and teaching and if home conditions are suitable. There is evidence that parents and children can accept and learn to cope with diabetes more quickly at home, provided an effective community team exists. At present, however, over 80% of children with newly-diagnosed diabetes are admitted for about 1 week, during which time parents can be supported through the shock of the initial diagnosis and introduced to basic diabetic care, involving nursing and medical staff, paediatric dietician and diabetes nurse specialist. They are taught about:

— diet
— insulin:
  • injection technique and sites
  • factors likely to alter requirements
  • what to do if the child develops an infection
— the interaction between food, insulin and exercise
— home blood and urine glucose monitoring, and recording of results
— recognition and management of hypoglycaemia, including use of a home glucagon kit
— 24 h telephone contact numbers for advice
— support groups such as local branch of British Diabetic Association (BDA)

Long-term management

Aims (a) Optimal control of blood glucose in context of minimal disruption of family and school life and normal growth.

(b) Encouragement of increasing understanding of the condition in the developing child and self-confidence in its management.

Children attending specialist paediatric diabetic clinics have been shown to achieve better control than those managed in general paediatric clinics. Achievement of good long-term control is helped by the multidisciplinary team available in such designated children's diabetic clinics. The team includes:

— paediatric dietician
— diabetes nurse specialist

— playworker and psychologist or child psychiatrist
— paediatrician with special expertise in care of diabetes

The team liaises with hospital social worker, paediatric ophthalmologist, chiropodist and dental hygienist. The family GP and School Medical Officer must be kept fully informed about the child's condition. The GP may find it helpful to have copies of information booklets supplied by the clinic and to discuss management of problems over the telephone with the liaison sister or paediatrician, so that consistent advice is given to the family. The BDA supplies pamphlets for school teachers and many diabetes nurse specialists visit schools.

The clinic may incorporate a diabetic stall or shop and provide written information to consolidate education about diabetic care. At the clinic, progress is monitored by:

(a) Assessment of emotional and physical well-being. Physical examination includes:

— monitoring growth and sexual development
— checking eyes for retinopathy or cataracts. Annual review by ophthalmologist
— blood pressure
— injection sites and technique
— test for microalbuminuria, the earliest sign of nephropathy

(b) Assessment of recorded results of home blood or urine glucose monitoring. Spring-activated lancets may be used to obtain capillary specimens. A variey of test strips and reflectance meters are available. Profiles based on capillary glucose test strips at intervals through the day are a helpful guide to the adequacy of control.

(c) Measurement of glycosylated haemoglobin (HbAlc) provides an index of glycaemic control over the preceding 2–3 months. Normal range depends on method, usually 3–7%.

Complications   1. *Early*:

— ketoacidosis
— coma
— hypoglycaemia
— skin lesions: moniliasis, necrobiosis lipoidica diabeticorum
— oedema
— neuropathy: symmetrical sensory or asymmetrical motor (diabetic amyotrophy)
— pneumomediastinum

2. *Later*:

— hepatomegaly ±dwarfism, obesity and hypogonadism (Mauriac syndrome)
— fat atrophy or hypertrophy

— joint contractures
— cataracts: rare (but lenticular opacities may occur within weeks of diagnosis)
— retinopathy — seen in: 10% after 5–9 years
                          70% after 15 years
                          90% after 25 years
— nephropathy: develops in approx. 40% of diabetics by 25 years after presentation in childhood
— psychological, including increased risk of suicide

Future developments   (a) Improved blood glucose control from miniaturized sub-cutaneous closed-loop infusion pumps linked to glucose sensors.
(b) Immunotherapy to prevent continuing β-cell destruction during the initial autoimmune process.
(c) Islet cell implants ('cytografts').

Calcium metabolism   Normal calcium homeostasis is critical for endocrine and neuromuscular functioning and growth in the developing child. Control of calcium and inorganic phosphate metabolism is complex. Calcium circulates in the plasma in three forms:

— combined with plasma proteins
— combined with citric and other organic acids
— ionized (65%). This form can diffuse through semi-permeable membranes and is metabolically active

Its concentration is controlled by parathyroid hormone (PTH), calcitonin and vitamin D, and is affected by acid–base changes.

Parathormone   Role of PTH is to maintain serum calcium in the normal range. It acts by:

— mobilizing calcium from bone (via vitamin D)
— reducing renal calcium losses
— increasing renal phosphate excretion
— increasing gastrointestinal calcium absorption (via vitamin D)

Calcitonin   Release of calcitonin by C-cells of thyroid gland is regulated by the plasma calcium concentration.

— reduces plasma calcium concentration by inhibition of bone resorption by osteoclasts
— at high levels, causes increased renal phosphate excretion

Vitamin D   Role is to promote bone mineralization by increasing calcium and phosphate concentrations in the extracellular fluid.

Vitamin D metabolism   (a) Vitamin D is obtained from two main sources:

— *skin*. UVL acts on 7-dehydrocholesterol in the deeper layers of the skin to produce cholecalciferol (vitamin D3).

— *diet*. Both ergocalciferol (D2) and cholecalciferol (D3) are efficiently absorbed from the intestine. Foods naturally rich in vitamin D include oily fish, eggs, butter and margarine. (Cow's milk and human milk have a low vitamin D content). Foods fortified with vitamin D include formula baby milks and some baby cereals

(b) After absorption, cholecalciferol is transported in the plasma to the liver where it is hydroxylated to 25-hydroxycholecalciferol.

(c) 25-hydroxycholecalciferol is transported in the plasma to the kidney where it is further hydroxylated:

— if serum calcium is low, it is hydroxylated to 1α, 25-dihydroxycholecalciferol (the active form)
— if serum calcium is high, it is hydroxylated to 24,25-dihydroxycholecalciferol (inactive form)

The active hormone 1α, 25-dihydroxycholecalciferol (1α, 25-diOH-D3) acts by increasing calcium absorption from the gut and increasing phosphate reabsorption from the gut and renal tubules. Calcium absorption from gut is also affected by upper intestinal pH and binding by dietary substances, e.g. phytates.

Rickets

Definition   Inadequate mineralization of new bone formation in growing bones, histologically characterized by accumulation of un-calcified osteoid tissue.

Causes   1. *Nutritional*. Major cause of rickets worldwide. Due to dietary deficiency of vitamin D combined with inadequate skin synthesis.

2. *Vitamin D-dependent*. Inherited condition (autosomal recessive). Type I: deficiency renal 1 hydroxylase enzyme; Type II: ?end-organ resistance to 1α, 25-diOH-D3. Treat with 1α, 25-diOH-D3.

3. *Renal osteodystrophy*. Seen in children with chronic renal failure. Cause complex, involving limited formation of 1,25-diOH-D3 due to renal damage and effects of secondary hyperparathyroidism. Treat by controlling hyperphosphataemia by oral phosphate binders, e.g. aluminium hydroxide, calcium supplements and vitamin D.

4. *Familial vitamin D–refractory hypophosphataemic rickets*. Inherited as an X-linked dominant trait. Main defect in proximal renal tubular absorption of phosphate. May also be a relative deficiency of active vitamin D due to a coexisting renal defect of 1-hydroxylation. Treat with massive doses of vitamin D, or with 1α, 25-diOH-D3 and phosphate supplements.

5. *Rickets associated with renal tubular disorders*:

— de Toni–Debre–Fanconi syndrome. Multiple defects proximal renal tubule with aminoaciduria, glycosuria and phosphaturia. Causes include:
  • inborn errors of metabolism, e.g. cystinosis, Lowe's syndrome
  • acquired, e.g. heavy metal poisoning
  • idiopathic

— renal tubular acidosis

6. *Rickets associated with anticonvulsant therapy.* Anticonvulsant induction of liver enzymes causes accelerated degradation of cholecalciferol to inactive metabolites. Serum calcium and phosphate should be checked periodically in children receiving anticonvulsants such as phenobarbitone and phenytoin.

Nutritional rickets

Incidence   The decline in rickets which followed the introduction of vitamin D supplements under the Welfare Food Scheme in the 1940s was halted in the 1960s when reports appeared of a significant incidence of rickets amongst immigrant families, particularly Asian. Factors predisposing to rickets in Asian children are:

— lack of exposure to sunlight: women and children tend to go out less, particularly in cold weather; girls and women are reluctant to uncover their limbs in public
— vegetarian diet. Gujerati Hindus are usually strict vegetarians and are at high risk
— maternal deficiency of vitamin D during pregnancy and lactation
— prolonged breast feeding or use of cow's milk for infant feeding

Clinical features   — thinning of skull bones (craniotabes)
— delayed closure of fontanelles
— frontal bossing
— delayed eruption of teeth
— Harrison sulci
— kyphoscoliosis
— bowing of legs, knock-knees (genu valgum)
— swelling at wrists and costo-chondral junctions (rickety rosary)
— muscular weakness, hypotonia, delayed walking
— rarely, tetany, hypocalcaemic convulsions

Radiological features   — loss of dense white lines at metaphyses with increased submetaphyseal lucency are early signs, seen best at distal ends of radius and ulna

— the next stage is widening of the metaphysis with cupping and splaying, irregularity and fraying
— in severe cases there is progressive rarefaction of the shaft, fractures of the cortex may occur and membrane bones are osteoporotic
— in treated cases, signs of healing include reappearance of the provisional zone of calcification as a transverse band at the end of the shaft and lamellated appearance of the cortex

Biochemical features
— increased plasma alkaline phosphatase
— calcium normal or low
— phosphate normal or low
— serum parathormone normal or increased

Prevention
Vitamin supplements should be given to infants and young children from 6 months (on cessation of fortified infant milks and cereals) until at least 2 years. Breast-fed infants should receive the supplements from 1 month.

Infants of Asian mothers should also receive early supplements which may need to continue up to 5 years, particularly if vegetarian.

Preterm infants should receive 20 µg (800 iu) of vitamin D daily for 3 months then 10 µg daily.

Standard children's vitamin drops supplied through child health clinics are free to families claiming family income supplement. The daily dose contains 10 µg (400 iu) of vitamin D.

Education
Campaigns to inform Asian communities about infant nutrition and prevention of rickets have been run by the DHSS and Save The Children Fund. The Health Education Council supplies leaflets in the main Asian languages on antenatal care, nutrition, rickets and breast feeding, and health education in schools has helped to reduce rickets in Asian adolescents.

Treatment
For nutritional rickets vitamin D 75 µg (3000 iu) daily for 4–6 weeks, then reduce to 10 µg (400 iu) daily with biochemical and radiological monitoring of response.

Thyroid disorders

Normal function
Production of thyroxine (T4) and tri-iodothyronine (T3) by the thyroid gland is stimulated by TSH from the anterior pituitary gland. Secretion of TSH is regulated by hypothalamic thyrotrophin-releasing hormone (TRH) and also by negative feedback of T4 and T3 levels.

Free T3 is the most active thyroid hormone fraction. Depending on metabolic demands, circulating T4 is converted either to active T3 or to an inert isomer, reverse T3 (rT3).

Neither thyroid hormones nor TSH cross the placenta in significant concentrations, so the fetal pituitary–thyroid axis is autonomous. After birth there is a surge of TSH release, provoked by cooling, which peaks at 30 min. This evokes release of thyroid hormones and there is also enhanced peripheral conversion of T4 to T3 within 4–6 h after delivery. TSH and T3 fall to basal levels after 3 days; T4 may not reach basal levels for 5–7 days.

Neonatal screening   Early diagnosis and prompt treatment are essential to prevent mental retardation in babies with congenital hypothyroidism. Diagnostic clinical features may not be recognized until the infant is several months old but the disease can be reliably detected biochemically in the newborn period. Such biochemical screening procedures result in clear benefit both in financial and human terms in the prevention of long-term handicap. The optimal time for screening is after the postnatal changes.

In Europe most programmes measure TSH by radioimmunoassay using a blood sample spotted onto filter paper between the 5th and 9th day of life, which can be combined with screening for phenylketonuria, usually on day 6. This assay fails to detect secondary hypothyroidism due to hypothalamic pituitary disease, but this is very rare (1 in 100 000); it may be suspected clinically due to physical signs, e.g. micropenis, hypoglycaemia, and is less likely to result in mental retardation. In parts of the USA, T4 is measured, with additional TSH assay when values are low.

Screening programmes worldwide have detected an incidence of permanent primary hypothyroidism of about 1 in 4000 births, most cases resulting from dysgenetic or ectopic thyroid tissue.

Hypothyroidism

Causes   1. Congenital:

— thyroid dysgenesis
  • total — 'athyreosis'
  • partial — hypoplastic, ectopic
— defect in thyroid hormone biosynthesis or action — dyshormonogenesis
— lack of pituitary TSH — secondary congenital hypothyroidism (Isolated or associated with other pituitary hormone deficiencies)
— maternal ingestion of goitrogens during pregnancy, e.g. PAS, iodine-containing cough mixtures, antithyroid drugs
— deficiency of iodine — endemic cretinism, e.g. New Guinea, Congo

2. Acquired:

— autoimmune thyroiditis (Hashimoto disease)
— post-thyroidectomy

— post-ingestion of goitrogens
— iodine deficiency

Clinical features of congenital hypothyroidism

— postmaturity
— lethargy
— large tongue, poor feeding, noisy breathing
— constipation
— hoarse cry
— prolonged unconjugated hyperbilirubinaemia
— hypothermia
— bradycardia
— coarse facies, low hairline, dry skin and hair
— short neck and goitre
— delayed closure of fontanelles, delayed bone age
— retarded development
— growth failure, infantile body proportions (upper/lower segment ratio increased)

Diagnosis

(a) In most cases, measurement of low serum T4 and TSH is sufficient to establish the diagnosis of primary hypothyroidism.

(b) Other tests distinguish between different causes of hypothyroidism, e.g. TSH response to TRH stimulation, serum T3 level, thyroid antibodies.

(c) Radioisotope scanning with technetium or ^{123}I helps to confirm whether thyroid tissue is present and whether it is ectopic.

(d) Radiological manifestations include retarded bone age, delayed irregular calcification of epiphyseal ossification centres, e.g. distal femoral epiphysis, usually calcified in term infants but not in cretins.

Treatment

Thyroxine, initially 10 µg/kg daily in congenital hypothyroidism. Dose adjusted to keep serum thyroxine in upper normal range for age. TSH levels take some months to fall.

In acquired primary hypothyroidism TSH levels are a guide to the adequacy of replacement together with monitoring of growth and skeletal maturation. Overtreatment may cause excessively rapid advance in bone age and early epiphyseal fusion, which will result in stunting.

Thyrotoxicosis

1. Congenital hyperthyroidism

Very rare. Due to transplacental passage of human thyroid stimulating immunoglobulins (HTSI) from a mother with active or treated Graves disease. Only about 1% of infants born to such mothers develop overt symptoms, with degree of risk relating to maternal HTSI levels.

Clinical features

— goitre
— irritability, jitteriness
— eye signs—lid retraction, oedema, proptosis
— tachycardia, cardiac failure

— voracious appetite with poor weight gain or weight loss
— diarrhoea, sweating, flushing

Treatment   Carbimazole or thiouracil. Propanolol if acutely thyrotoxic to reduce tachycardia and treat high-output cardiac failure.

Usually recover spontaneously by about 6 months. Persistence suggests early onset autonomous Graves disease.

2. Acquired hyperthyroidism   Much rarer than hypothyroidism. Autoimmune disease with familial tendency. Commoner in girls.

Postulated mechanism is defect in suppressor T lymphocytes permitting synthesis of thyroid stimulating immunoglobulins.

Clinical features   Onset usually insidious with behavioural changes (emotional lability, restlessness, deterioration in school performance), weight loss, diarrhoea and palpitations. Prominent glittery staring eyes and goitre develop. May be a thyroid bruit.

Diagnosis   Confirmed by finding increased T3 and T4 levels.

Treatment   1. *Medical.* Carbimazole; propanolol for acute manifestations. (Monitor for side-effects, e.g. neutropenia.)

After 2 euthyroid years treatment can sometimes be stopped. Monitoring should continue as relapse is not uncommon.

2. *Surgery* is considered if medical control is not satisfactory. Subtotal thyroidectomy with subsequent thyroxine replacement therapy gives good results.

3. Radioiodine ablation is *not* used in children because of long-term risk of thyroid carcinoma.

Causes of thyroid enlargement   1. *Congenital goitre*:

— maternal ingestion of goitrogens: antithyroid drugs, iodides
— congenital hyperthyroidism (maternal Graves disease)
— dyshormonogenesis

2. *Endemic*:

— iodine deficiency.

3. *Acquired sporadic goitre*:

— autoimmune thyroiditis
— drug-induced — iodide, lithium carbonate, PAS

4. *Simple (colloid) goitre.* Euthyroid. More common in girls, peak incidence around puberty. Aetiology unknown.

5. *Adenomatous goitre.*

6. *Tumours.*

7. *Other*

— Sarcoid, TB, syphilis

Thyroid carcinoma   Very rare in the UK. Higher incidence in the USA, particularly post-irradiation to head and neck in infancy.

Presentation   Solitary thyroid nodule or more often as generalized nodular thyroid enlargement. Any nodularity in a goitre is suspicious; thyroid scan and biopsy are indicated.

Histology   Usually well differentiated papillary or follicular in children. Up to 10% from para-follicular (C) cells (medullary carcinoma). May secrete calcitonin, ACTH, 5HT. In some families this is associated with:

phaeochromocytoma parathyroid hyperplasia ±mucosal neuromas skeletal anomalies	Sipple syndrome (multiple endocrine adenomatosis)

Treatment   Autosomal dominant inheritance.
(a) Complete thyroidectomy as far as possible.
(b) Radioactive iodine if complete surgical removal impossible, or distant metastases.
(c) Postoperative radiotherapy to neck.
(d) Thyroxine to maintain euthyroidism and suppress TSH production (this promotes regression of any remaining tumour).

The adrenal gland   The adrenal glands form from two sources: the medulla develops from neural crest cells and the cortex from a thickening of the coelomic epithelium between the mesentery and the mesonephros.

The fetal adrenal cortex is well developed and physiologically active but after birth the central (fetal) cortical zone involutes and the gland becomes smaller.

The adrenal cortex has three histologically distinct zones, the outer zona glomerulosa and two inner zones: zona fasciculata and reticularis. It secretes three types of hormone:

— mineralocorticoids (MC), principally aldosterone
— glucocorticoids (GC) (many of which have significant MC activity)
— Androgens and oestrogens.

Aldosterone secretion is controlled mainly by the renin–angiotensin system, plasma sodium and potassium concentrations and ACTH. Secretion of the other hormones is stimulated by ACTH.

Congenital adrenal hyperplasia (adrenogenital syndrome)   Biosynthesis of adrenocortical hormones is controlled by a series of enzymes. Defects in any of these enzymes may be inherited (autosomal recessive) and present as life-threatening neonatal emergencies. They are the commonest cause of ambiguous genitalia in the newborn.

Incidence   In UK, 1 in 5000, of which >95% are due to 21α-hydroxylase deficiency. Gene frequency for heterozygosity is 1 in 35. Heterozygote detection (by HLA typing and hormonal studies)

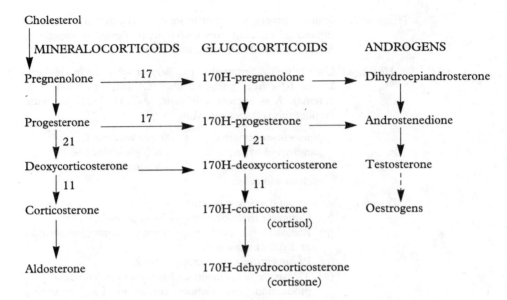

Enzymes: 17 = 17 α-hydroxylase, 21 = 21 α-hydroxylase, 11 = 11 β-hydroxylase

Fig. 4 Pathways of steroidogenesis

and antenatal diagnosis (by amniotic fluid 17α-hydroxy-progesterone (17P) at 17–18 weeks and/or chorionic villus biopsy) are possible.

21α-hydroxylase deficiency   Commonest type of congenital adrenal hyperplasia (CAH). 21-hydroxylation in MC and GC pathways are under separate genetic control and there are two clinical variants:

— hydroxylation defect affects GC pathway alone (milder form, non-salt losing)
— hydroxylation defect affects both pathways (salt-losing form)

In both types there is compensatory adrenocortical hyperplasia causing excess androgen production, resulting in virilization of the female, with ambiguous genitalia at birth, and macrogenitosomia developing in the male though not evident at birth.

If not recognized at birth, the condition may be diagnosed in the following situations:

(a) Loss of >10% of birth weight and failure to regain it by 7th day.
(b) Salt-losing crisis: often collapse with dehydration and salt loss ± hyperkalaemic cardiac arrest by 10th–14th day of life.
(c) Sick infant with family history of CAH or unexplained infant illnesses or deaths.

(d) Diarrhoea, vomiting and poor feeding in the neonatal period.

(e) Hypertension.

(f) Early puberty with advanced bone age.

(g) Hirsutism or virilism inappropriate for age or sex.

(h) Primary amenorrhoea.

Investigations

(a) Low serum sodium, high potassium and urea.

(b) Increased urinary excretion of sodium chloride. Fantus silver nitrate test for urinary chlorides is rapid; a high level in a vomiting infant helps to exclude gastroenteritis and pyloric stenosis.

(c) Immunoassay for plasma 17α-hydroxyprogesterone (17P) levels. Plasma ACTH raised in all forms of CAH (normally falls rapidly due to clearance of placental-derived 17P in first 24 h so best measured after 1st day of life. (Plasma 17P levels may be elevated in sick infants, particularly preterm babies who may be hyponatraemic due to a combination of inappropriate fluid replacement and transient renal tubular unresponsiveness to MC.)

(d) 24-h urine collection — gas chromatography patterns of urinary steroid metabolite excretion can confirm diagnosis and distinguish between some forms of enzyme deficiency.

Treatment

(a) If serum and urine biochemistry suggest the diagnosis in an acutely ill infant, take blood sample for 17P then start treatment without waiting for confirmation of diagnosis.

(b) Rehydrate carefully with normal saline, monitoring serum sodium and blood glucose.

(c) Once sodium balance is restored start MC replacement treatment with aldosterone (short-acting) and DOC pivalate (long-acting).

(d) In the extremely sick infant it may be necessary to give hydrocortisone i.v. 25–50 mg stat but efficacy of this treatment is thought to be due mainly to MC effects. Aldosterone is more effective than cortisol, and administration of the latter may make establishing a diagnosis more difficult.

(e) Long-term management:

— Oral fludrocortisone; monitor BP, urine and plasma sodium, plasma renin activity

— Hydrocortisone; dose is titrated against plasma ACTH, 17P profile and androgen levels. Height and skeletal maturation are carefully monitored

— dose must be increased 2–3 fold during stress, e.g. sepsis, surgery

— a Medicalert bracelet should be worn

— surgical correction of clitoromegaly in girls with virilizing CAH is usually done before 18 months. Vaginoplasty is more successful if delayed until after 16 years of age

— girls with genital ambiguity and their parents may need psychotherapy to help deal with confusion over gender identity

Screening for CAH Pilot screening programmes have employed blood spot 17P immunoassays which can be combined with screening for PKU and hypothyroidism. Problems potentially avoidable by screening for CAH include:

— life-threatening salt wasting crises
— inappropriate gender assignment
— incorrect diagnosis of 'pyloric stenosis'
— precocious puberty
— stunted growth
— sudden death

However, there are technical problems with the assay, including a high false positive rate, particularly in preterm infants, and debate continues as to whether screening is justified to detect the small number of infants where the diagnosis is missed on clinical criteria.

Inborn errors of metabolism (IEM) IEM are genetically inherited enzyme defects resulting in the accumulation of toxic metabolites which may cause neurological damage and death. Many can be detected antenatally and screening programmes have been developed for a few, but most are too rare for screening of the whole population to be practical.

Clinical clues *Infancy* — persistent or recurrent vomiting
— weight loss, poor feeding
— jaundice, hepatomegaly
— lethargy
— unusual smell of body or urine

especially if accompanied by metabolic acidosis, ketosis and/or hyperammonaemia, or if there is a family history of unexplained infant deaths

Older children — mental retardation, self-multilation, microcephaly
— renal calculi
— coarse facies, dislocated lenses, abnormal hair
— hypopigmentation
— osteoporosis
— failure to thrive

Disorders of amino acid metabolism

Phenylketonuria (PKU) Frequency: 1 in 7000 in UK. Enzyme defect: L-phenylalanine hydroxylase and variants.

Clinical features   Commonest IEM causing mental retardation. If untreated, present with global developmental delay, mainly between 6 and 12 months. May be hypertonic; 1 in 4 have seizures, usually starting after 6 months. Characteristic musty or mousy odour due to metabolite phenylacetic acid. Many patients are fair haired, blue eyed and 20% have eczema.

Screening   National programme using Guthrie test since 1974 (technique first described in 1963). β2-thienylamine, an antimetabolite analogue of phenylalanine, inhibits the growth of *Bacillus subtilis* in an agar medium. If phenylalanine is added in sufficient amounts it will overcome the effect of the inhibitor and the organism will grow. In screening, capillary blood is taken by heelprick onto thick filter paper discs which are sent to the regional screening centre and incubated with the special medium. The size of the growth zone of the organism is a function of the concentration of phenylalanine in the sample. Guthrie tests detect levels >0.25 mmol/1. There are several causes of hyperphenylalaninaemia and diagnosis of classical PKU must be confirmed by finding serum phenylalanine levels >1.2 mmol/1 on a normal diet.

Treatment   Restriction of dietary phenylalanine. In infancy, diet is based on special milks such as Lofenalac (Mead–Johson) or Minafen (Cow & Gate), which have low levels of phenylalanine and added tyrosine. Weaning is started as usual about 4 months with low protein foods. As the child grows, it is important to ensure the diet is nutritionally complete; a phenylalanine-free formula such as Albumaid X-P (Scientific Hospital Supplies, SHS) is used as protein and calorie source, and measured amounts of cereal, milk and vegetarian foods are added.

Blood phenylalanine should be monitored frequently and maintained between 0.15–0.5 mmol/1. Clinical status, growth and intellectual development are assessed regularly. The diet should be continued until the child is at least 10 years old; some believe it ·should be continued into adult life, particularly in women during the reproductive years.

Maternal PKU   There is a high risk of fetal damage with maternal hyperphenylalaninaemia. Phenylalanine restriction started before conception improves outcome.

2. Homocystinuria   Second commonest disorder of amino acid metabolism (1 in 20–40 000). Enzyme defect: cystathione synthetase.

Clinical features   Variable:

— tall with arachnodactyly, osteoporosis, kyphoscoliosis, pectus excavatum
— downward dislocation of lenses usually develops by 10 years. Also myopia, glaucoma, retinal detachment, cataracts and optic atrophy

— brittle fair hair, coarse skin, acne
— neuropsychiatric symptoms: 50% mentally retarded, schizoid personality disorders reported
— vascular; tendency to intravascular thromboses may manifest as superficial or deep vein thrombosis, renal artery stenosis, pulmonary embolism, intracranial thrombosis or early coronary artery disease.

Treatment   50% of patients respond to treatment with large doses of the coenzyme pyridoxine. Non-responders are treated with a low methionine diet supplemented with cysteine.

3. Branched-chain amino   — maple syrup urine disease   ⎫   Disorders of branched-
   acid disorders   — methylmalonic acidaemia   ⎬   chain amino acids
   — propionic acidaemia   ⎬   leucine, isoleucine,
   — isovaleric acidaemia   ⎭   valine

Frequency: 1 in 250 000.

Clinical features   Vomiting, poor feeding, acidosis, ketonuria. May be associated with thrombocytopaenia, hypoglycaemia. Severe cases present in 1st week of life and severe retardation ensues unless treated promptly.

Treatment   Strict dietary treatment with individual adjustment of the three branch-chain amino acids can prevent brain damage if started early. Thiamine helps some cases of MSUD and vitamin B12 (cobalamin) should be tried in methylmalonic acidaemia.

Urea cycle defects   Enzyme defects are described for all stages in the urea cycle; the common feature is high blood ammonia, and some of the defects also cause orotic aciduria.

Clinical features   — failure to thrive
— mental retardation, seizures, ataxia

Infection can precipitate hyperammonaemic crises with coma.

Treatment   In crises, high carbohydrate protein-free diet, gut sterilization, anabolic steroids and dialysis may be required.

Disorders of carbohydrate
metabolism

1. Galactosemia   Frequency: 1 in 50–70 000; Enzyme defect: galactose-1-phosphate uridyltransferase or variants.

Clinical features   — vomiting, diarrhoea and failure to thrive
— jaundice, anaemia, purpura, cirrhosis
— cataracts, hypoglycaemia
— septicaemia
— mental retardation

Treatment   Lactose- and galactose-free diet for life. Suitable milk substitutes include Pregestimil, Nutramigen (Mead – Johnson), Galactomin (Cow & Gate). Medicines and supplements must be lactose free. Monitor by erythrocyte galactose-1-phosphate levels.

Glycogen storage disorders

Eponym (type)	Enzyme defect	Clinical features
von Gierke (I)	Glucose-6-phosphatase	Failure to thrive, short stature hepatomegaly, platelet defect, xanthomata, bleeding problems, hypoglycaemia, hyperuricaemia.
Pompe (II)	α1,4-glucosidase	— *Infantile*: After 1 month progressive hypotonia, macroglossia, cardiomegaly with heart failure and death in 2nd year. — *Childhood*. Slower progression, death in 2nd decade — *Adult*. Chronic myopathy
Cori (III)	Amylo-1,6-glucosidase (debrancher enzyme)	Hepatomegaly, poor growth, hypoglycaemic seizures. Abates with age
Andersen (IV)	α1,4-glucan-6-glucosyl transferase	Failure to thrive, hypotonia, hepatosplenomegaly, liver failure. Survival 6 months to 5 years
McArdle (V)	Muscle phosphorylase	Muscle weakness and pain on exercise with myoglobinuria
Hers (VI)	Hepatic phosphorylase	Similar to mild form of type I. Hepatosplenomegaly, hypoglycaemia
Tarui (VII)	Muscle phosphofructokinase	Similar to type V + haemolytic anaemia
Huijing (VIII)	Hepatic phosphorylasekinase	Mild, hepatomegaly

2. Mucopolysaccharidoses (MPS)

(a) *Hurler syndrome (MPS I)*. Frequency: 1 in 100 000; Enzyme defect: αL-iduronidase.

Clinical features: Manifest from 6 months. Large macrocephalic infant, recurrent URTI, hepatosplenomegaly, coarse facies, corneal clouding, inguinal and umbilical hernias, claw hand, contractures, hirsutism, lumbar gibbus. Progressive psychomotor retardation. Cardiomyopathy. Death 6–10 years.

Treatment: Symptomatic and supportive. Role of BMT under evaluation.

(b) *Hunter syndrome (MPS II)*. Enzyme defect sulphoiduronide sulphatase. Similar to Hurler phenotype but X-linked inheritance and no corneal clouding.

(c) *Sanfilippo syndrome (MPS III)*. Mental deterioration predominates with hyperkinetic aggressive behaviour and mild Hurler-like physical features.

(d) *Morquio–Brailsford syndrome (MPS IV)*. Mainly skeletal abnormalities: contractures, dwarfism, odontoid hypoplasia and myelopathy. May be valvular heart disease. Intelligence usually normal.

Disorders of lipid
metabolism

1. Mucolipidoses   Lysosomal storage disorders in which mucopolysaccharides
and sphingolipids are presumed to accumulate.
   Clinical features include variations of Hurler type skeletal
manifestations, hepatosplenomegaly and mental deterioration
but no excess mucopolysacchariduria.

2. Sphingolipidoses   Lysosomal enzyme deficiency resulting in excess accumulation
of a normally synthesized product. Autosomal recessive in-
heritance.

Eponym	Enzyme defect	Clinical features
Tay-Sach's disease	Hexosaminidase A	Macrocephaly, blindness, macular cherry-red spot Dementia, fits, tetraplegia
Gaucher's disease	β-glucosidase	*Acute* infantile form — psychomotor deterioration, cyanotic attacks, tetraplegia *Chronic* childhood form — hepatosplenomegaly, normal IQ
Niemann–Pick disease	Sphingomyelinase	Fits, blindness, cherry-red spot, pulmonary infiltrates, hepatosplenomegaly, foamy lymphocytes

18. Haematology

Physiology of blood formation

Haematopoesis is extramedullary in the fetus (yolk sac, liver, spleen); bone marrow progressively takes over during last trimester. Extramedullary haematopoesis may persist or recur after birth if there is excessive blood destruction or loss.

Normal neonatal blood count

(a) Hb rises to mean 19 g/dl (17–22 g/dl) in cord blood at term.

(b) Hb values are lower in preterm infants, with macrocytosis and nucleated red blood cells.

(c) Changing pattern of Hb synthesis up until:

36/40	~90% HbF
40/40	50–85% HbF
6/12	5% HbF
12/12	0–2% HbF

HbF ($\alpha_2\gamma_2$) can be detected by its resistance to denaturation with acids and alkalis, e.g. Kleihauer film, Singer test.

(d) Neutrophil leucocytosis peaking at 12 h, disappears by 2 days. Thereafter preponderance of lymphocytes (~60% of total) until age 4 years.

(e) Coagulation times in newborn are slightly prolonged with lowest levels of coagulation factors around 3rd day, probably due to low stores of vitamin K at birth.

Causes of neonatal anaemia

1. Haemorrhage
   — twin–twin transfusion
   — feto-maternal transfusion
   — intrapartum — external
      • placenta praevia
      • placental abruption
      • placental incision during CS
      • umbilical cord rupture
                    — internal
      • intracranial
      • intra-abdominal
   — postpartum — haemorrhage disease of the newborn (HDN), vitamin K deficiency
   — bleeding from alimentary tract
   — iatrogenic

2. Haemolysis — transfer of maternal antibodies:
  - blood group incompatibility e.g. Rhesus/ABO/Kell, Lewis, Duffy
  - maternal autoimmune haemolytic anaemia
  - maternal SLE
— transfer of maternal drugs to infant with G6PD deficiency, e.g. sulphonamides, dapsone, quinine
— associated with infection
— vitamin E deficiency in preterm infants
— congenital defects of red cell:
  - membrane disorders, e.g. hereditary spherocytosis, elliptocytosis, stomatocytosis
  - red cell enzyme disorders, e.g. glucose-6-phosphate dehydrogenase deficiency, pyruvate kinase deficiency
  - Hb abnormalities:
    structural, e.g. sickle cell disease ⎤ both β-chain
    synthesis, e.g. thalassaemia major ⎦ defects — rarely
    cause problems
    <3–6 months

3. Impaired production — congenital red cell aplasia (Blackfan Diamond syndrome)
— haematinic deficiency

Anaemia in childhood

Iron deficiency   Commonest cause of anaemia; maximum incidence at 6 months to 3 years.
  Increased susceptibility in infants because:
(a) >75% of total body iron in newborn is in circulating Hb. Stores are dependent on Hb concentration at birth and blood volume (body weight).
(b) Human milk has low iron content (1.5 mg/l).

Stores in mature infant at term are sufficient for ~4 months' normal requirements. From 4–12 months a daily oral intake of at least 1 mg/kg/day elemental iron is needed (assuming absorption efficacy ~10%).

Preterm and low-birth-weight infants will have inadequate stores at birth and will need supplements until established on a mixed diet.

Predisposing conditions — low birth weight
— prematurity
— feeding with cow's milk (iron content 0.5 mg/l)
— blood loss
  - perinatal
  - GI, e.g. oesophagitis, PU, varices, Meckel's diverticulum, IBD, reduplication, HSP, drugs (e.g. aspirin, steroids), parasites (e.g. hookworm)
  - epistaxis

- renal
— malabsorption, e.g. coeliac, IBD, giardia, blind-loop syndrome

Investigations
— Hb, Hct
— MCHC <30%, MCV <80 fl, MCH <29 pg
— film
  - microcytosis (cells with low MCV)
  - hypochromia (reduced staining due to iron deficiency)
  - anisocytosis (cells of variable size)
  - poikilocytes (pencil cells)
  - codocytes (target cells)
— iron studies will show:
  - low serum iron (normal range by 3 years 10–31 mmol/l)
  - high serum TIBC (normal range after 6 months 45–90 mmol/l)
  - % transferrin saturation <16%
  - low serum ferritin
    (normal range 16–70 ng/ml at 1 year)
    10–40 ng/ml 5–15 years
  - raised erythrocyte protoporphyrin (normally <40 ng/dl erythrocytes)

Other causes of hypochromic anaemia
— chronic infection (low Fe, high ferritin, normal TIBC)
— chronic inflammation, e.g. JCA
— malignancy
— thalassaemia (high Fe, high ferritin, normal TIBC)
— sideroblastic anaemia — rare in childhood, e.g. lead poisoning, dietary pyridoxine deficiency
— copper deficiency

Treatment
(a) *Correct underlying cause*: dietary advice is often needed. Red meat is the best source; in a vegetarian diet iron is obtained from eggs, cereals and leguminous vegetables (pulses, 'dahl').
(b) *Iron supplementation*. Preferably oral administration as ferrous salt in liquid form, e.g. ferrous sulphate, gluconate or succinate. If symptoms of intolerance occur, chelated preparations may be better tolerated, e.g. Sytron (iron EDTA), Niferex (polysaccharide iron complex).

Prophylactic dose 2 mg elemental Fe/kg/day in three divided doses between meals; therapeutic doses 5 mg elemental Fe/kg/day in three divided doses. (Severe symptomatic anaemia (Hb usually <4–6 g/dl) indicates need for blood transfusion.)

Response rate to iron therapy:
— reticulocyte peak between 5–10 days
— increase Hb by 2 g/dl every 3 weeks
— treatment should be continued for ~8 weeks then check Hb

Reasons for *failure to respond* to iron therapy:

— poor compliance
— inadequate dosage
— impaired absorption
— continued blood loss
— coexisting disease, e.g. renal failure
— coexisting folate deficiency
— incorrect diagnosis

Folic acid
— deficiency rare in children; causes a megaloblastic anaemia
— occurs as polyglutamates in green vegetables, human and cow's milk (not goat's milk)
— absorbed in duodenum and jejunum
— daily requirement in infants — 20–50 µg/day
                      children — up to 2 mg/day

Factors associated with depletion
— preterm and low-birth-weight infants
— overheating milk; overcooking vegetables
— malabsorption syndromes
— increased demand, e.g. increased cell turnover (malignancy or chronic haemolysis)
— drugs
   • anticonvulsants: phenobarbitone, phenytoin
   • methotrexate, azothioprine
   • nitrofurantoin, cotrimoxazole
— maternal folate depletion

Vitamin B12
— deficiency rare in children; causes a megaloblastic anaemia
— occurs in milk, eggs, meat and fish
— hepatic stores at birth sufficient for 8-12 months
— absorbed in terminal ileum complexed with intrinsic factor (IF) and subsequently transported in portal circulation bound to transcobalamin II (a β-globulin). (Transcobalamin I is a circulating B12 storage complex)

Causes of deficiency

1. *Nutritional*:

— secondary to maternal deficiency
— strict vegetarians, e. g. vegans

2. *Impaired absorption*:

— true juvenile pernicious anaemia. Autoimmune disease with antibodies to gastric parietal cells and IF. Rare before 2nd decade. May be other endocrine abnormalites
— congenital absence of IF
— transcobalamin II deficiency; early presentation, usually in 1st month
— short bowel syndrome — after extensive gut resection
— malabsorption syndromes, e.g. tropical sprue (rare in coeliac disease)

| Vitamin E | Antioxidant essential for normal red cell membrane function. VLBW infants may need supplements. |

Vitamin E — Antioxidant essential for normal red cell membrane function. VLBW infants may need supplements.

Other rare deficiency anaemias
— pyridoxine
— copper
— vitamin C
— thyroxine

Haemolytic anaemias

General features   (a) Red cell changes:

— spherocytes — reflect damage to red cell membranes, e.g. hereditary or drug-induced spherocytosis, red cell trauma
— red cell fragmentaion — burr cells (schistocytes)
— decreased red cell survival

(b) Marrow response:

— increased reticulocytes >2%, may be up to 30%
— erythroid: myeloid ratio >1:1 in haemolysis (normally 1:5)

(c) Intravascular haemolysis. Free Hb is liberated into the circulating blood and bound to circulating haptoglobins, then removed by reticulo-endothelial system. Plasma haptoglobins then fall (but are low or absent in the normal neonate).

Once Hb–haptoglobin complex is saturated, the Hb is oxidized to haematin and combines with albumin to form methaemalbumin (detected by Schumm's test).

Causes   1. *Hereditary*:

— red cell membrane defects
  • spherocytosis
  • elliptocytosis
  • stomatocytosis
— red cell enzyme defects
  • G6PD deficiency
  • pyruvate kinase deficiency
— defects in Hb synthesis or structure
  • thalassaemias
  • sickle cell disease

2. *Acquired*:

— immune haemolytic anaemias:
  • HDN
  • cold agglutinins — IgM, e.g. mycoplasma
  • Autoantibodies — IgG, e.g. SLE, rheumatoid, malignancy, idiopathic
  • drugs, e.g. methyl dopa
— trauma:

- cardiac–prosthetic valve, open heart surgery
- microangiopathic haemolytic anaemia — haemolytic uraemic syndrome, thrombotic thrombocytopenic purpura, acute glomerulonephritis, SLE, burns
— infection: • malaria
  - toxoplasmosis
  - clostridia
  - typhoid
  - cholera
— Chemicals: • napthalene
  - sulphonamides

Haemolytic disease of the newborn

Rhesus antigen system consists of three red cell membrane antigens (Cc, Dd and Ee), controlled by three gene pairs. 85% of Caucasians have 'D' antigen, i.e. are Rhesus positive. If exposed to 'D', Rhesus negative individuals will make antibodies to red cells bearing 'D' and haemolysis will ensue. If a sensitized Rhesus negative mother gives birth to a Rhesus positive infant, haemolytic disease of the newborn will occur.

Sensitization may occur after:

(a) Prior transfusion of mother with Rhesus positive blood

(b) Fetomaternal blood leak in previous pregnancy at abortion or delivery.

There is an amplified response in production of these IgG antibodies in the second and each subsequent exposure. Thus significant HDN is rare in first pregnancy and increases in incidence and severity with increasing parity.

Prevention of rhesus haemolytic disease (RHD)

(a) Blood group of all mothers checked at booking antenatal visit.

(b) Rhesus negative mothers at risk (Rh. pos. father) checked regularly in pregnancy for antibodies.

(c) If increasing antibody titre:

— before 28–32 weeks amniocentesis: measure amniotic fluid antibody titres and bilirubin. If high or increasing bilirubin consider foetal transfusion. Maternal plasmapheresis in 2nd trimester may be effective

— after 32 weeks with increasing titre consider elective preterm delivery

(d) If antibodies not detected/low titre not increasing, give human Rhesus hyperimmune gammaglobulin ('anti D') within 72 h of birth (or after amnio/TOP).

ABO haemolytic disease

Infants of blood group A (or more rarely B) born to mothers with blood group O may develop jaundice early (within first 24 h) due to transplacental passage of maternal antibodies directed against the A (or B) antigen.

Maternal circulating antibody levels do not correlate well with the severity of haemolysis. These antibodies are usually large IgM molecules which cannot cross the placenta.

— usually causes only mild/moderate early jaundice
— occasionally treatment with phototherapy or exchange transfusion may be required
— continuing low-grade haemolysis may lead to late anaemia after 10–14 days

Hereditary haemolytic anaemias

Glucose-6-phosphate dehydrogenase deficiency

This is the commonest known enzyme deficiency worldwide (West Africa, Mediterranean, SE Asia, M East).

Cause: Diminished activity of the enzyme G6PD which results in impaired reduction of glutathione so that the red cell is more susceptible to oxidant stress.

Inheritance: X-linked. Homozygote females may be as severely affected as males. Heterozygote females have intermediate enzyme activity levels. Wide range of genetic variants; three main types, i.e. Mediterranean, African, Oriental.

Clinical Manifestations include:

— neonatal jaundice, usually develops 2/3rd day
— acute episodes of haemolysis causing pallor, dark urine and sometimes jaundice, precipitated by drugs, infection or consumption of fava beans
— congenital non-spherocytic haemolytic anaemia

Precipitants of acute haemolysis

— infections and other acute illnesses, e.g. diabetic ketoacidosis
— drugs:
  • antimalarials, e.g. primaquine, pyrimethamine, chloroquine, dapsone
  • analgesics, e.g. acetylsalicylic acid
  • antibacterials, e.g. sulphonamides, nitrofurantoin, penicillin
  • miscellaneous, e.g. vitamin K, napthalene
— Fava beans (broad beans): Mediterranean and Oriental types

Diagnosis

(a) *Between crises:*

— blood count and film are normal
— enzyme deficiency may be detected by direct red cell enzyme assay or screening tests, e.g. brilliant cresyl blue decoloration

(b) *During crisis:*

— Hb may fall to 2–5 g/dl
— film: crescent cells, spherocytes and Heinz bodies (oxidized, denatured Hb)
— may be features of intravascular haemolysis
— screening tests and enzyme assay may be falsely

normal because reticulocytes produced in response to haemolysis have higher enzyme levels

Treatment
— identify and avoid precipitants
— maintain good hydration and high urine output.
— blood transfusion for severe anaemia
— analgesia
— occasionally, antioxidants — methylene blue, vitamin C

Hereditary spherocytosis

Commonest hereditary haemolytic anaemia in N Europeans. *Cause*: defective red cell membrane sodium transport. Red cells accumulate fluid and have increased osmotic fragility. *Inheritance*: autosomal dominant with variable expression. *Clinical features*:

— anaemia, presenting at any age
— mild jaundice, often fluctuating
— splenomegaly
— gallstones
— leg ulcers
— aplastic crises, usually precipitated by viral infections, particularly parvovirus

Management: Splenectomy if severe.

Defects in haemoglobin synthesis: thalassaemias

There are three main types of Hb normally produced after birth:

	% normal adult type
$F(\alpha_2\gamma_2)$	0.5
$A(\alpha_2\beta_2)$	97
$A_2(\alpha_2\delta_2)$	2.5–3.5

In thalassaemia, a defect in genes organizing globin chain synthesis results in unbalanced production of α and β chains.

β-Thalassaemia (Mediterranean anaemia, Cooley anaemia)

Incidence: As the name suggests found mainly in Mediterranean races with incidence ~20% in Turkey and Greece, ~10% in Sicily, also in Burma, Thailand and less commonly in China, India and C Africa.
Inheritance: β-Chain synthesis controlled by a pair of allellomorphic genes. In thalassaemia *major*, both are replaced by β-thalassaemia genes (homozygous). In thalassaemia *minor*, only one is replaced by a β-thalassaemia gene. In addition there are two types of β-thalassaemia gene:

— no synthesis of β chains — β°
— decreased synthesis of β chains — β^+

Pathophysiology of β-thalassaemia major:
(a) Decreased β-chain synthesis leads to defect in HbA + ↑HbA2 $(\alpha_2\delta_2)$ and HbF $(\alpha_2\gamma_2)$.
(b) α-chain excess tetramers cause RBC damage and haemolysis.

Clinical features:
Thal. minor:

— mild anaemia. No treatment required
— occasional splenomegaly
— differential diagnosis from iron deficiency (NB: may coexist)
  • fasting serum iron normal/increased
  • TIBC   ⎫
  • % saturation   ⎬ normal
                    ⎭

Thal. major: Rarely symptomatic before 6 months:

— progressive pallor
— poor feeding, failure to thrive
— hepatosplenomegaly
— characteristic facies — 'mongoloid', with frontal bossing
  and prominent malar eminences
— bone changes due to marrow hyperplasia:
  • skull 'hair on end' appearance
  • delayed bone age
  • generalized osteoporosis; pathological fractures may
    occur

Management thal. major:
(a) Programme of regular and frequent blood transfusions
    with iron chelating regimens using subcutaneous desferi-
    oxamine given nightly at home to prevent haemosiderosis.
(b) Splenectomy if there is evidence of hypersplenism, i.e.
    excess transfusion requirement, gross splenomegaly,
    thrombocytopenia.
(c) Folic A supplements.
(d) Prophylactic penicillin post-splenectomy (because of in-
    creased risk of pneumococcal infection) + Pneumovax.

Defects in haemoglobin structure: haemoglobinopathies

Many abnormal Hb variants have been described; the
majority are asymptomatic. By far the most important is
sickle cell anaemia.

Sickle cell anaemia

Cause: Synthesis of an abnormal Hb chain with substitution
of valine for glutamic acid in position 6 on the β-polypeptide
chain (HbS).
Inheritance: Autosomal recessive.
Incidence: Common in Negro races. Carriage of HbS up to
40% in Africa, 8% in American Negro, 10% in Afro-
caribbeans in UK.
Clinical features:
(a) *Heterozygotes* HbS 35–45% (sickle cell trait).
    Asymptomatic, except rare vaso-occlusive crises if
    severely hypoxic, e.g. flying at high altitude in
    unpressurized aircraft.
(b) *Homozygotes*: HbS 90–95%, HbF 5–10%, no HbA.
    Chronic haemolytic anaemia (Hb 6–8 g/dl) with
    frequent painful crises of sickling and acute haemolysis

from ~6 months. Capillary obstruction by abnormal shape of erythrocytes leads to vaso-occlusive phenomena affecting any organ.

Common symptoms: abdominal pain, chest pain, fits, hemiplegia, haematuria.

+ Effects of chronic anaemia: delayed puberty, destructive bone changes with periosteal reaction, pigment gall stones, leg ulcers.

+ Susceptibility to infection, particularly *salmonella*, *Staph. aureus*, *pneumococcus*, parvovirus.

Management:

(a) Treat precipitating cause.
(b) Supportive treatment with fluids, oxygen, analgesia.
(c) Antibiotics.
(d) Blood transfusion or red cell exchange transfusion indicated:

— prolonged/extreme pain
— extensive involvement lungs/CNS
— prior to GA
— in late pregnancy
— in sequestration or aplastic crises.

(e) Splenectomy — only if recurrent sequestration crises/hypersplenism.
(f) Prophylaxis — dental care, pneumovax, penicillin.

Typical laboratory profile

	SC trait (Homozygous)	SC disease (Heterozygous)
Hb	Normal	6–8
Film	Normal	Hypochromia Target cells Howell Jolly bodies Occasional sickle cells
Sickledex screen	Positive	Positive
Hb electrophoresis	Two bands, A and S	One band in S region

Combination of HbS with other Hb abnormalities

For example:

1. *HbSC disease*: HbC has lysine substituted in the 6 position on β-chain. Moderately severe anaemia and may have vaso-occlusive crises but usually milder than sickle cell disease. Tendency to thrombosis and pulmonary embolism, aseptic necrosis of femoral head.

2. *HbS-thalassaemia*: Moderately severe anaemia with microcytosis, mild–moderate vaso-occlusive crises, splenomegaly.

Antenatal diagnosis

(a) Fetal blood sampling by fetoscopy: globin chain synthesis measured in circulating normoblasts. Cannot be used before ~18/40.

(b) Fetal DNA analysis of cells obtained from either amniotic fluid or trophoblast biopsy. Can be done in 1st trimester utilizing radioactive gene probes (see p. 10). Can be used in the antenatal diagnosis of thalassaemia and haemophilia.

Aplastic anaemia

Bone marrow stem cell failure in infants and children is uncommon but occurs in several important disorders. The diagnosis is suspected when there is progressive anaemia with:

— no evidence of haemolysis or blood loss
— accompanying neutropenia and thrombocytopenia
— no reticulocyte response

and confirmed on bone marrow biopsy, which shows hypocellular fatty marrow with reduced haematopoesis in all cell lines. There may be replacement of marrow by infiltrating substance, e.g. malignant cells, lipid.

Causes

1. *Congenital*:

— pure red cell aplasia (Blackfan–Diamond syndrome)
— Fanconi anaemia
  • autosomal recessive: presents 18 months to 3rd decade
  • associated features
    • skeletal anomalies inc.absent radii/thumbs
    • renal anomalies inc. absent/horseshoe kidneys
    • short stature
    • chromosomal fragility
  • treatment: androgens, BMT

— constitutional aplastic anaemia without associated anomalies.

2. *Acquired*:

— idiopathic ~50%
— drugs, e.g. antineoplastics-cyclophosphamide, MTX, chloramphenicol, phenylbutazone
— chemicals, e.g. benzene, glue
— ionizing radiation
— viral infections, e.g. hepatitis A, IMN, *H. simplex*
— secondary to marrow infiltration, e.g. leukaemia, neuroblastoma, lipid storage disorder

Management

Variable success according to aetiological type:

— androgens
— high-dose methyl prednisolne
— antilymphocyte globulin
— BMT

Haemorrhagic disorders

When taking history about suspected bleeding disorder, note especially:

— family history of bleeding disorder
— history of bleeding after previous surgery
— child's previous medical history, e.g. congenital heart disease, renal disease, drug ingestion
— antecedant illness prior to development of bleeding tendency
— trauma

Causes of purpura and bleeding

1. *Platelet deficiency* — thrombocytopenia <150 000/mm^3:
(a) Decreased production by megakaryocytes e.g.

— drug-induced
— aplastic anaemia
— acute leukaemia
— congenital-intrauterine viral infections, congenital amegakaryocytic thrombocytopenia (TAR syndrome)

(b) Increased destruction e.g.

— maternal antiplatelet antibodies
— maternal ITP
— drug-induced autoantibodies
— ITP
— consumption coagulopathy, e.g. Waterhouse–Friedrichson syndrome
— microangiopathic haemolytic anaemia
— Wiskott–Aldrich syndrome:
  • usually presents 1st months of life
  • defects of cellular and humoral immunity
  • recurrent pyogenic infections
  • eczema
  • small platelets

2. *Defective platelet function*:
(a) Congenital, e.g. Von Willebrand Disease
    Thrombasthenia (Glanzmann disease)
    Bernard–Soulier syndrome
    May-Hegglin anomaly
(b) Drugs — aspirin, indomethacin.
(c) Uraemia.
(d) Advanced liver disease.
3. *Capillary damage*:
(a) Henoch-Schönlein purpura.
(b) Infection

— bacterial: meningococcal, typhoid, rickettsiae
— viral: IMN, CMV

(c) drugs — salicylates, high-dose penicillin.
(d) Mechanical, e.g. pertussis.
(e) Inherited — Hereditary haemorrhagic telangiectasia, Ehrler–Danlos syndrome.

4. *Coagulation deficiency*:
(a) Inherited
  • haemophilia (factor VIII deficiency)
  • Christmas disease (factor IX deficiency)
  • Von Willebrand disease
(b) Acquired:

— impaired hepatic production of vitamin K dependent factors: II, VII, IX and X, e.g. in HDN, liver disease, malabsorption
— increased consumption of clotting factors I, II, V, VIII and platelets (disseminated intravascular coagulation). Features:
  • low platelet count
  • low fibrinogen and prolonged PT
  • low factor V and sometimes VIII and II
  • elevated fibrin degradation products (FDP) due to sepsis, asphyxia or localized lesion, e.g. giant haemangioma

Haemophilia
— due to deficient Factor VIII coagulation
— X-linked, i.e. only occurs in males, transmitted by females
— ~20% occur by spontaneous mutation

Diagnosis
— factor VIII level low — <50%
  0–1% Severe
  1–5% Moderate
  5–50% mild
— bleeding time normal

Clinical features
Tendency to haemorrhage
  • bruising
  • haemarthroses
  • after dental extraction/surgery
  • retro-peritoneal

Management
Should be supervized by a haemophilia centre but can largely be based at home.
(a) In acute episodes prompt replacement treatment with freeze-dried FVIII concentrate (or cryoprecipitate/FFP). 1 u/kg raises FVIII by ~2%. Many children learn to give their own injections.
(b) Must never be given aspirin.
(c) Must never be given intramuscular injections (Routine childhood immunizations may be given by deep subcutaneous injection with pressure on the site for several minutes afterwards.)
(d) Prophylactic dental care.
(e) All operative procedures in consultation with haemophilia centre.

Von Willebrand's disease — incidence 1 in 150 000
— autosomal dominant inheritance
— platelet dysfunction with prolonged bleeding time, reduced adhesion to glass beads, absent aggregation to ristocetin + FVIII deficiency (all components VIIIc, VIIIvw, VIIIag low)

Clinical features — very variable severity between patients and over time
— usually affects mainly skin and mucosa
— in severely affected, haemarthroses and haematuria may occur

Treatment — cryoprecipitate (2 u/kg body weight) or FFP (15 ml/kg)
— watch for development of iron-deficient anaemia
— never give aspirin

Haemolytic uraemic syndrome (HUS) See p. 232.

Henoch-Schönlein purpura See p. 330.

19. Oncology

Malignant disease occurs in 1 in 10 000 children per year. A child has a 1 in 600 risk of developing malignant disease by the age of 15 years, compared with a 1 in 5 chance in adult life. The types of malignancy affecting children differ from those occurring in adults; approximately one-third are leukaemias, one-third brain tumours and the remainder include Wilms' tumour, neuroblastoma and retinoblastoma, occurring mainly in the first 2 years of life; Hodgkin's lymphoma and bone tumours are more frequent in older children.

Aetiology

Genetic   1. *Familial*. The only tumour with clearly defined inheritance is retinoblastoma:

— unilateral — rarely inherited
— bilateral — autosomal dominant trait. Often multifocal, may be associated with pineal tumour. Bilateral multifocal forms of Wilms' and nephroblastoma may also be inherited.

2. Pre-neoplastic genetic disorders with high risk of cancer:

— DNA repair defects, e.g. xeroderma pigmentosum, ataxia-telangiectasia
— hamartomatous disorders, e.g. neurofibromatosis, polyposis of colon
— immunodeficiency syndromes, e.g. subacute combined immunodeficiency (SCID)

3. *Chromosomal aberrations*:

— anomalies: Down syndrome — 14 fold increased risk of leukaemia, Philadelphia chromosome in CML
— fragility: Fanconi aplastic anaemia, Bloom syndrome

4. Cancer-malformation syndromes:

— Wilms' tumour + congenital anirida, mental retardation, genitourinary anomalies (partial deletion of short arm chromosome 11)
— Wilms'
adrenocortical hyperplasia } + hemihypertrophy
liver cancer

Environmental   About 30 environmental agents are known to cause human neoplasms; their carcinogenicity may be influenced by host factors

1. *Physical*

— solar radiation
— ionizing radiation
  • atomic bomb survivors
  • Chernobyl explosion
  • abdominal X-ray exposure in pregnancy
  • possible relationship between occupational exposure to radiation in fathers and leukaemia in their offspring
— asbestos

2. *Chemicals*, e.g. diethylstilboestrol given to pregnant women associated with risk of vaginal cancer in daughters. An association has been reported between childhood cancer and i.m. administration of vit K after birth for prevention of haemorrhagic disease.

3. *Viruses.* Association with Epstein-Barr virus in African children and Burkitt lymphoma (+ chromosomal translocation in most cases).

Leukaemia

Acute lymphoblastic leukaemia (ALL)   85% of childhood leukaemia.

Incidence   This is the commonest malignancy in childhood. Peak incidence 2–6 years. Slight male predominance (55%).

Clinical features   — fatigue and pallor, irritability
— bleeding, bruising, petechial rash
— bone pain
— fever, infections
— lymphadenopathy, hepatosplenomegaly

Diagnosis   Blood film shows anaemia, thrombocytopenia and circulating blast cells in most cases. Bone marrow aspiration performed to characterize the leukaemia by morphology, cytochemistry, cell surface markers and cytogenetic tests.

Subtypes   Classified according to immunological surface membrane markers:
— common — most frequent; best prognosis
— null cell
— T-cell — more common in older boys, associated with high blast count and anterior mediastinal mass; poor prognosis
— B-cell — worst prognosis
or Alternative French–American–British (FAB) classification according to blast cell morphology L1/L2/L3, claimed to correlate with prognosis (L1 best–L3 worst).

Treatment   Prehydration, urine alkalinization and allopurinol for 24 h prior to chemotherapy help to prevent uric acid nephropathy.

1. *Induction of remission.* Steroids + vincristine (VCR), asparaginase and adriamycin. Remission means <5% blast cells in bone marrow and regression of clinical signs. Achieved in 95% within 4 weeks.

2. *Intensification and CNS prophylaxis.* Value of further blocks of intense chemotherapy to 'consolidate' remission under study.

CNS treatment essential to prevent development of meningeal leukaemia. Intrathecal MTX and cranial irradiation; high dose i.v. MTX under evaluation.

3. *Maintenance treatment.* Most protocols use cycles of drugs such as 6-MP and MTX combined with pulses of prednisolone, VCR and cytosine for 2–3 years.

Prognosis   Most children with leukaemia and other cancers are now treated according to protocols under evaluation by national and international study groups, e.g. MRC, UICC. This has led to better understanding of childhood cancer and improvement in outcome. Late sequelae of treatment (see p. 308) are increasingly important as the number of survivors to adult life rises.

5-year disease-free survival rates for ALL are 50–75%. After completion of maintenance treatment about 10% relapse, usually within the 1st year. A small proportion of children with a second bone marrow relapse benefit from BMT. *Unfavourable prognostic factors* include:

— <2 years and >10 years
— CNS disease at presentation
— presence of anterior mediastinal mass with T-cell markers
— high presenting WCC (>20 000/mm^3)
— cell surface markers
  • 'T' (thymus) cell markers 10–20%; poor prognosis
  • 'E' (bursa) cell markers <1%; worst prognosis
— enzyme markers — high acid phosphatase in T-cell leukaemia correlates with poor prognosis

Acute myeloblastic   More common in teenagers or children <2 years. Includes
leukaemia (AML)   myeloblastic, myelomoncocytic and monocytic.

Clinical features   Haemorrhagic symptoms; local leukaemic infiltrations (chloromas) of skin or palate. Periorbital infiltrates may cause proptosis.

Diagnosis   — bone marrow reveals myeloblasts (histochemistry: Sudan black and peroxidase +ve, PAS −ve, terminal deoxynucleotidyl transferase (TdT) activity low
— may be associated with chromosomal anomalies
— may transform to AML from CML with Philadelphia chromosome positive

Treatment   Vigorous chemotherapy including cytosine arabinoside and anthracyclines achieves remission in 60–70% but median survival is only about 12 months. If there is a suitable donor, BMT is the treatment of choice once remission is achieved.

Other treatment modalities such as immunotherapy are under study.

Chronic leukaemia

Only 3% of cases are chronic in childhood.

Chronic myeloid leukaemia (CML) adult type

Usually presents with marked hepatosplenomegaly and leucocytosis. Philadelphia chromosome (t(9:22) translocation) positive. Treatment with Busulphan. Conversion to AML (blast crisis) is usual within 1–3 years of presentation, with poor response to treatment.

Juvenile chronic myeloid leukaemia (myeloproliferative syndrome)

Presents with eczematoid rash, hepatosplenomegaly and recurrent infections. Bone marrow shows myeloid proliferation; evidence of fetal erythropoiesis (e.g. raised fetal Hb). Philadelphia chromosome negative. Do not respond well to treatment. Median survival about 6 months, death due to marrow failure.

Lymphomas

Hodgkin's disease

Uncommon in children, particularly <5years. Male preponderance. Four histological subtypes:

— lymphocyte predominant
— nodular sclerosing
— mixed cellularity
— lymphocyte depleted with diffuse fibrosis and Reed–Sternberg cells

Prognosis becomes worse from type 1 to type 4.

Clinical features

Painless lymphadenopathy, usually cervical. Systemic symptoms (fever, night sweats, pruritus) in one-third, usually with advanced disease.

Must establish histological subtype and extent of disease, as these determine treatment and outlook.

Investigations may include lymphangiography, CAT or radioisotope scans and staging laparotomy with splenectomy.

The Ann Arbor Staging System is widely used:

Stage I: limited to one lymph node region or one extra-lymphatic site

Stage II: involvement of two or more lymph node regions on same side of diaphragm

Stage III: involvement of lymph nodes or extra-lymphatic sites on both sides of diaphragm

Stage IV: Diffuse involvement of extra-lymphatic organs or tissues with or without nodal involvement.

		5-year survival rate
Treatment Stage I — involved field radiotherapy		>90%
II		
III } chemotherapy ± radiotherapy		70–90%
IV		

Several successful chemotherapeutic regimens, e.g. MOPP — nitrogen mustard, VCR, prednisolone and procarbazine; Ch1VPP — chlorambucil, vinblastine, prednisolone and procarbazine.

Non-Hodgkin's lymphoma (Lymphosarcoma)

All malignant tumours of lymphoid system except Hodgkin's. Difficult to classify but in children are usually diffuse with poorly differentiated histology. High frequency of marrow and CNS involvement. The distinction between lymphosarcoma with marrow involvement and ALL is blurred.

This group includes Burkitt's lymphoma. This lymphosarcoma, involving the jaw, occurs in Africa, but the same histological type in Caucasians usually presents as an abdominal tumour.

Staging systems for NHL include the St Jude's Children's Research Hospital system.

Treatment

Varies with side and extent of disease. Combination chemotherapy programmes include:

— CHOP–VCR, cyclophosphamide, MTX and prednisolone
— COMP–cyclophosphamide, VCR, MTX and prednisolone

Lymphosarcoma is radiosensitive and radiotherapy is sometimes added.

Prognosis

Stage I and II — 2 year disease free survival rate 80%; III and IV 30–50%.

Brain tumours

See p. 258.

Wilms' tumour (Nephroblastoma)

Accounts for 4% of childhood malignancies. Peak incidence 2–6 years. Associated with congenital anomalies in >10% cases, e.g., hemihypertrophy, aniridia (with deletion of short-arm chromosome 11), genitourinary anomalies, Beckwith-Wiedemann syndrome (macroglossia, gigantism and umbilical hernia).

Stage (National Wilms' Tumour Study Group)		Treatment	% survival
I	Tumour limited to kidney and completely resected	Surgery + VCR, actinomycin-D	80–90
II	Extends beyond kidney but completely resected	As above + abdominal irradiation	80
III	Residual non-haematogenous tumour; LN and peritoneal involvement		
IV	Haematogenous metastases — most frequent to lung (20% at diagnosis)	As above + lung irradiation Actinomycin-D	50
V	Bilateral renal involvement	? Wedge resection of less involved kidney + chemotherapy as above	40

Prognosis also depends on age of patient (children <2 years, higher response rate) and histology; about 10% of tumours contain anaplastic or sarcomatous elements which carry a worse prognosis.

Clinical features   Usual presentation is with an abdominal mass; may be associated pain, vomiting or haematuria. Hypertension in 30–60%. Tumours bilateral in 10%. Histology and staging of extent of spread determine optimal treatment.

Neuroblastoma   Mainly affects young children (75% under 4 years); can be congenital. Can arise anywhere in the sympathetic nervous system, e.g. adrenal, coeliac axis, cervical ganglia. A high proportion of children have widespread dissemination at diagnosis, with metastases to bone, particularly orbits and liver.

Clinical features   Abdominal mass crossing midline, anaemia, bone pain, skin nodules (blueberry muffin baby), proptosis, periorbital haemorrhage, Horner's syndrome and raised intracranial pressure. Acute encephalopathy with oculogyric crises (rare).

In most children this is an extremely aggressive malignancy with poor response to treatment, but in infants under 12 months with disseminated disease there is a spontaneous regression rate around 60%.

Diagnosis   Because of its protean presentation, this tumour is part of the differential diagnosis of several common presenting symptoms, e.g. anaemia, PUO, failure to thrive, limp, refusal to walk.

Investigations   — FBC, ESR
— Bone marrow: densely packed small round cells in clumps, 'pseudorosettes', neurofibrils
— abdominal X-ray: tumour may be calcified ± ^{131}I-MIBG scan, IVP, CT scan, myelography
— skeletal survey, isotope bone scan
— urinary catecholamine metabolite assay, e.g. vanillyl mandelic acid (VMA), homovanillic acid (HVA)

Treatment   (a) Complete excision of localized tumours.
(b) Chemotherapy disappointing, but new combinations under study (especially for advanced stages) using high-dose melphelan, total body irradiation and autologous bone marrow rescue.

Prognosis   In the early stages with localized disease the prognosis is good, but for the majority with disseminated disease, 2-year survival rate is between 10–25% (although improving with new protocols).

Retinoblastoma   This tumour is most often diagnosed in children <2 years. In about one-third, the tumour is bilateral; these children have a dominantly inherited predisposition to retinoblastoma (probably deletion of long-arm chromosome 13) and are also at risk of other tumours, particularly osteosarcoma. Usually presents with absence of red reflex, white pupil (leukokoria) or squint.

Treatment depends on extent and includes enucleation, craniospinal irradiation and combination chemotherapy. An ocular prosthesis is fitted within 6 weeks of enucleation and changed as child grows.

Parents and patients need genetic counselling.

Soft tissue sarcomas 4–8% of childhood malignancies. Arise in embryonic mesenchymal tissue in many sites. More than half are rhabdomyosarcomas, which occur with peak incidence between 1 and 7 years, then a further peak in adolescence. May present as an asymptomatic swelling, or with symptoms depending on site. One-third occur in head and neck region. Tend to metastasize early and used to have a high mortality but advances in multimodal treatment, including adjuvant chemotherapy, have resulted in considerable improvement in survival rates.

Bone tumours Constitute 10–12% of childhood malignancies. Maximum incidence in 2nd decade.

— osteosarcoma
— Ewing's sarcoma

Both commoner in boys. Present with pain, swelling or pathological fractures. 90% occur in long bones; osteosarcoma in the metaphyseal region, Ewing's in the shaft.

Radiological features (a) *Osteosarcoma*: destruction and new bone formation seen as radiolucent and sclerotic areas. 'Sunburst' appearance where radiating spicules of new bone elevate the periosteum.

(b) *Ewing's* causes localized rarefaction and periosteal reaction resembling onion skin layers.

Treatment (a) *Osteosarcoma*: urgent amputation used to be advocated but approach to treatment has changed over the last decade: cytotoxic drugs have proved effective in shrinkage of tumour and metastases (e.g. high-dose MTX with folinic acid rescue, cisplatinum) and are used as adjuvant to surgical excision of affected bone with bridging prosthesis.

(b) *Ewing's*: chemotherapy and resection of tumour where possible. Irradiation to pulmonary metastases and residual disease.

5 year disease-free survival rates vary 40–70%, depending on site and stage.

Side effects of cancer treatment

Chemotherapy

1. *General*

— immunosuppression
— nausea and vomiting
— alopecia
— hypersensitivity reactions
— fever
— diarrhoea, malabsorption, lactase deficiency
— stomatitis

2. *Specific*

— hepatotoxicity, e.g. 6MP, MTX
— pancreatitis, e.g., 6MP, L-asparaginase
— cardiotoxicity, e.g. daunorubicin
— pulmonary toxicity, e.g. busulfan
— neurotoxicity, e.g. MTX, vincristine

Radiotherapy

1. *Acute*

— skin erythema and desquamation
— diarrhoea
— headache
— marrow depression

Delayed

— cranial:
  • neuropsychological effects, developmental and learning difficulties
  • impaired growth hormone production
— bone: necrosis, impaired growth, asymmetry, exostoses
— skin and soft tissue effects; loss of subcutaneous or muscle tissue
— pneumonitis
— hypothyroidism
— radiation nephritis/hepatitis
— sterility
— second malignancies

Family support and psychological care

The diagnosis of cancer comes as a profound shock to parents, siblings, extended family and friends of an affected child. The future is suddenly full of anxiety and uncertainty, family life is disrupted and parental priorities and expectations are radically altered. Emotional support and practical help are needed in coming to terms with the diagnosis and understanding the nature of the illness.

Following the diagnosis a prolonged hospital stay often ensues, during which time strong links are built up between the family and the specialist paediatric oncology team. The

Chemotherapeutic agents

	Mechanism of action	Side-effects
Vincristine/vinblastine	Vinca alkaloids, inhibit mitosis (metaphase arrest)	Neurotoxicity (peripheral neuropathy) Abdominal and jaw pain Alopecia
Daunorubicin (anthracycline)	Antibiotic derived from Streptomyces sp. — inhibits DNA and RNA synthesis	Cordiotoxicity Myelosuppression Nausea and vomiting Alopecia
L-Asparaginase	Enzyme obtained from E. coli, induces asparaginase deficiency and so inhibits cells which require this AA for growth.	Anaphylaxis Liver dysfunction Myelosuppression
Methotrexate	Folic acid antagonist; inhibits DNA synthesis	Mucosal and gut ulceration Hepatitis Osteoporosis Encephalopathy
6-Mercaptopurine	Inhibits purine and DNA synthesis	Myelosuppression Mouth ulcers Hepatitis
Cyclophosphamide	Alkylation of DNA and RNA	Myelosuppression Haemorrhagic cystitis
Ifosfamide	Structural isomer of cyclophosphamide	Haemorrhagic cystitis (given with Mesna (sodium 2-mercaptoethane sulphonate), a uroprotective agent)
5-Fluorouracil	Inhibition of thymidine synthesis	Mucosal and gut ulceration Myelosuppression
Procarbazine	Inhibits DNA/RNA synthesis	Gut ulceration Neurotoxicity Myelosuppression
Actinomycin-D	Inhibits RNA synthesis	Myelosuppression Gut ulceration Radiosensitization

GP should keep abreast of the situation by telephone and letters; some oncology units send out information packs to aid the GP in dealing with children with cancer and their families.

Parents need:

(a) Honest, accurate and consistent information.

(b) Encouragement to ask questions and to discuss fears and uncertainties.

(c) To know that their cultural and religious beliefs are respected.

(d) Time, counselling and occasionally medication for symptoms of anxiety, depression, etc.

(e) 'Permission' to spend time away from hospital at home with their family.

(f) A clear picture of the roles of the various members of the health care team and where to turn for help if needed.

(g) Guidance in understanding changes in the child's behaviour and defensive coping mechanisms employed by partners, relatives and friends.

(h) Advice about what to tell siblings and how to deal with their reactions.

(i) To be prepared as much possible for what may happen.

The *child* needs

(a) To be able to trust those looking after him.

(b) To feel secure, with the family around him as much as possible. A period of emotional separation from the parents and concealment of feelings may follow the diagnosis and the child often feels isolated. He needs to be helped to express his anxieties either verbally or through drawing or play, and to have his questions answered honestly in a way that he can understand.

(c) Simple and direct explanations about the illness and treatment.

(d) Investigations and procedures to be kept as pain-free as possible, and unnecessary interventions avoided.

(e) To maintain contact with friends and keep up with school-work to reduce isolation and facilitate return to school if possible.

(f) Limits for acceptable behaviour; excessive over-indulgence confuses and disturbs the child, but special events and treats within reason are a pleasant distraction, provide something to look forward to and allow non-verbal expressions of love.

Care of the dying child   Despite the improving prognosis in many childhood cancers, treatment fails in a significant proportion. The emphasis of care then changes to ensuring that the remainder of the child's life is as comfortable and happy as possible. This is usually best achieved by providing terminal care at home, which is possible in most cases with the combined support of the GP and primary health care workers. Some oncology units have a 'home terminal care team', comprising a domiciliary family support nurse, a specialist social worker, a clinical assistant and the consultant paediatric oncologist, who work together with the GP to offer support for terminal care at home. Daily visits are needed and the family must have round-the-clock access to medical help. Charities, such as the Malcolm Sargent Cancer Fund, can often support provision of home nursing for a limited period.

GPs involved in the care of such children must be familiar with the management of potential problems:

(a) Relief of distress:

— pain control: good analgesia is essential. Opiates such as diamorphine or the Brompton cocktail (morphine, alcohol, syrup, chloroform water ± cocaine) are usually effective if given regularly. It is often necessary to increase the dose to control pain in the final stages, and a change in administration route may also be needed (e.g. from oral to nasogastric, subcutaneous or intravenous).

— other palliative drugs may be needed, e.g. antiemetics, steroids, anticonvulsants, laxatives and haemostatic agents

— palliative radiotherapy is sometimes helpful in relief of obstruction or bone pain

(b) Risk of infection:

— children receiving chemotherapy must not receive live vaccines and potentially infectious contacts should be kept away

— unexplained fevers in immunosuppressed children must be investigated and treated urgently (although once the decision has been made that a terminal stage has been reached, it will usually be inappropriate to treat infection aggressively).

(c) Awareness of possible late effects of treatment, see p. 308.

(d) Practical aids to nursing at home which may be needed include ripple mattresses, suction machines, mouthcare packs, sheepskins and syringe pumps.

(e) Family support and counselling, including after the child's death. Parents may feel abruptly cut off from a team of professionals with whom they have had daily contact for months or years. Visits back to see the hospital team may help, but the GP has an ongoing relationship with the whole family which is an essential source of support in their bereavement.

20. Sudden infant death syndrome

Definition Sudden unexpected death of an infant which remains unexplained by careful clinical history and where thorough postmortem examination fails to demonstrate an adequate cause of death.

Incidence Very wide variation in incidence worldwide. Marked seasonal variation, always increased in the colder months.

Incidence in 1000 live births:

UK 1.44 (approx. 1100 babies/year)

Sweden 0.9

Hong Kong 0.3

Asia 0.1

New Zealand 6.3

SIDS is the commonest recorded cause of postneonatal death in the western world, accounting for about 20% of the total in this age group in England and Wales.

Aetiology Unknown but there are two consistent features:

— 80% occur between the ages of 1–6 months
— 66% of cases occur in the winter months

Risk factors — male sex
— low birth weight
— respiratory infection
— young mother
— high parity
— multiple birth
— bottle feeding
— social class IV and V
— previous history of sibling dying of SIDS ($\times$ 10)
— maternal drug use ($\times$ 30)
— illegitimacy
— short interpregnancy interval
— prone sleeping position

Theories about possible causes 1. *Viral infections.* SIDS is commonly associated with evidence of an upper respiratory infection. The incidence has shown a simultaneous increase with the occurrence of epidemics of whooping cough and RSV.

2. *Hyperthermia.* Several studies have shown a marked increase in immediate postmortem body temperature. The face is important for cooling in babies. The combination of too many clothes, high tog-rated duvets and the prone

sleeping position (see below) may combine to cause a dangerous degree of overheating.

3. *Prone sleeping position.* Different sleeping position is suggested as an explanation for the very low incidence of SIDS in Hong Kong and other eastern countries, where it is usual for parents to be advised to place babies supine. This may help with temperature control as babies seem to move more in this position and are free to kick off bedclothes. The incidence of SIDS in the Netherlands increased 3 fold after public policy was changed to encourage mothers to place their babies in the prone position. In 1992, UK national guidelines were changed to advise parents to place babies in the supine or side position (except for babies with micrognathia or reflux problems). This has resulted in a marked decline in SIDS (although there are peaks and troughs).

4. *Apnoea.* Various mechanisms for the cause of sudden apnoea have been suggested, including:

— a hypothalmic defect leading to central apnoea
— seizure-induced apnoea
— obstructive apnoea due to subglottal thickening and narrow airways
— developmental immaturity of cardio respiratory control, especially in preterm infants

5. *Intrapulmonary shunting.* Recent studies with babies who have suffered a 'near miss' cot death have demonstrated the occurrence of a sudden intrapulmonary shunt, most commonly triggered by infection, resulting in a rapid fall in PaO_2 and a prolonged expiratory effort. It has been postulated that this might be due to pulmonary vasoconstriction and therapy with pulmonary vasodilators may provide effective prophylaxis.

6. *Lack of environmental stimuli.* The practice of putting babies to sleep on their own in a quiet room resulting in low levels of environmental stimuli may be a factor in prolonged fatal apnoea.

7. *Inherited metabolic disorders.* A small percentage of affected infants have been shown to have rare enzyme defects of fatty acid metabolism causing increased risk of hypoglycaemia, especially if stressed, e.g. by infection.

8. *Mattresses.* Old polyvinyl chloride mattresses may discharge toxic gases. It has been suggested that these may poison the sleeping infant.

9. *Immune defects.* Increased levels of IgG, IgM and IgA have been found in the lungs of some victims, suggesting an abnormal response to a minor respiratory infection.

Immediate management of a sudden unexpected infant death

Most babies are discovered dead in their cots and are generally taken directly to the local hospital:

(a) The paediatrician should examine the baby to confirm

death and to look for any physical signs which may help to establish the cause of death (e.g. rash, evidence of URTI, trauma).

(b) Bloods, urine, CSF and swabs should be taken for culture and serology. Further metabolic studies of CSF, urine, liver and skin biopsies are necessary if underlying inherited metabolic disease is suspected.

(c) A detailed history should be taken from the parents. If there is no clue as to the cause of death, they should be informed that their child has probably died of SIDS and that there was nothing they could have done to prevent the death. The need for a postmortem should be explained.

(d) The parents must be given the opportunity to hold their baby for as long as they wish in a private room. Photographs of the infant or other keepsakes such as footprints or locks of hair should be taken for the parents.

(e) Religious support should be offered as appropriate.

(f) Ensure that siblings are being cared for and that the family has transport home.

(g) Inform coroner, GP, health visitor, family social worker if applicable, CMO, other hospitals or clinics where infant has been attending.

(h) Later appointment with the paediatrician should be made to discuss postmortem results and to give parents time to raise further questions. Risk of recurrence and possible monitoring of the next infant should be discussed.

GP's role (a) The GP should visit the parents the same day.

(b) The parents must be informed about procedures such as postmortem examination and possibility of police interview. They may also need help to arrange the funeral and inform relatives and family friends.

(c) Time to listen and answer questions is one of the most important priorities. The family needs the opportunity to discuss their feelings; most parents have strong feelings of guilt that they 'did something wrong' and thereby caused the death. The feelings and reactions of siblings should be discussed.

(d) Mothers may need bromocriptine to suppress lactation.

(e) The Foundation for the Study of Sudden Infant Deaths supplies a booklet with useful explanatory information about cot death, as well as a telephone 'help line'.

(f) The GP should undertake regular visits to the family in the ensuing weeks. Depression is often at its worst after about 1 month when the initial period of shock is over.

The Care of the Next Infant (CONI) scheme operates in many areas nationally, providing guidance and support for recently bereaved parents, with a system of increased surveillance by health visitors and GPs for the next infant.

Families who have lost a baby tend to consult more readily over minor symptoms in their next child. The GP should examine the infant carefully and reassure the parent if all is well, emphasizing that they were right to bring the baby to be checked.

Parents should be taught how to assess signs of illness in their children. Monitoring systems such as the Baby Check score have been devised to help parents decide whether their baby is ill and needs medical attention. Current national guidelines to parents include: supine sleeping position, avoiding overheating, advice to contact GP if illness suspected.

Monitoring and SIDS   1. Use of *apnoea monitors* (controversial — no study has shown a decrease in SIDS associated with their use):

(a) Infants who have had a 'near miss' cot death (those found apnoeic, cyanosed or pale, and hypotonic) and subsequent siblings may be supplied with an apnoea monitor in an attempt to prevent undetected apnoea a second time.

(b) Parents should be instructed in the use of the alarm, and how to perform cardiopulmonary resuscitation in the event of a second attack being detected.

(c) The full support of the health visitor, GP and paediatrician is essential.

Advantages	Disadvantages
Easy to use	High rate of false alarms
Provides parental reassurance	Expensive
Portable	Do *not* detect hypoxia
	May increase anxiety levels in parents

2. *Transcutaneous oxygen monitoring.* There is evidence that some cases of SIDS are due to sudden profound hypoxaemia with or without apnoea. In this instance an apnoea monitor would alarm too late.

PO_2 monitors modified for home use have been tried. This involves changing an electrode 6 hourly but has been shown to be helpful in identifying life-threatening events at an early stage when resuscitation is effective. Other methods of monitoring such as pulse oximetry, inductance plethysmography and airflow detectors are being evaluated.

Prevention of SIDS   Several studies have tried to use established risk factors to predict high risk babies. Professor Emery in Sheffield produced a scoring system which identified those at high risk and instituted a programme of increased surveillance by the health visitor with daily weighing, and early referral to the paediatrician in cases of unexplained fall in weight gain. The incidence of SIDS in the area was much reduced subsequently. The CONI scheme incorporates this approach in an attempt to reduce the incidence of SIDS nationally.

Southall and Samuels at the Brompton Hospital, London, are testing the use of transcutaneous oxygen monitors in the prevention of SIDS in high-risk babies and siblings of children who have died of it. They have proposed a series of measures which may reduce the incidence of SIDS:

(a) Early immunization against pertussis (this is now national policy).

(b) Segregation of infants from older children attending surveillance clinics to reduce the risk of cross infection.

(c) Health care workers with respiratory infection should avoid contact with healthy infants.

(d) Continuing education to encourage parents to stop smoking and to teach them to recognize signs of illness in their babies.

21. Dermatology

Eczematous eruptions Characterized by erythema, vesicles, weeping, crusting, scaling and intense itching. Chronic lesions thickened, dry, scaly, with coarse skin markings (lichenification) and altered pigmentation.

Atopic eczema
— very common under 2 years
— incidence increasing, affects up to 12% of children
— usually family history of atopy (70%)

Presentation
(a) Usually before 6 months, but can be any age.
(b) Often starts on face and neck, behind ears, but may occur anywhere. Flexural lesions are more common in older children.
(c) 50% remit by 5 years, 80% by 10 years. In more persistent cases, skin becomes dry and thickened, with eczema confined to antecubital and popliteal fossae.

Management
(a) Rehydration of skin with regular use of emollients. Start with simple aqueous cream on the skin and emulsifying ointment when bathing.
(b) Stop use of soaps, bubble baths and detergents.
(c) Cotton clothes.
(d) Exposure to sunlight usually helps (although sweating generally aggravates).
(e) Topical steroids (low potency preferred, e.g. hydrocortisone) applied sparingly to more severely affected areas.
(f) May need antibiotics for secondary infection.
(g) Itching at night may be helped by antihistamines, e.g. trimeprazine.
(h) Emotional factors are important. Eczema is often worse in an unhappy or stressed child.
(i) For difficult cases consider:

— coal tar occlusive bandages
— potassium permanganate soaks (1:8000); useful for infected eczema
— evening primrose oil
— exclusion diets (under dietician's supervision)
— potent flourinated steroids may be applied sparingly over a few days to severe lesions. Prolonged application *must* be avoided because of risk of striae, dermal atrophy and systemic absorption

Prevention (a) Breast feeding or hypoallergenic formula milks have both been shown to reduce risk and severity of eczema in infants with a positive family history of atopy. (Lucas 1991 suggests that early artificial feeding increases risk of atopy at 18 months 2–3 fold if there is a positive family history of atopy.)

(b) Mothers with strong atopic family history should be advised to breast feed only; avoidance of common food allergens (e.g. cow's milk and eggs) may also help. Specialist dietary advice will be necessary to avoid calcium depletion.

Complications (a) Infection: staphylococcal, streptococcal. This may necessitate oral antibiotic therapy.

(b) Eczema herpeticum: primary infection of eczematous skin with herpes virus. Lesions may be widespread and cause severe systemic upset. Refer to hospital for treatment with i.v. acyclovir.

Seborrhoeic dermatitis (a) Usually begins in infancy with thick scales on scalp (cradle cap). Tends to improve after the first 6 months.

Treatment — apply baby oil for 30 min then comb hair with a fine toothed comb, followed by shampooing
— wash hair regularly with antiseborrhoeic shampoo

(b) May involve nappy area — where rash is characteristicaly very red and extensive with clearly demarcated margins.

Treatment — mild cases — more frequent nappy changes and barrier creams
— topical corticosteroids — hydrocortisone 0.5–1.0% is effective. May need combined antifungal cream because of candidiasis.

Irritant contact dermatitis 1. *Nappy rash*. Caused by ammonia released by breakdown of urea in urine by bacteria. Produces widespread erythema with ulceration sparing flexures (contrast with atopic eczema).

— prevent by regular nappy changing and cleaning of skin
— superadded infection with candida is common in extensive nappy rash, so treatment should include an anti candida agent. Common combinations include barrier cream (zinc or silicone) together with weak topical steroid and antifungal
— severely affected areas may need exposure to the air to allow drying and subsequent healing

2. *Lip-licking dermatitis*. Sharply demarcated perioral rash. Common in 5-10-year age group, caused by repeated licking of the lips due to dryness.

Treatment	Regular application of vaseline or soft paraffin to the lips.

3. *Juvenile plantar dermatosis.* Caused by 'trainers', where excessive sweating followed by drying leads to fissuring of the soles.

Treatment	Directed at improving foot hygiene. Advise children to wear cotton socks and to go barefoot indoors wherever possible.
Allergic contact dermatitis	Caused by type IV hypersensitivity cell-mediated inflammatory reaction. Sensitizing agents include:

— plants, e.g. primula, chrysanthemums
— jewellery, especially nickel
— creams containing perservatives
— topical medicaments, e.g. antibiotics, antihistamines
— shoes: chromium salts in leather, dyes
— bubble baths
— biological washing powders/liquids

Infestations

Head lice (Pediculosis capitis)	— common problem, particularly amongst school children — spread by direct contact, combs, hairbrushes and occasionally via infested clothing — adult female lives 40 days and lays 10 eggs/day, which are cemented to hair shaft and laid near scalp, hatching in about 8 days
Presentation	— itchy scalp and nape of neck; empty egg cases (nits) visible on close examination of hairs — secondary infection often with occipital lymphadenopathy
Treatment	— Malathion 0.5% left on for 12 h before shampooing off — Permethrin creme rinse needs only to be applied for 10 min and kills both eggs and lice — after all treatments a 'nit' comb must be used to remove eggs from hair. With long hair application of dilute (1:1) vinegar or lemon juice before combing helps to breakdown the attachment of the nits to the hair shaft — treat contacts
Body lice (Pediculosis corporis)	Flourish in overcrowded and unhygienic conditions, especially if clothing not removed during sleep. Eggs laid in seams of clothing and killed by hot water so do not withstand normal laundering.
Presentation	— itchy wheals, papules, excoriations with or without secondary infection — may be asymptomatic
Treatment	— hot wash and dry clothing — apply 1% gamma benzene hexachloride to whole body

Crab lice (Pediculosi pubis)
Colonize pubic hair, eyebrows, eyelashes and beards. In adults, spreads as venereal infection. In children, usually around scalp margins and eyelashes. Not usually related to sexual abuse; can easily be transmitted from hairy chest. Examine parents.

Treatment
— 1% gamma benzene hexachloride to whole trunk and limbs. Leave for 12 h, then wash off
— alternatively a 10 min application of Permethrin is effective. May need to repeat treatment after 10 days. Nits should be removed with a fine-toothed comb

Scabies
Infestation with Sarcoptes scabiei mite. Transmitted by direct contact and occasionally by clothing. Incubation 1 month.

Presentation
— intensely itchy rash, worse at night
— burrows most likely to be found in interdigital webs or flexor aspects of wrists in older children. Papular excoriated rash usually widespread. With infants face and scalp often involved as well; burrows may be absent

Treatment
1% gamma benzene hexachloride lotion. Apply from neck down and leave for 12 h (6–8 h in infants). Reapplication after 7 days. Treat whole family and launder clothes, bedding and towels.

Ringworm
Superficial fungal infections usually confined to skin, e.g.

— tinea pedis (athlete's foot)
— tinea capitis (scalp ringworm)
— tinea corporis (skin infection)
— tinea cruris

Caused by filamentous fungi (hyphae):

— microsporum canis (usually acquired from cats, or less often from dogs)
— trichophyton
— epidermophyton

Presentations
1. *Athlete's foot*:

— usually caused by tricophyton infections, but can be candidal
— uncommon in young children under 5 years
— very common in adolescents. Often associated with prolonged wearing of trainers
— itching, macerated, peeling skin between toes with an unpleasant odour

2. *Scalp ringworm*. May present with concern about hair loss. Circular patches of alopecia with scaling of the skin and broken hairs. Trichophyton violaceum most likely organism in Asian children from Indian subcontinent.

3. *Skin infection.* May only present with itching, but commonly causes scaly circular lesions anywhere on the body. Ringworm lesions have a typical annular appearance due to clearing of the central area. May have small vesicles at the periphery.

Differential diagnosis:

— eczema
— psoriasis
— pityriasis versicolor
— herald patch of pityriasis rosea

4. *Tinea cruris.* Presents with a bilateral, red, scaly, irregular-shaped patch around the groin and upper thighs. Common in adolescents, rare in young children.

5. *Cattle ringworm.*
May be picked up by children visiting farms. Causes a severe inflammatory reaction which looks bacterial. May only involve scalp in children, producing a boggy swelling or kerion which is often mistaken for an abscess.

Diagnosis   (a) Microsporum canis infections fluoresce under Wood's light
(b) Skin scrapings and plucked hairs should be examined microscopically for hyphae and spores.
(c) The fungi can also be cultured on agar plates.

Treatment   (a) Small areas — clotrimazole cream; large areas — griseofulvin orally for 4–6 weeks.
(b) The family should also be examined and treated (including pets).

Pityriasis versicolor   Lightly pigmented irregular rash which does not tan, or hypopigmented patches on black skin. Due to skin spread of Malassezia furfur (commonsal yeast-like fungus normally found in hair follicles).

Treatment   Selsun shampoo (selenium sulphide) 3 times a week for 3 weeks or half-strength Whitfield's ointment.

Pityriasis rosea   Cause unknown, probably viral.

Presentation   (a) Initial solitary 'herald patch' 2–3 weeks before main eruption. 1–5 cm round or oval lesion, often mistaken for ringworm.
(b) Main rash small red ovoid scaly macules, incline down to midline — Christmas tree pattern, especially on back — in lines of skin cleavage. Slightly itchy, affects trunk and limbs proximally. Lasts about 6 weeks.

Treatment   Symptomatic only; topical emollients, antihistamines.

Granuloma annulare

Circular lesion, usually on dorsum of hand or foot. Ring of raised papules with normal centre, gradually enlarges to 1–4 cm diameter. May persist for several months.

Treatment

Spontaneous resolution is usual. If painful or disfiguring, can be treated with intralesional hydrocortisone or triamcinolone.

Alopecia

1. Traction alopecia — ponytails, plaits and pigtails, child abuse.
2. Toxic — radiation, drugs, e.g. chemotherapy.
3. Alopecia areata. Complete loss of hair in round patches on the scalp, with 'exclamation mark' hairs at periphery of lesions. Probably autoimmune disorder, may also be related to stress or emotional factors. Often starts in childhood. 20% have family history.

Spontaneous resolution is usual but may recur. Corticosteroid injections may be used to stimulate hair growth if recovery is slow.

Trichotillomania

Compulsive hair pulling, may be precipitated by psychological factors. Can result in large areas of hair loss. Close examination shows broken hairs of differing lengths. Causes permanent hair loss if persistent.

Differential diagnosis

— scalp ringworm
— alopecia areata

Acne vulgaris

Very common skin disorder in the 12–18-year age group. It affects males more than females and may continue into the 20s. Rarely occurs in infancy (check for associated sexual precocity).

Onset usually triggered by pubertal changes. Androgenic hormones promote sebum production with blockage and inflammation of pilosebaceous follicles, causing comedones ('blackheads'). Follicles are colonized by *Corynebacterium acnes* and yeasts which break down sebum releasing free fatty acids which cause an inflammatory reaction in the dermis. Pustules and cystic lesions can develop and lead to scarring. Lesions mainly on face, chest and back, also deltoid area. Emotional stress and menstruation are common aggravating factors.

Treatment

(a) Sunlight usually helps.
(b) Cleansers and desquamating agents.
(d) Retinoic acid (aids in eliminating keratin plug).
(e) Topical antibiotics, clindamycin, erythromycin.
(f) Oral antibiotics, e.g. tetracycline (> 12 years) or erythromycin. Bacteriostatic and reduce free fatty acid concentrations in sebum. Maximum effect not achieved before 3–6 months; treatment should be continued for at least 6–12 months.
(h) Antiandrogens, e.g. cyproterone, spironolactone are sometimes helpful in refractory cases.

(i) Roaccutane (a vitamin A derivative) may be used under hospital supervision only.

Staphylococcal infections

Impetigo
— Infection with staphylococcus phage type 71 in 80% of cases. Secondary streptococcal infection may occur.
— Causes honey-coloured crusting lesions anywhere on the skin, particularly exposed areas.
— Spreads very easily on and between children. Nasal carriage important source of infection.

Treatment
— Child should stay away from school until lesion is dry and healing.
— Send skin swabs for culture and sensitivities.
— Apply topical antibiotic, e.g. mupiricin, fusidic acid after soaking off crusts with liquid paraffin.
— Systemic antibiotics may be necessary, e.g. for secondary infection.
— Launder clothing thoroughly.

Scalded skin syndrome (Toxic epidermal necrolysis, Lyell's disease)
— Commonest in children <10 years.
— Caused by group 2 phage type 71 *Staphylococcus aureus*.
— Exotoxin causes large bullae which burst, causing peeling of the epidermis with rapid spread over the body.
— Usually febrile. May also have pharyngitis and conjunctivitis. Can develop septicaemia.
— High mortality if untreated, especially in neonates.

Treatment
(a) Admit to hospital.
(b) i.v. penicillinase-resistant penicillins.
(c) Fluid replacement if lesions large.

Streptococcal infections

Erysipelas
Streptococci enter break in skin causing area of hot indurated erythema with dermal oedema and palpable spreading border. High fever and rigors.
Treat with systemic penicillin.

Cellulitis
Painful, shiny, erythematous area of infected skin with poorly defined border. Regional lymph nodes enlarged and tender; may be damage to lymphatic drainage. Usually child is pyrexial and systemically unwell.
Treat with i.v. penicillin (or erythromycin) followed by oral therapy for a total of at least 10 days.

Viral infections

HIV
Dermatological manifestations of HIV infection (see also p. 150):

— fungal infections, particularly candidiasis

— herpes
— molluscum contagiosum
— warts
— impetigo
— alopecia
— folliculitis

Warts   (a) Human papilloma infection is very common in all age groups, especially 5–10 years.
(b) Lesions may be solitary or multiple.
(c) Transmitted by direct contact, although generally of low infectivity.
(d) Antibody response is poor, then increases suddenly after several months leading to spontaneous resolution after months or years.
(e) Lesions on soles (veruccae) can be painful, otherwise warts are usually asymptomatic but cosmetically unacceptable.

Treatment   (a) Wart paints containing keratolytic, e.g. salicyclic acid topically, applied daily.
(b) Cryocautery with CO_2 or liquid nitrogen.
(c) Electrocautery.
(d) Curettage.

Molluscum contagiosum   Pox virus infection causing small pearly, umbilicated lesions, occurring anywhere on the body.
Tendency to spread as satellite lesions around the original lesion. Easily spread to family contacts via water when sharing baths. Rapid spread in some children, especially if atopic or immunocompromized.

Treatment   Spontaneous resolution occurs after several months. If treatment is considered desirable on cosmetic grounds the lesions are pierced with a sharpened orange stick dipped in phenol. Alternatively application of liquid nitrogen is effective.

Psoriasis   A common chronic inflammatory skin disorder of unknown aetiology. Often familial. In children most common type is guttate psoriasis, with widespread small scaly red macules. Last several weeks, similar to pityriasis rosea, but usually round not ovoid. Often follows follicular tonsillitis. Good prognosis. Chronic psoriasis with plaque or annular lesions less common in childhood. Plaques — especially found on knees, elbows and scalp.

Treatment   (a) Coal tar derivatives, salicyclic ointments and bath additives daily. Shampoos are helpful to relieve itch and scaling.
(b) Sunlight usually helps (artifical UV light may be used under hospital supervision).
(c) Dithranol in Lassar's paste for severe cases.

22. Rheumatology and orthopaedics

Rheumatology

Joint pains in children are mostly due to trauma and are self-limiting. Post-viral arthropathies are usually easy to distinguish by history.

Causes of arthritis in childhood

— infective: • viral — rubella • bacterial — haemophilus
        mumps   staphylococcus
        chickenpox   salmonella
        adenovirus • other — Lyme disease
        parvovirus   rickettsia
                mycoplasma
— post-infective: rheumatic fever, Kawasaki, dysentery
— post-traumatic
— allergic: food and drug allergy, Henoch-Schönlein purpura
— synovitis
— haematological: leukaemia, haemophilia, sickle cell anaemia
— collagen/autoimmune diseases: juvenile chronic arthritis, SLE, dermatomyositis
— gastrointestinal: Crohn's disease, ulcerative colitis
— gout
— hypogammaglobulinaemia
— neoplasia, e.g. neuroblastoma
— mucopolysaccharidoses

Juvenile chronic arthritis (JCA)

This is a generalized disorder characterized by chronic synovitis occurring in association with extra-articular manifestations. Diagnostic criteria include onset under 16 years of age and minimum duration of 3 months.
 Classification by presentation at onset:

— systemic (30%)
— polyarticular (35%)
— pauciarticular (45%)

Systemic

Still's disease; juvenile rheumatoid arthritis.
— Presents with intermittent high spiking fever, generalized aches and pains in muscles and joints, and coppery-red flitting maculopapular rash. Usually involves knees, wrists and ankles.
— Lymphadenopathy, weight loss, anaemia.
— May have splenomegaly, lymphadenopathy, pericarditis, pleurisy.
— Usually <5 years, when sex incidence is equal. Later, girls are more commonly affected.

       — Investigations show ESR usually high, >100, with poly-morphonucleocytosis. All Igs may be raised but IgM rheumatoid factor usually negative.

Polyarticular More common in girls (F:M 8:1). Presents at any age with any joint affected, although usually wrists and hands, knees and ankles. Other features may include weight loss, fever and general malaise. Two subgroups:
(a) Rheumatoid factor positive. ANA-positive in 75%. Present later in childhood. >50% progress to severe chronic arthritis. May have subcutaneous nodules.
(b) Rheumatoid factor negative. ANA-positive in 25%. Better prognosis; only 10% develop severe chronic arthritis

Pauciarticular Commonest type. Involvement of 1–4 joints in first 3 months, usually knee/ankle. Three sub-groups:
(a) Type I: young girls, +ve ANF, iridocyclitis in 50%.
(b) Type II: older boys, HLA B27 +ve, develop ankylosing spondylitis later in many cases. Usually present with hip or knee involvement. Family history in 50%.
(c) Type III: monoarticular. Usually female, >8 years. Knee joint most commonly affected. ANA and RF negative. ESR often normal.

Differential diagnosis — juvenile ankylosing spondylitis
       — enteropathic arthritis
       — psoriatic arthritis
       — SLE
       — sarcoidosis
       — dermatomyositis

Management of JCA (a) Control pain with aspirin and non-steroidal anti-inflam-matory drugs, e.g. naproxen, ibuprofen.
(b) Rest. During periods of systemic illness or when joints are acutely painful, bed rest is required, but it is essential to maintain functionally good posture, using appropriate splints and mobilize as soon as possible. Prone-lying during a daily rest period helps prevent or treat hip-flexion contractures but prolonged bed rest must be avoided.
(c) Physiotherapy to encourage movement and retain strength and mobility.
(d) Daily exercise programme may include walking, hydro-therapy and cycling. Vigorous contact sports are discouraged.
(e) Other anti-inflammatory drugs sometimes used in JCA include:
       — steroids: prednisone or ACTH, preferably alternate day regimen to minimize toxicity
       — for refractory cases, gold salts, penicillamine, anti-malarials or immunosuppressives may be used. All

have significant adverse effects and require close monitoring

(f) Slit lamp examination 4 monthly for young girls with pauciarticular JCA with +ve ANF to look for early irido-cyclitis and to exclude cataracts. Annual examination for other types.

(g) Good diet with adequate calorie and protein intake.

(h) Psychosocial support including patient and parent education, involvement of psychologist and/or psychiatrist, genetic and vocational counselling.

Prognosis
— 70% achieve normal function
— 50% resolve completely
— mortality from infection or amyloidosis: 2–7%

Septic arthritis   Infection of single or multiple joints, most often due to staphylococci, streptococci, *Haemophilus influenzae*, salmonella, or gonococcus. Arthritis results due to blood-spread infection or penetration of the joint. Usually acute onset with hot, swollen and tender joint in febrile child.

Management
(a) Admit to hospital, bed rest, immobilize joint by splinting in functional position.

(b) Investigations:

— FBC, ESR
— culture blood and joint aspirate
— X-ray affected joint (and opposite side for comparison)

(c) Intravenous antibiotics for minimum of 3 weeks, complete 6 week course orally.

(d) Continue daily joint aspiration if pus under tension in joint, and consider open surgical drainage if aspirate not reducing after 3–4 days.

Osteomyelitis   Haematogenous spread of bacterial infection to metaphyses of long bones. Infecting organism is *Staphylococcus aureus* in at least 70% of cases. Others include *Haemophilus influenzae* and *Streptococcus pneumoniae*. Salmonella infections complicate sickle cell anaemia.

Presentation
— Painful, immobile limb with swelling and erythema.
— 30% femur, 30% tibia, but any bone may be affected. Multiple foci not uncommon, especially in infants.
— May have sterile effusion of adjacent joint.

Diagnosis
(a) FBC, ESR.
(b) Blood cultures.
(c) X-ray changes take 10–14 days to develop, after which the typical appearance of subperiosteal new bone forma-tion and localized rarefaction may be seen.
(d) Technetium bone scan may reveal area of osteitis before it becomes evident on X-ray.

Management

(a) Admit for bed rest and splinting if necessary.

(b) i.v. antibiotics for at least 10–14 days, continuing orally for at least 2 weeks after all signs of infection have resolved.

(c) Physiotherapy in recovery stage.

Complications of osteomyelitis and septic arthritis

— irreversible bone necrosis
— chronic osteitis with persistent discharging sinus
— limb shortening or deformity
— amyloidosis

Infantile cortical hyperostosis (Caffey disease)

— Presents as unhappy irritable baby with fever and tender soft tissue swelling overlying thickened bone. Commonest sites are mandible, clavicle, ulna, humerus, ribs.
— Aetiology unknown. Rarely familial.
— X-ray changes differentiate this from osteomyelitis. There is no bone necrosis but new bone formation can be seen.
— May run a prolonged course, with hyperostosis persisting for months after acute signs subside.
— Steroids are used to relieve symptoms in severe cases.

Henoch-Schönlein purpura

This is a diffuse self-limiting allergic vasculitis, often following a viral infection.

Features

— Transient large joint arthritis.
— Usually associated with purpuric rash, especially affecting buttocks and legs (extensor surface).
— Renal involvement, see p. 229.
— Occasionally abdominal pains and signs of bleeding. Intussusception is a rare complication.

Management

(a) Bed rest while purpura persists.

(b) Analgesia.

(c) Admit if renal or gastrointestinal involvement.

Intoeing

Three causes:

1. *Foot.* Metatarsus varus: adduction deformity of highly mobile forefoot. Heel is in normal position, no treatment needed.

2. *Lower leg.* Medical tibial torsion associated with bowing of tibia. Corrects within 5 years, no treatment necessary (forward bowing is pathological, e.g. rickets).

3. *Upper leg.* Femoral neck anteverted in relation to shaft. Usually corrects by age 8 years. No treatment in most cases; femoral derotation osteotomy rarely needed for persistent anteversion.

Flat feet

Loss of the medial longitudinal arch. Physiological in infancy and common in growing children. May be familial. Providing feet are pain free, mobile and medical arch restored on dorsiflexion of hallux or standing on tip toe, no treatment necessary.

Pathological causes
— congenital vertical talus
— cerebral palsy, muscular dystrophy, spina bifida
— JCA
— infection sub-talar joint
— joint laxity, e.g. Ehler–Danlos syndrome
— peroneal spastic flat foot

Knock knees (Genu valgum)   Normal up to about 5 years. If marked, exclude rickets.

Bow legs (Genu varum)   Normal in infant. Corrects usually by age 3 years. Medial tibial torsion (see above) often presents with bow legs and pigeon toes. May be secondary to:

— rickets
— infantile tibia vara (Blount disease)
— osteogenesis imperfecta
— chondrodysplasia

Painful knees   Knee pain is not uncommon in childhood. It is important to examine both the knee and the hip carefully, as hip pain is often referred to the knee.

Osgood-Schlatter's disease   Inflammation of the tibial tuberosity at the insertion of the patellar tendon. The pull of the quadriceps muscle then results in a traction apophysitis. Onset often after starting strenuous sporting activity. Commoner in boys.

Management   (a) Rest until pain free.
(b) May need to restrict sports at school if slow to resolve.
(c) Long-term prognosis excellent, always resolves when apophysis fuses to metaphysis.

Chondromalacia patellae   Softening of the patellar cartilage. Causes pain on going up and down stairs, also on squatting and standing up from sitting. On examination there may be crepitus of the knee, tenderness and effusion.

Management   (a) Rest the knee. Analgesia if required.
(b) Usually resolves spontaneously.

Osteochondritis dissecans   Avascular necrosis of the cartilage of the distal femur. Occasionally fragments break off becoming 'loose bodies' within the knee joint. These may cause pain and locking of the knee.

Management   (a) X-ray to confirm diagnosis.
(b) Arthroscopy may be necessary to remove loose bodies.
(c) Large fragments may need to be pinned.
(d) Prognosis good.

Scoliosis

Innocent postural scoliosis   This corrects naturally on flexion of the spine. May cause low back pain.

Structural scoliosis   1. *Idiopathic adolescent scoliosis* (85% of cases). Incidence 3 in 1000, commoner in girls, usually convex to the right. Usually presents after age 10 years, during the growth spurt, with progressive rotation of the vertebral bodies resulting in a rib hump. Severe scoliosis may cause cardiorespiratory problems as well as cosmetic deformity.

Management   (a) Prevention may be attempted by screening at the start of secondary school. Examination of the spine on forward bending is a sensitive test but is not specific, resulting in referral of up to 15% of children screened, many of whom have mild non-progressive curves. The British Scoliosis Society does not recommend routine screening in the UK.

(b) Treatment by bracing helps if started early.

(c) Later treatment involves operative corrections.

2. *Congenital scoliosis*. Vertebral anomalies, e.g. hemivertebrae.

3. *Secondary scoliosis*:

— muscular dystrophy
— neurofibromatosis
— Marfan's syndrome
— poliomyelitis

Hip disorders   — 0–5 years — congenital dislocation, see p. 27
— 5–10 years — Perthes' disease
— 10–15 years — slipped upper femoral epiphysis

Irritable hip (transient synovitis)   This is the commonest cause of hip pain in children, particularly boys 2–12 years. Usually unilateral and self-limiting. May follow upper respiratory tract infection.

Presentation   — Sudden onset of limp and hip or knee pain.
— Well, a febrile child.
— Decreased abduction, internal and external rotation of hip.

Investigations   To exclude serious causes of hip pain.
(a) FBC, ESR.
(b) Serology, blood cultures.
(c) X-ray.

Management   — Analgesics and bed rest on traction.
— Generally resolves spontaneously within days or weeks.

Perthes' disease   Due to avascular necrosis of the femoral head, followed by revascularization and reossification over 18–24 months. Avoidance of weight-bearing prevents flattening of the femoral head but distortion of the epiphysis may lead to residual deformity if left untreated. Commoner in boys (M:F 5:1), mainly between 5 and 10 years.

Presentation   (a) Sudden onset of limp and pain, may be indistinguishable from a transient synovitis in the early stages.

(b) Examination shows similar restriction of abduction and internal rotation of hip.

Investigation (a) Blood tests to exclude arthritis, etc.

(b) X-ray initially shows increased density of the femoral head, then fragmentation and irregularity. If more than half the epiphysis is involved there is more likely to be deformity of the femoral head and metaphyseal damage. Following revascularization the femoral head reossifies and X-rays may gradually return to normal in treated cases.

Treatment — Aim of treatment is to minimize the distortion of the femoral head by containing it within the acetabulum. This is achieved by bracing the hip in abduction, e.g. broomstick plaster, pattern caliper.
— If detected in the early stages, may need only bed rest and traction.
— Severe cases may need osteotomy.
— Treatment may need to be continued for 2–4 years.

Complications — muscle wasting
— abnormal growth

Slipped upper femoral epiphysis Displacement of the femoral head postero-inferiorly. Common during adolescent growth spurt (10–15 years), especially in obese individuals; more common in boys than girls.

Presentation (a) Limp, hip pain, restricted abduction and internal rotation.
(b) May present acutely, especially after trauma.

Management (a) X-ray confirms diagnosis; NB ask for lateral views otherwise may be missed.
(b) Treatment is operative; manipulation and internal fixation is usually required.

Pulled elbow Traumatic subluxation of the radial head. Common injury caused by pulling on the arm whilst the child is resisting and rotating it, so that radial head slips out of annular ligament. May be recurrent.

Presents with sudden onset of pain and child holding the arm flexed, pronated and immobile. X-ray normal.

Treatment Reduce by holding child's hand and fully supinating forearm with your thumb over the head of the radius. The child will usually start moving the arm immediately but may take up to 30 min.

23. Ophthalmology

Causes of painful red eye
— conjunctivitis
— acute iritis
— trauma, foreign body
— acute keratitis ('corneal ulcer')
— acute glaucoma

Conjunctivitis Irritation, mild photophobia, blepharospasm.

Causes   1. *Infection*
(a) Viral:

— epidemic keratoconjunctivitis: adenovirus
— blepharoconjunctivitis: herpes simplex
— associated with systemic infection, particularly measles

(b) Chlamydia:

— inclusion conjunctivitis, transmitted in swimming pools, by sexual contact in adolescents and intra-partum in the newborn. Usually mild in Britain
— trachoma, transmitted by flies. Major cause of blindness in tropical areas

(c) Bacterial:

— acute purulent conjunctivitis, e.g. *Staphylococcus aureus*, pneumococcus
— ophthalmia neonatorum. May be due to *Neisseria gonorrhoeae* or more often to chlamydia. See p. 19
— membranous conjunctivitis: *Corynebacterium diphtheriae*. Now rare.

2. *Allergic*
(a) *Atopic* conjunctivitis, often associated with asthma or hayfever.
(b) *Vernal* conjunctivitis, seen in young children, commoner in boys, in spring. Attributed to airborne allergens such as pollen.
(c) *Phlyctenular* conjunctivitis. Now rare. Localized nodular conjunctival inflammation, probably due to local allergy. In developing countries seen as reaction to tuberculoprotein in malnourished children.

3. *Associated with systemic disorders*, e.g. Kawasaki disease, Reiter's disease, Stevens–Johnson syndrome.

4. *Chemical*. Irritants include silver nitrate in newborn, smoke, sprays and industrial pollutants.

Treatment   (a) Clean the eye; irrigation with sterile saline may be soothing.

(b) Antibiotic drops for bacterial infection. Chloramphenicol treats most bacterial eye pathogens, but in neonates, use systemic and topical penicillin for gonococcus or systemic erythromycin for chlamydia.

(c) For allergic conjunctivitis:

— avoid allergen if possible
— topical sodium chromoglycate
— brief course of topical corticosteroids or systemic antihistamines occasionally necessary

Uveitis   Inflammation of the uveal tract (i.e. iris, ciliary body and choroid) is comparatively rare in children.

Anterior uveitis (iritis or iridocyclitis)

Presentation   Tender painful red eye with photophobia and lacrimation. Contracted pupil with circumcorneal injection. Pus cells may collect at bottom of anterior chamber (hypopyon) and adhere to back of cornea (keratic precipitates) causing blurred vision.

Causes   — often undetermined
— collagen disorders, e.g. JCA, ankylosing spondylitis
— infections (herpes simplex, TB, syphilis, brucellosis)
— sarcoidosis

Management   Refer to hospital. Treatment:

— atropine to dilate pupil
— local corticosteroid drops
— eye pad
— treatment of underlying disease

Complications   Secondary cataract or glaucoma.

Posterior uveitis

Presentation   Painless, impaired vision. Retina often also involved. Choroidoretinitis.

Causes   — viral: herpes simplex, CMV
— toxoplasma
— TB, syphilis, brucellosis
— histoplasma
— toxocara

Treatment   Specific treatment depending on cause. Systemic corticosteroids.

Lacrimal disorders

Congenital obstruction of naso-lacrimal duct   Occurs in about 2% of term infants. Usually due to delay in canalization; occasionally due to blockage by debris or membrane at lower end. May cause epiphora and mucoid conjunctival discharge; the lacrimal sac may become infected with a tender swelling or mucocele at the medial canthus. Congenital obstruction of the tear duct usually clears spontaneously.

Treatment   (a) Bathe with sterile saline.
(b) Massage tear passages gently to express mucopus.
(c) Antimicrobial drops.
(d) If infection is severe or obstruction persists for longer than a few months, probing of nasolacrimal ducts may be necessary. If this is unsuccessful dacryo-cystorhinostomy may be performed.

Acute dacryocystitis   May be due to congenitally obstructed lacrimal duct as above, or to ascending infection from nasopharynx (usually pneumococcus) when it is treated with systemic and topical antibiotics.

Dry eyes   Absent or undersecreting lacrimal glands.

Causes   — congenital absence lacrimal glands, e.g. in cryptophthalmos
— anhydrotic ectodermal dysplasia
— familial autonomic dysfunction (Riley–Day syndrome)
— collagen vascular disorders

Orbital cellulitis   Marked orbital oedema and limitation of ocular movement in an unwell febrile child.

Causes   Spread from:
— adjacent sinusitis (commonest organisms are *Staph. aureus*, streptococcus, *Haem. influenzae*)
— bacteraemia
— other contiguous sites, e.g. orbit wound, conjunctiva, lacrimal apparatus

Treatment   Prompt intravenous antibiotics as serious risk of damage to eye or other complications, including cavernous sinus thrombosis, meningitis, brain abscess.

Blepharitis   1. *Seborrhoeic* (squamous). Usually responds to improved hygiene with vigorous bathing: corticosteroid ointment in resistant cases.
2. *Infective*:

— staphylococcal: hard to eradicate. Clean and treat with combined antibiotic–steroid drops or ointment
— angular blepharitis, often associated with conjunctivitis, usually due to *Moraxella*. Treat with antibiotic ointment
— viral, e.g. herpes simplex, zoster, molluscum contagiosum, vaccinia
— fungi

3. *Contact dermatitis*: irritants include cosmetics, soaps, poison ivy, etc. Treat by avoiding irritant, systemic antihistamines and topical corticosteroids.

Glaucoma Uncommon in childhood but should be considered in any child with apparently very large eyes.

Primary buphthalmos (infantile glaucoma) Congenital anomaly in the anterior chamber interfering with drainage of aqueous humour. May be associated with other abnormalities, e.g. Sturge–Weber syndrome, aniridia. Eye enlarges due to raised intraocular pressure and photophobia is an early symptom. More common in boys. Urgent surgery (goniotomy) is needed to prevent visual loss.

Secondary buphthalmos May be due to:

— uveitis
— intraocular haemorrhage or tumour
— trauma
— rubella
— retinopathy of prematurity
— corticosteroid therapy

Cataracts

Presentation (a) Leucocoria — parents or doctor note white pupillary reflex.
(b) Impaired vision; may present with searching nystagmus.
(c) During investigation for failure to thrive or in children with other signs of systemic disorders.

Causes 1. *Infants appearing otherwise healthy*

— hereditary — autosomal dominant with variable penetrance
— intrauterine infections
  • toxoplasmosis
  • rubella
  • CMV
  • herpes simplex
  • varicella
— galactokinase deficiency
— retinopathy of prematuriry
— idiopathic

2. *Infants with other signs providing clues to aetiology*

— intrauterine infections
— metabolic disorders, e.g.
  • classical galactosaemia
  • hypoparathyroidism
  • diabetes mellitus

- avitaminosis D
- mucopolysaccharidoses
— trauma
— chromosomal disorders
  - trisomies including Down's
  - Turner's syndrome
— ocular abnormalities, e.g. microphthalmia, coloboma, aniridia
— rare syndromes, e.g. Smith-Lemli-Opitz, Stickler
— systemic corticosteroid treatment

Eye injuries   Trauma causes one-third of blindness in children.

1. *Blunt trauma*. Often causes periorbital haemorrhage, which resolves spontaneously, but the eye must be carefully examined for accompanying more serious injury such as intraocular haemorrhage or orbital fracture.

2. *Corneal abrasion*. Causes pain or foreign body sensation, redness, epiphora and blepharospasm. Diagnosis is facilitated by fluoresceine staining. Treat with antibiotic eye drops and eye pad; refer for ophthalmological opinion, preferably the next day. May be associated foreign body or iritis.

3. *Penetrating injuries*. Emergency referral to ophthalmologist for evaluation and surgical repair.

4. *Chemical injuries*. Immediate copious irrigation and urgent referral.

5. *Child abuse*. Major cause of ocular injuries (see p. 129). Consider NAI in any child with:

— bruising or haemorrhage in or around the eye
— subluxated lens or cataract
— retinal detachment
— fracture of the orbit

(Retinal haemorrhages seen in high percentage of normal newborns but usually clear within 3 weeks.)

Retinoblastoma   See p. 306.

Causes of some ocular signs

Ptosis   1. *Congenital*:

— familial (autosomal dominant)
— syndromes: fetal alcohol, Sturge–Weber, Moebius

2. *Acquired*:

— progressive intracranial lesions compressing oculomotor N (complete ptosis)
— cervical sympathetic lesions (Horner syndrome) (partial ptosis)

— myasthenia gravis
— myopathy, e.g. myotubular
— trauma
— progressive external ophthalmoplegia
— botulism

Nystagmus   1. *Ocular*:

— defects of vision: refractory errors, astigmatism, optic atrophy, cataracts
— congenital nystagmus
— albinism

2. *Vestibular lesions:*

— infection, e.g. mumps, encephalitis, vestibular neuronitis
— drugs, e.g. gentamicin

3. *Brain stem lesions,* e.g. infection, tumour.
4. *Cerebellar,* e.g. tumour, degenerative disorders, drugs (e.g. phenytoin).

Diplopia   Due to malalignment of visual axes, usually because of muscle imbalance. Causes include:

— encephalitis
— space-occupying intracranial or orbital lesion
— iridocyclitis
— drugs, e.g. antihistamines, phenytoin, vincristine
— botulism
— lens subluxation
— myasthenia gravis

Proptosis   — tumours: neuroblastoma, retinoblastoma, rhabdomyosarcoma, neurofibroma
— thyrotoxicosis
— trauma: fractured base of skull
— cystic swellings: encephalocele, dermoid
— cellulitis of orbit
— cavernous sinus thrombosis
— craniostenosis

Visual handicap   See p. 97.

24. Alternative paediatrics

Parents are increasingly turning towards alternative therapies to treat some common childhood ailments for which conventional medicine has little to offer, e.g. frequent viral infections.

Advantages
(a) Can treat many symptoms and disorders where prolonged use of conventional medicines has possible side-effects, e.g. steroids.
(b) Avoidance of surgery, e.g. glue ear.
(c) 'Natural' method of healing which involves stimulating the body's natural defences.
(d) Unlikely to cause adverse reactions; will either have a positive response or none at all.
(e) Cheap.
(f) Child may benefit in several ways from a holistic approach to treatment.

Homeopathy
Homeopathy is the most commonly used alternative medicine for children. The decision as to which medicine or 'remedy' to prescribe involves taking a detailed history, paying special attention to specific aggravating and relieving factors, e.g:

— effect of temperature changes, sleep, time of day
— marked likes and dislikes of certain foods
— general health and temperament of the child

Homeopathy attempts to treat disease using the 'Simile principle' of 'like treating like'. Hence Alium cepa (onion extract) can be used to treat the common cold — streaming nose, sore eyes.

Homeopathic remedies are prepared by serial dilution of the mother tincture, which is usually derived from a plant extract. The dilutions are of the order of 10^6 or more, which makes all remedies safe, even those prepared from poisons like arsenic or lead and even if taken in overdose.

Homeopathic medicines can be used in two ways:

1. As *symptomatic treatment*, e.g.

— belladonna for fever
— chamonilla for teething
— arnica for injury of any kind, especially with bruising
— Rhus tos for itching vesicles in chickenpox
— ipecacuanha and Arsenicum album for asthma

2. As *constitutional treatment for chronic disease,* when a fine match is made between symptom picture and drug effects. Different remedies may be used for children with the same disease because each child's reaction to the disease is unique.

Doctors sometimes fear that homeopaths will interfere with conventional treatments. Medical homeopaths, however, will usually suggest that the homeopathic remedy be used in addition to other drugs; e.g. in asthma, it may be suggested that parents try giving the homeopathic drug early in an attack, before bronchodilators, to try to abort it.

Dosage   There are many different strengths or dilutions of remedies. In homeopathy, frequency of administration is more important than dosage. Commonly a 6 c strength is used for acute conditions and a 30 c strength for chronic. If there has been a sudden onset of symptoms, e.g. fever, belladonna 6 c may be given every 10–15 minutes until the fever is controlled. Chronic conditions like asthma may be treated with, for example, Tuberculinum bovinum 30 c once a month.

Homeopathic treatment is available on the NHS in one of the four regional Homeopathic Hospitals in London, Bristol, Tunbridge Wells and Glasgow. GPs may prescribe homeopathic remedies on an FP10 in the same way as other drugs.

Vaccination   The Faculty of Homeopathy recommends routine vaccination as per the National Schedule.

Acupuncture   Rarely used in children as they do not like needles! They do however respond well and need only infrequent needling.

Any condition may be treated by acupuncture; it is commonly used for:

— control of pain
— asthma
— nausea and vomiting

Hypnotherapy   — Good for relaxation especially in stress-related disorders, e.g. stammer, enuresis, asthma.
— Can be used to relieve pain in chronic conditions.
— Creative visualization: a useful technique which helps children express feelings and fears at a subconscious level and often resolves them spontaneously. The child is encouraged to close his eyes and allow his mind to wander, describing what he sees. Children will usually embark on a colourful journey of adventure during which they meet apparently insurmountable problems. With non-directional guidance they will often overcome these and in so doing seem to help themselves resolve current problems.

Cranial osteopathy   Cranial osteopaths claim to alter the flow of CSF through gentle manipulation, with a beneficial effect on abnormal posture and musculoskeletal pain. It is also claimed to stimulate the immune system and is tried as a treatment for recurring infections or asthmatic attacks.

25. Pharmacology

Safe and effective prescribing for children depends on knowledge of the way they handle and respond to drugs; there is much variation according to age and between individuals.

Pharmacokinetics   The processes which determine the time-dependent changes in serum concentrations of drugs and their metabolites:

— absorption
— distribution
— elimination

1. Absorption

Depends on:

— route of administration
— physicochemical properties of the drug
— site and area of absorbing surface

Bioavailability means the percentage of the dose administered reaching the systemic circulation. Different preparations of the same drug may vary in bioavailability. By definition, drugs administered intravenously have 100% bioavailability; most drugs administered topically have low bioavailability (varies with skin thickness, local inflammation, tissue perfusion, etc.).

2. Distribution

Depends on:

— tissue mass
— fat content
— membrane permeability
— blood flow
— protein binding

Age related changes affecting these factors include:

(a) Relative proportions of body water compartments. The ratio of total body water and extracellular water volumes to weight are highest in the first few months then fall throughout childhood. (Total body water accounts for 80% of a newborn infant's body weight, compared with 60% at 1 year and 55% in adults.) Most drugs are water-soluble so are diluted through a relatively larger compartment in infants; larger doses — relative to weight — are therefore required to achieve similar concentrations as in older children.

(b) Lower drug protein binding in the first few months of life results in increased amounts of unbound (pharmacologically active) drug, but also more free drug available for breakdown and excretion.

3. Elimination

(a) *Biotransformation:* whereby drugs are made more water-soluble to enhance their elimination. Mainly occurs in the liver. Depends on:

— size of liver
— efficiency of hepatic enzymes, particularly microsomal cytochrome P450 sytem

In neonates, particularly if preterm, the microsomal enzyme system is immature and some drug metabolism is inefficient. This is responsible for the fatal cardiorespiratory collapse (grey baby syndrome) in infants given similar weight-related doses of chloramphenicol as older children.

After the first few months, the relatively large size of the liver compared with body weight in small children is associated with more rapid drug metabolism, so that the most rapid clearance rates for many drugs occur in early childhood, e.g. diazepam, theophylline, phenobarbitone, carbamezepine.

(b) *Excretion*: depends on:

— glomerular filtration and tubular secretion, which both increase with age, so renal excretion of drugs, e.g. penicillins, is slower over the first few months until GFR reaches adult values by 3–5 months and tubular secretion by 5–7 months
— disease-related changes in renal function

Pharmacodynamics

The mechanism of drug action and the relationship between drug dose and effect. Drugs may have different effects in children compared with adults, e.g. some sedatives have paradoxical stimulatory effects in children.

Adverse effects

Undesirable effects of drugs or their metabolites.

Incidence: at least 10–15% of children given drugs suffer adverse effects, usually in the 1st week or 2 of therapy.

May be — concentration-related, e.g. deafness with toxic concentrations of gentamicin
— idiosyncratic (unrelated to dose)
— allergic, e.g. penicillin anaphylaxis

Drug interactions

There are many potential drug interactions but only a few are clinically relevant in children. Drug levels are helpful in monitoring the interactions of drugs, especially anticonvulsants, chloramphenicol and theophylline.

Frequently observed drug reactions

System	Effect	Drug
Gastrointestinal	Nausea and vomiting	Most drugs
	Diarrhoea	Ampicillin
	Moniliasis	Ampicillin
	Stained teeth	Tetracycline
Haematological	Marrow depression	Cytotoxics, Chloramphenicol
	Megaloblastic anaemia	Cotrimoxazole, Phenytoin
Cutaneous	Maculopapular rash	Ampicillin, Carbamezepine, Phenytoin
	Urticaria	Penicillin
	Alopecia	Sodium valproate, Cytotoxics
Neurological	Nystagmus	Carbamezepine, Phenytoin
	Drowsiness	Antihistamines, Carbamezepine, Phenobarbitone
	Tremor	β_2-agonists
	Ataxia	Phenytoin Carbamezepine
	Dyskinesia	Metaclopromide, Prochlorperazine
	Hyperkinesis	Phenobarbitone
Metabolic	Hypokalaemia	Frusemide
	Hyperglycaemia	Steroids, Thiazides
	Cushingoid syndrome	Steroids
Cardiovascular	Bradycardia	Digoxin
	Hypertension	Prednisolone
	Tachycardia	β_2-agonists

Mechanisms of drug interactions

Mechanism	Drugs	Result
1. *Pharmacodynamic*:		
— competition for receptor sites	Atropine and acetylcholine	Increased effect
— drug-induced changes in electrolyte balance altering response to another drug	Diuretic-induced hypokalaemia and digoxin	Increased risk of digoxin toxicity
2. *Pharmacokinetic*:		
— induction of hepatic enzymes	Carbamezepine, Phenobarbitone Rifampicin	Decrease blood level of concurrently used hepatically-metabolized drugs, e.g. chloramphenicol
— inhibition of hepatic enzymes	Chloramphenicol, Erythromycin, Cimetidine, Isoniazid	Increased effect of concurrently used hepatically-metabolized drugs, e.g. theophylline
— displacement of another drug from its protein binding site	Sodium valproate	Displaces phenytoin

Route of administration

Oral   Liquid preparations are generally preferred for younger children. Sucrose-based liquid medicines cause dental caries and gingivitis; their use should be avoided in favour of sugar-free medicines. Some preparations contain lactose or colouring agents which may cause reactions in sensitive children.

Rectal   Generally unpopular with parents and children but some uses in paediatrics include diazepam for convulsions, paracetamol for febrile children who are vomiting.

Inhalation   Very useful in respiratory disorders, see p. 167. Mode of delivery depends on age and ability of child.

Topical   For skin conditions. NB, if skin broken or inflamed, drug absorption is increased with a risk of systemic side-effects, e.g. topical corticosteroids.

Injection   i.m. injections hurt and should be avoided. The i.v. route is generally indicated in sick children.

Dosage   (a) Because infants and younger children have a higher proportion of body water, they have larger volumes of distribution for most drugs. Therefore, the younger the child, the larger will be the weight-related single dose of a drug.

(b) Drug doses related to surface area are similar throughout childhood.

(c) It is generally preferable to use drugs which need to be given only once or twice daily; more frequent dosages are likely to be forgotten. The interval between doses depends on the half-life of the drug. Slow release preparations allow longer dose intervals.

(d) A steady-state concentration is not reached until 5-6 elimination half-lives have elapsed. If treatment is urgent, a loading dose must be given for drugs with long half-lives, e.g. phenobarbitone, digoxin.

(e) Doses must be modified in children with hepatic or renal failure.

(f) Calculation of doses should be based on body weight (kg) or body surface area estimated using a nomogram. The Percentage method may be used for those drugs which have a wide margin between the therapeutic and the toxic dose.

Compliance   The overall non-compliance rate for children is estimated at ~50%.

Steps which may improve compliance include:

(a) Use as few drugs as possible.

(b) Prescribe the minimum number of doses necessary, based on drug kinetics.

Percentage method for dosage estimation

Age	Mean body wt (kg)	Mean surface area (m^2)	% of adult dose
Newborn (term)	3.5	0.23	12.5
4 months	6.5	0.34	20
1 years	10	0.47	25
3 years	15	0.62	33
7 years	23	0.88	50
12 years	37	1.25	75
Adult (M)	68	1.8	100

(c) Use palatable preparations in easy unit sizes or volumes.

(d) Explain to patient and parent:

— what medication is for and how it works

— how and when to take it—in relation to sleep/meal/school times

— what problems may arise

— how long treatment is likely to be required for

(e) Give written as well as verbal instructions, especially if more than one drug is prescribed.

(f) Discuss consequences of not taking medication.

(g) Encourage older children to assume responsibility for remembering to take their medication themselves.

(h) Ask parents to bring all medications to consultations to avoid confusion about which preparations are being used, check techniques of administration and also make sure medication is disappearing at an appropriate rate.

Drugs in pregnancy

Prescription of drugs in pregnancy has decreased considerably since the thalidomide tragedy in the early 1960s. Drugs cross the placenta by passive diffusion and can harm the fetus at any stage in pregnancy.

In the 1st trimester there is a risk of teratogenesis and congenital malformations, particularly associated with cytotoxics, lithium, phenytoin, valproate, warfarin, trimethoprim, isotretinoin, progestagens, alcohol and live vaccines.

Drugs which may affect the fetus if taken in the 2nd or 3rd trimester:

Drug	Effect on fetus
Aminoglycosides	VIII N damage
Amiodarone	Goitre
Antithyroid drugs, iodine	Goitre
Chloramphenicol	Cardiovascular collapse Cleft lip/palate
Sulphonamides	Kernicterus, prolonged jaundice

Tetracyclines	Tooth discoloration, bone growth retardation
Aspirin	Haemorrhagic tendency
	Neonatal pulmonary hypertension
Indomethacin	Neonatal pulmonary hypertension
	Cleft lip/palate
Warfarin	Haemorrhagic tendency
Diazoxide	Fetal diabetes
Hypoglycaemic agents	Hypoglycaemia
Propanolol	Bradycardia, hypoglycaemia
Quinine	Thrombocytopenia
Thiazides	Thrombocytopenia

Drugs in breast milk Most drugs are excreted in breast milk, but in amounts that are too small to harm the baby. The amount available for absorption by the infant is usually <1–2% of the maternal dose. The milk/plasma ratio for most drugs is between 0.35 and 1.0, varying with drug pH, milk pH, dose interval, protein binding and lipid solubility.

Breast feeding is contraindicated during maternal treatment with the following drugs:

— cytotoxics
— radiopharmaceuticals
— lithium
— ergot alkaloids
— chloramphenicol

26. Hints on passing the DCH

The DCH is designed to test for knowledge and competence in the primary care of children.

The syllabus includes:

(a) Diagnosis, management, epidemiology and prevention of the common and important disorders of childhood.
(b) Pre-and perinatal care; preparation for parenthood; care of the newborn.
(c) Infant feeding.
(d) Normal and abnormal growth and development.
(e) Principles of health surveillance.
(f) Immunization and screening; criteria, evaluation.
(g) Effects of social environment on child health including accident prevention, child abuse.
(h) Principles of cooperation with social and educational agencies. Legislation relevant to children.

The Royal College recommends that candidates complete 12 months' experience in the care of children before sitting the examination, although this is not obligatory.

The examination can only be attempted four times.

The written examination

Paper I (3 hours)

— 10 short notes questions (50% total marks)
— 2 case commentaries (25% each)

Paper II (2 hours)

— MCQs

Copies of past papers can be obtained from the Examinations Office, the Royal College of Physicians, 11 St Andrew's Place, Regent's Park, London NW1 4LE. It is useful to go through papers to gain an idea of the format and emphasis of the type of questions asked.

(a) Practising MCQ papers is a good way to test your knowledge and helps you to train yourself to read questions carefully to make sure you have understood what is being asked. It will also help in judging how good your hunches usually are — the MCQ paper is negatively marked so it is not advisable to guess if you have absolutely no idea of the answer. You must pass the MCQ paper in order to attend the clinical section of the examination.
(b) It is compulsory to complete all the questions in the short notes section so it is important to divide your time

carefully and make sure you answer every question. Organize your answer into sections or lists if this helps you to be concise. Make sure your hand-writing remains legible and define any abbreviations used.

The clinical examination   Consists of:

— 1 long case (40 min and examination 20 min)
— several short cases (25 min, of which 10 min will be devoted to developmental testing, including vision and hearing)

Passing any clinical examination depends as much on tactics and technique as on knowledge.

Practice   It is always more stressful to examine patients under examination conditions when time is limited and the examiner may be observing your performance. It is advisable, therefore, to practise both long and short case presentation with a critical colleague.

Equipment   Take a watch with a second hand and your own paediatric stethescope. Other necessary equipment should be made available to you, but you may prefer to take items with which you are familiar, e.g. ophthalmoscope, bright pen torch, small cubes or toys, tape measure. Equipment for vision and hearing assessment will be provided; it is essential that you are proficient in performing age-appropriate tests (see Chapter 4).

Long case   Be sure you know how much time you have and divide it up before you start, allowing for history, examination and thinking time at the end.

(a) Spend a few minutes introducing yourself to the child and the parents and chatting rather than bombarding them with a stream of questions straight away. If you are friendly and sympathetic, parents are usually keen to be helpful.

(b) Make sure you have covered all relevant social and educational considerations when taking the history (e.g. housing conditions, diet, progress at or time off school, social services involvement, do the family have a car/telephone/sick cat?). You will not usually need to include all of this information when presenting the case, but should have it up your sleeve if requested.

(c) Much useful information may be gained from asking the parents what they have been told about the illness and what investigations and treatment the child has had.

(d) Your examination should be thorough and systematic as per your usual clinical practice, but concentrate on the affected system(s). Check whether the child is growing normally: measurements of height, weight and head circumference are usually provided but if they are not obviously displayed, either ask for them or measure the child yourself. Plot on the correct centile chart.

Always check the blood pressure if possible; in a smaller child who may be uncooperative, the BP may be recorded for you if it is relevant. Also consider whether you need to check the urine; again, if it is at all likely to be relevant, a specimen will usually be put aside somewhere waiting for you to ask for it.

(e) Be sure to leave 5–10 min to memorize the main points and prepare a concluding summary, including your diagnosis or differential diagnosis. Formulate a plan of management and try and anticipate the sort of questions the examiners are likely to ask. You may have a good knowledge of some possible discussion areas but be less happy to talk about others — so try to guide the direction the discussion is taking, steering away from your weak spots.

(f) When presenting your findings, be concise and fluent. Remember the examiner has heard most of it eight times already and try to maintain his/her interest and attention. Speak clearly, injecting some expression into your voice and avoid droning on in a monotonous mechanical fashion. Maintain eye contact, and refer to your notes as little as possible. Try to deliver the whole story without interruption and come to a confident conclusion, rather than fading away into apologetic mumblings.

(g) Do not try to be too clever and never argue with the examiner.

Short cases   Eliciting physical signs and suggesting diagnoses without much, if any history, is not the usual way of examining patients and practice is particularly important with short cases. You will often be directed to examine one system or part of a system ("listen to the heart", "examine the eyes"). Start by speaking to the children and do not frighten them by suddenly attacking the indicated part. Make sure you use correct gender when referring to the child. Do not be rude, and choose your words carefully; never say a child looks 'abnormal'.

— Facilities and time may limit handwashing between each short case but you should always wash your hands before examining babies.

— Always be systematic; e.g. if requested to listen to the heart, rapidly assess general appearance, size for age, check colour, clubbing, thoracic asymmetry, scars, palpable thrills/heaves, apex beat and pulses before auscultating. All of this can be done in seconds and demonstrates that you are thorough — but avoid exasperating the examiner by taking too long before concentrating on the area specified.

— Explain clearly to the child what you want him to do; ask him if there are any sore areas and watch his reactions during the examination to make sure you are not hurting him. Using distracting toys may help you to complete your examination without distressing small children.

— Your examination should be slick, progressing rapidly from one test to the next, without stopping to scratch your head and look mystified in between. Try to tie your findings together mentally as you proceed, so that you remember to look for associated relevant signs in other systems and can present a rational summary at the end, together with the inferred diagnosis, or differential diagnosis. (Some candidates prefer to comment on findings as they go along but this does carry a risk of committing yourself too quickly without sufficient reflection about the clinical picture as a whole.)

— When you have finished, thank the patient and say goodbye.

— Never give up half way through — you may feel sure you've failed already when you haven't!

Recommended reading

Behrman RE, Vaughan VC (eds) 1987 Nelson's textbook of pediatrics, 13th edn. Philadephia: WB Saunders

Campbell AGM, McIntosh N (eds) 1992 Forfar and Arneils's textbook of paediatrics, 4th edn. Edinburgh: Churchill Livingstone

Dept. of Health, Welsh Office, Scottish Home & Health Department, DHSS (N. Ireland) 1992 Immunisation against infectious disease. London: HMSO

Hall DMB 1984 The child with a handicap. Oxford: Blackwell Scientific Publications

Hall DMB (ed) 1991 Health for all children — a programme for child health surveillance. A report of the Joint Working Party on Child Health Surveillance. Oxford: Oxford University Press

Harvey D, Kovar I (eds) 1991 Child health: A textbook for the DCH, 2nd edn. Edinburgh, Churchill Livingstone

Illingworth RS 1987, The development of the infant and young child, normal and abnormal; 9th edn. Edinburgh Churchill Livingstone

Nicoll A, Rudd P (eds) 1989 Manual on infections and immunisations in children. Oxford: Oxford Medical Publications

Glossary of abbreviations

AC	acetylcholine
ACTH	adrenocorticotrophin
AFP	alphafetoprotein
AIDS	acquired immunodeficiency syndrome
ALL	acute lymphoblastic leukaemia
AML	acute myeloblastic leukaemia
AoR	aortic regurgitation
APH	antepartum haemorrhage
ARF	acute renal failure
ASD	atrial septal defect
ASOT	antistreptolysin O titre
ATNR	asymmetric tonic neck reflex
AV	atrioventricular
AXR	abdominal X-ray
BCG	Bacille-Calmette-Guerin
BMT	bone marrow transplant
BP	blood pressure
BVH	biventricular hypertrophy
CAH	congenital adrenal hyperplasia
CCF	congestive cardiac failure
CDH	congenital dislocation of the hip
CHD	congenital heart disease
CHS	child health surveillance
CF	cystic fibrosis
CML	chronic myeloid leukaemia
CMV	cytomegalovirus
CMO	Community Medical Officer
CP	cerebral palsy
CPAP	continuous positive airway syndrome
CRP	C-reactive protein
CRS	congenital rubella syndrome
C&S	culture & sensitivities
CSA	child sexual abuse
CSF	cerebrospinal fluid
CVP	central venous pressure
CVS	cardiovascular system
CXR	chest X-ray
CTG	cardiotocography
DIC	disseminated intravascular coagulopathy

DKA	diabetes ketoacidosis
DOC	deoxycorticosterone
EBV	Epstein-Barr virus
ECG	electrocardiogram
EDH	extradural haemorrhage
EEG	electroencephalogram
EM	electron microscopy
ESM	ejection systolic murmur
ESR	erythrocyte sedimentation rate
FBC	full blood count
FDP	fibrin degradation products
FFP	fresh frozen plasma
FSH	follicle stimulating hormone
GA	gestational age
GFR	glomerular filtration rate
GH	growth hormone
GN	glomerulonephritis
GnRH	gonadotrophin releasing hormone
GV	growth velocity
HCG	human chorionic gonadotrophin
Hct	haematocrit
HD	haemodialysis
HDN	haemorrhagic disease of the newborn
HIE	hypoxic-ischaemic encephalopathy
HIV	human immunodeficiency virus
HMD	hyaline membrane disease
HNIG	human normal immunoglobulin
HSP	Henoch-Schönlein purpura
HUS	haemolytic-uraemic syndrome
ICD	International Classification of Disease
ICP	intracranial pressure
ICS	intercostal space
IDDM	insulin-dependent diabetes mellitus
IEM	inborn errors of metabolism
IF	immunofluorescence
IPPV	intermitent positive pressure ventilation
IPV	inactivated polio vaccine
ITP	idiopathic thrombocytopaenic purpura
ITT	insulin tolerance test
IUCD	intrauterine contraceptive device
IVF	in vitro fertilization
IVU	intravenous urogram
IUGR	intrauterine growth retardation
JCA	juvenile chronic arthritis
JOD	juvenile onset diabetes

JVP	jugular venous pressure
LA	left atrium
LAD	left axis deviation
LBW	low birth weight
LFT	liver function tests
LH	luteinising hormone
LIP	lymphoid interstitial pneumonitis
LMN	lower motor neurone
LP	lumbar puncture
LRTI	lower respiratory tract infection
L:S	lecithin:sphingomyelin
LSE	left sternal edge
LTB	laryngotracheobronchitis
MCH	mean cell haemoglobin
MCU	micturating cysto-urethogram
MCV	mean cell volume
MMR	measles, mumps, rubella
MOD	maturity onset diabetes
MPS	mucopolysaccharidoses
MSAFP	maternal serum AFP
MSU	midstream specimen of urine
MSUD	maple syrup urine disease
NAI	non-accidental injury
NBM	nil by mouth
NEC	necrotising enterocolitis
NGT	nasogastric tube
NG	nasogastric
NICU	neonatal intensive care unit
NMR	nuclear magnetic resonance imaging
NS	nephrotic syndrome
NTD	neural tube defect
OC	oral contraceptive
OFC	occipitofrontal circumference
OPV	oral polio vaccine
ORS	oral rehydration solution
PAS	para-aminosalicylic acid
PCV	packed cell volume
PEFR	peak expiratory flow rate
PD	peritoneal dialysis
PDA	patent ductus arteriosus
PFC	persistent fetal circulation
PFT	pulmonary function tests
PGE	prostaglandin E
PKU	phenylketonuria
PMN	polymorphonuclear (leucocyte)

PNMR	perinatal mortality rate
PR	pulmonary regurgitation
PROM	prolonged rupture of membranes
PS	pulmonary stenosis
PT	prothrombin time
PTH	parathyroid hormone
PTT	partial thromboplastin time
PU	peptic ulcer
PUO	pyrexia of unknown origin
PVH	periventricular haemorrhage
PVR	pulmonary vascular resistance
RA	right atrium
RAD	right axis deviation
RBBB	right bundle branch block
RBC	red blood cells
RDS	respiratory distress syndrome
RFLP	restriction fragment length polymorphism
RHD	Rhesus haemolytic disease
ROP	retinopathy of prematurity
RS	respiratory system
RSV	respiratory synctical virus
RTA	road traffic accident
RTI	respiratory tract infection
RVH	right ventricular hypertrophy
SAH	subarachnoid haemorrhage
SBR	serum bilirubin
SCID	severe combined immunodeficiency
SD	standard deviation
SDH	subdural haemorrhage
SG	specific gravity
SGA	small for gestational age
SLE	systemic lupus erythematosus
SOL	space occupying lesion
SPA	suprapubic aspiration
SR	slow release
SSPE	subacute sclerosing panencephalitis
STD	sexually transmitted disease
SVR	systemic vascular resistance
SVT	supraventricular tachycardia
TB	tuberculosis
TFT	thyroid function tests
TGA	transposition of great arteries
TIBC	total iron binding capacity
TLE	temporal lobe epilepsy
TNF	tumour necrosis factor
TPN	total parenteral nutrition
TSH	thyroid stimulating hormone

| TT | thrombin time |
| TTN | transient tachypnoea of the newborn |

UAWO	upper airways obstruction
U&E	urea & electrolytes
UMN	upper motor neurone
URTI	upper respiratory tract infection
US	ultrasound
UTI	urinary tract infection

| VSD | ventriculoseptal defect |
| VUR | vesico-ureteric reflux |

| WBC | white blood cell |
| WCC | white cell count |

Index